Pulmonary Blood Volume
in Health and Disease

PAUL N. YU, M.D.

Professor of Medicine and Head, Cardiology Unit, University of Rochester School of Medicine; Physician, Strong Memorial Hospital, Rochester, New York

Lea & Febiger · *Philadelphia, 1969*

Published in Great Britain by
  Henry Kimpton, London

Library of Congress Catalog Card
  Number 68:18860

Printed in the United States of America

Gratefully Dedicated to

DOCTOR WILLIAM S. MCCANN
Professor and Chairman, Emeritus

and

DOCTOR LAWRENCE E. YOUNG
Professor and Chairman

Department of Medicine, University of
Rochester School of Medicine and
Dentistry and Strong Memorial Hos-
pital, Rochester, New York

PREFACE

It is generally recognized that complete assessment of pulmonary hemodynamics requires adequate and precise measurement of blood flow, pressure, and volume in the pulmonary circulation. The pioneering work of Cournand and Dexter and their respective associates made possible our present understanding of blood pressure and flow in the human pulmonary circulation in health and disease. Study of pulmonary blood volume, however, was limited until feasible and safe techniques for left atrial catheterization and more sophisticated applications of the indicator-dilution techniques were developed. With refinements in methodology during the past decade, so much new information about pulmonary blood volume and pulmonary circulatory dynamics has accumulated that review, analysis, and correlation of the available data seem appropriate. Accordingly, this monograph is an attempt to review and summarize current knowledge and understanding of pulmonary blood volume in man under normal and abnormal conditions. The data are presented in a manner intended to serve the needs of clinicians, cardiologists, cardiopulmonary physiologists, and clinical pharmacologists.

The historical background, methodology, and general principles of estimating pulmonary blood volume are described and appraised. Quantitation of pulmonary blood volume is derived from the published data of others as well as data from our own studies of more than 600 patients using indicator-dilution techniques. Special attention is directed toward the pulmonary blood volume in disease and its relation to the many physiologic factors which it affects and which affect it. Changes in pulmonary blood volume under various physiologic and mechanical stresses and in response to a variety of pharmacologic agents in particular are also emphasized. Observations of changing pulmonary vascular pressure-volume relationships have permitted demonstration of active and passive pulmonary vascular activity and assessment of the distensibility characteristics of the pulmonary vascular bed. In patients with congestive heart failure evidence is presented that alterations of the pulmonary vascular pressures are the predominant effect, while the magnitude of the pulmonary blood volume is of secondary importance.

A section on the measurement of pulmonary capillary blood volume in man is included. Pulmonary blood volume and pulmonary capillary blood volume were measured and correlated in a series of more than 100 patients. Notwithstanding differences in the techniques and principles used in estimating these two parameters, the data provide preliminary information concerning the distribution of blood in the various compartments of the human pulmonary vascular bed and permit speculation regarding the implications and significance of this distribution in a number of clinical conditions.

The references cited have not been exhaustive, and I apologize for the many omissions and oversights.

Paul N. Yu

ROCHESTER, NEW YORK

Acknowledgments

I should like to express my deep appreciation and gratitude to Professor Sir John McMichael, formerly Chief of the Medical Service, London Postgraduate School and Hammersmith Hospital, London. It was largely through his inspiration and guidance that I became interested in cardiology and the pulmonary circulation. I am especially indebted and grateful to my previous Chief, Dr. William S. McCann, and my present Chief, Dr. Lawrence E. Young. During the past 18 years they not only have been a constant source of personal counsel and encouragement, but also have provided adequate financial support for the investigative work. It is indeed most fitting to dedicate this monograph to them. I also wish to express my thanks and appreciation to Drs. Nolan L. Kaltreider, Robert A. Bruce and Frank W. Lovejoy, Jr. for their continued interest and advice. Throughout the years they have remained loyal and inspiring friends. I am indebted to Dr. Bernard F. Schreiner, Jr., colleague and friend, who has given generous support and made many contributions to the development and planning of this monograph.

Many thanks also are due to Dr. Celia Oakley, who has graciously permitted me to use freely data from her M.D. thesis, entitled "Pulmonary Blood Volume in Man." This material was largely based on work carried out in our laboratory during her tenure as a Medical Research Council Fellow (Lederle International) in 1960-61. Drs. Gerald W. Murphy, Kuddusi M. Gazioglu, Jules Cohen, Arthur J. Moss, David H. Kramer, Herbert J. Marx, Pravin M. Shah, and W. Bromley Clarke, my present associates in the laboratory, have helped me in collecting and interpreting the data. Dr. Elliot O. Lipchik of the Departments of Radiology and Medicine has kindly provided me with the data on volume measurements by angiocardiographic technique. I am grateful to Drs. Lewis Dexter and William R. Milnor for their encouragement and valuable suggestions.

I also would like to acknowledge my appreciation to many of my previous associates for their interest and stimulation. Among these are Drs. Julian M. Aroesty, Paul L. Bleakley, Jr., Herbert Constantine, Deji Femi-Pearse, F. Joseph Flatley, James K. Finlayson, Gerald Glick, Douglas H. James, Howard A. Joos, Raymond J. Lipicky, Milton N. Luria, Anweruddin Masood, Richard M.

McCredie, Robert E. Nye, Peter T. Perkins, James M. Perry, C. Alpheus Stanfield, and W. David Westinghouse.

I wish to thank Dr. Arthur M. Dutton, Mr. Kurt Enslein, and Mr. James W. Pifer for their help in the computer programming and statistical study, and to Mr. Gerald Cooper, Mrs. Martha Strain and Mr. Robert C. Wabnitz for the preparation of medical illustrations. The technical assistance of Mr. Dennis Edwards, Mr. Nicholas J. Vasile, Mr. Theodore Oleksyn, Mrs. Patricia Rosone, and Mrs. Susan White is greatly appreciated. I am indebted to Mrs. Bonnie Sollie, Miss Sharon Frederick, Mrs. Edith Witt, Mrs. Florence Friedland, Miss Cynthia Stebbins, Miss Maureen Bishop and Miss Donna Dogoda for their time and effort in the preparation of the manuscript.

Deep appreciation is expressed to Dr. Howard A. Joos for his time and assistance in reviewing the whole manuscript.

It gives me great pleasure to acknowledge my profound indebtedness and gratitude to my wife Iling and our children Pauline, Diane, Lorraine and Corrine for their sacrifice, tolerance, and encouragement.

In the past 15 years our laboratory has been generously supported by various research and training grants from the National Heart Institute, the American Heart Association, the New York State Heart Assembly, the American Trudeau Society, the Genesee Valley Heart Association, the Hochstetter Fund, and the Ernest L. Woodward Fund.

Finally, I am glad for the opportunity to thank Mr. R. Kenneth Bussy and Mr. John F. Spahr of Lea & Febiger for their kindness, encouragement, and consideration shown to me during the production and publication of this monograph.

Paul N. Yu

CONTENTS

Section I

CHAPTER 1

Historic Review

Use of the indicator-dilution technique was first reported by Hering in 1829.[1] In a series of papers published between 1894 and 1921 Stewart described the principles of the indicator-dilution techniques in the measurement of several circulatory parameters in animals, including cardiac output, pulmonary circulation time and blood volume.[2-4] For determination of the mean pulmonary circulation time, the following paragraph is quoted from his paper published in 1894.

"The mean pulmonary circulation time is the time in which the whole of the blood in the lungs passes from pulmonary artery to pulmonary veins. In other words, it is the time in which the right ventricle throws into the former a quantity of blood equal to that in the pulmonary circulation. Supposing then that the ventricle up to a certain limit is able to force through the lungs all the blood it receives, independently of the vascular resistance, the pulmonary circulation time must vary inversely as the quantity of blood flowing into the right side of the heart per unit of time and directly as the quantity of blood in the pulmonary circulation at the beginning of observation. In any case if Q represents the capacity of the pulmonary circulation, Q' the average output of the right ventricle during the measurement, r the number of beats of the heart per second and T the pulmonary circulation time, we get $T = \frac{Q}{rQ'}$."

Three years later he published a paper concerning the measurement of cardiac output.[3] The principle of the method described is quoted as follows.

"A solution of a substance which can be easily recognized and quantitatively estimated in the blood is permitted to flow for a definite time at an approximately uniform rate into the heart. The injected substance mingles with the blood, and passes out with it into the circulation. At a convenient point of the vascular system, a sample of blood is drawn off just before the injection and another during the passage of the substance; and the quantity of solution which must be added to a given volume of the first sample, in order that it may contain as much of the injected substance as the second sample, is determined. This determination, it is evident, gives us the means of estimating the extent to which the injected solution has been mixed with blood in the heart, and therefore, knowing the quantity of the solution which has run into the heart, we can calculate the output in the given time."

In 1921 Stewart described in detail the principle and calculation of cardiac output determination in dogs by indicator-dilution technique after injection of a salt solution into the left ventricle.[4] Later he also reported methods for measuring the circulation time of the spleen, kidney, intestine, heart (coronary artery), and retina.[5] He fully recognized the limitations and potential errors of the methodology, particularly the problems of non-uniform mixing and of preferential flow (axial streaming).

In 1927, employing an active deposit of radium, Blumgart and Weiss[6] determined "the crude pulmonary circulation time" in normal human subjects. The material was injected into an arm vein and its time of arrival was determined over the right heart as well as in the brachial artery. The difference between the time of arrival of the material in the right heart and that in the brachial artery was referred to as "the crude pulmonary circulation time." "The actual pulmonary circulation time" was obtained by subtracting 4 3/10 seconds from "the crude pulmonary circulation time." The 4 3/10 seconds was the time required for the active deposit to travel through the heart and from the heart to the brachial artery. The pulmonary blood volume could then be estimated by multiplying the cardiac output by "the actual pulmonary circulation time."

It should be pointed out that the methods used both by Stewart and by Blumgart and Weiss were based upon the assumption that the most rapid circulation time does not differ significantly from the mean circulation time. Actually, however, the mean circulation time is considerably longer than the most rapid circulation time, as demonstrated conclusively by Hamilton and associates, who reported their classical work on indicator-dilution technique during the period between 1927 and 1933.[7-10] They developed a method of determining cardiac output from analysis of the dye concentration curve. Studying models they also validated Stewart's formula for estimating regional blood volume between points of injection and sampling of dye. The validity of the methodology for measuring blood flow and volume by indicator-dilution technique has been further affirmed on mathematical and theoretical grounds by Meier and Zierler.[11]

With the introduction of cardiac catheterization, the feasibility of determining cardiac output accurately by the Fick procedure was established.[12,13] Although many reports compared favorably the results of cardiac output determination by indicator-dilution technique with those obtained by the Fick procedure,[14-21] the latter method has been widely used for a number of years in most medical centers. Prior to 1950 one major reason for lack of interest in the use of indicator-dilution technique in clinical and investigative medicine was the required tedious and time-consuming procedure, which included the collection of multiple blood samples, analysis of the concentration of the dye, and plotting its time-concentration curve. Furthermore, tissue staining caused by Evans blue dye (T-1824) and the unreliability of estimating its concentration in unsaturated blood made limited its use in investigative study, particularly in the study of congenital heart disease.

Interest in indicator-dilution technique was renewed after Wood and co-workers demonstrated its feasibility and its contribution to the accuracy of diagnosis in congenital and acquired cardiac disease.[22-25] The reports of Schillingford stimulated extensive study of the magnitude of valvular regurgitation.[26,27] The introduction of radioisotopes made possible determination of cardiac output without arterial sampling and was another step toward bringing the indicator-dilution technique closer to clinical medicine.[28-32]

Many contributions have enhanced the utilization of indicator-dilution technique in the diagnostic and investigative study of cardiovascular disease. Representative examples might include (a) more sophisticated instrumentation resulting in reliable and direct inscription of the dye time-concentration curve for determining cardiac output and mean circulation time;[23,33-36] (b) the introduction of radioisotopes and a more stable and rapidly excreted dye (indocyanine green) as indicators;[28-30,37-39] (c) extensive application of the technique in the detection of intracardiac shunts and of valvular regurgitation;[26,27,40-50] (d) delineation and expansion of the theory and principles underlying the mathematical validity of the dilution method and the sampling system;[11,51-56] (e) the estimation of regional blood flow of the lung;[57-59] and (f) estimation of pulmonary blood volume[60-63] and of left ventricular volume.[64-68]

Blood volume in the lungs could not be estimated by indirect methods until blood leaving the lungs could be sampled and the mean transit time through the pulmonary vascular bed measured accurately. In 1917 Kuno measured the pulmonary blood volume in dogs by the method of direct exsanguination of the lungs and found it to be approximately 9% of the total blood volume.[69] This figure is surprisingly close to results obtained by the more sophisticated indicator-dilution method subsequently used in normal human subjects.[61-63]

Prior to 1949 nearly all measurements of the so-called "central" or intrathoracic blood volume were made after the injection of dyes into a peripheral vein or, rarely, the right atrium. Utilizing pulmonary artery catheterization, Ebert and associates in 1949 reported (a) the circulation time from the pulmonary artery to the femoral artery, and (b) the estimated blood volume from the pulmonary artery to a systemic artery in normal subjects, in patients with mitral stenosis, and in those with left ventricular failure[70,71] (see Chapter 3).

Since then, many workers have reported measurements of "central" blood volume by various techniques at rest, under physiologic stress, and after the administration of pharmacologic agents.[16,18,72-84] The validity of the measurement of "central" blood volume has been questioned when arterial blood is sampled, particularly after exercise.[85,86] Indeed, because of the unknown amount of blood in the left heart, aorta, or various arterial segments, changes in the so-called "central" blood volume in patients with cardiac disease cannot reflect accurately alterations of blood volume in the lungs. The history of the use of indicator-dilution technique for the estimation of cardiac output and central blood volume up to 1954 has been admirably summarized and critically evaluated by Dow.[87]

The advent of left atrial catheterization brought closer the measurement of true pulmonary blood volume in man by indicator-dilution technique.[88-90] In 1955 Kunieda and associates utilized simultaneous right heart and left atrial catheterization and published a paper in Japanese entitled "Evaluation of Pulmonary Blood Volume in Mitral Valve Disease by T-1824 Method."[60] Subsequently, a paper of identical content was published in English.[91] In it the author described the estimation of pulmonary blood volume by both what we now refer to as the double-injection and the single-injection methods.

The double-injection method used by Kunieda and associates consisted of sequential injections of T-1824 into the pulmonary artery and left atrium and sampling arterial blood at intervals of two seconds. The mean transit time (T_M) from the pulmonary artery to the left atrium was the difference between the T_M from the pulmonary artery to the systemic artery and the T_M from the left atrium to the systemic artery. Pulmonary blood volume was estimated by multiplying the cardiac output by the T_M from pulmonary artery to the left atrium.

In 1960-61 Dock and co-workers[62] and Milnor and associates[61] independently published their work on the measurement of pulmonary blood volume in man using a double-injection method similar to those described earlier by Kunieda and associates. Dock *et al.* adopted the procedure of injecting Evans blue dye and radioactive iodinated human serum albumin (RISA) respectively into the pulmonary artery and left atrium simultaneously and sampling from the brachial artery at 2-second intervals. Milnor *et al.* injected indocyanine green into the pulmonary artery and the left atrium sequentially and inscribed the arterial dilution curves with a cuvette densitometer.

Kunieda and associates[60] also employed the so-called single-injection and single-sampling method by injecting dye into the pulmonary artery and sampling blood from the left atrium. Levinson and co-workers[92] later applied the single-injection single sampling method to estimate pulmonary blood volume. Subsequently, Freitas and associates[93] used a third method by injection of indocyanine green into the inferior vena cava and simultaneous sampling from the pulmonary artery and the left atrium. The T_M from the pulmonary artery to the left atrium was the difference between the T_M from the inferior vena cava to the pulmonary artery and the T_M from the inferior vena cava to the left atrium.

Notwithstanding the variations in methodology used in different laboratories, the values for pulmonary blood volume in normal subjects and in patients with mitral valve disease estimated by various groups of workers were in general remarkably close. Recent studies by many workers include observations of changes in pulmonary blood flow, pressure and volume under physiologic stress and the effects of pharmacologic interventions.[94-102]

Pulmonary blood volume also has been estimated by precordial radioisotope counting. The radioisotope used is usually RISA. The first report of pulmonary blood volume estimated by such technique in a large series of normal subjects was published by Lammerant.[77] This was followed by studies reported by many other workers.[78,80,81,83,84] The mean transit time was generally measured from the peak of the right heart curve to that of the left heart curve, causing the "pulmonary blood volume" to be grossly overestimated. A portion of both right and left heart volume is necessarily included. Recently, utilizing the radioisotope precordial curves, two groups of investigators have devised special formulae for the calculation of pulmonary blood volume.[103-107] The results reported compare favorably with those obtained from dye dilution curves. A description of these methods appears in Chapter 7.

In parallel with these investigations of pulmonary blood volume in man, methods have been made available for the estimation of pulmonary capillary blood volume by the determination of the pulmonary diffusing capacity for carbon monoxide at two or more concentrations of oxygen.[108-114] These methods have enabled studies of changes in the pulmonary capillary bed in normal subjects and in patients with relevant disease under various physiologic and experimental conditions. These methods and results will be discussed in Chapters 13 to 15.

REFERENCES

1. Hering, E.: Experiments on the velocity of the circulatory motion of the blood and on the quickness with which secretions are formed. Edinburgh Phil. Trans., 6, 78, 1828.

2. Stewart, G.N.: Researches on the circulation time in organs and on the influences which affect it. II. The time of the lesser circulation. J. Physiol., 15, 31, 1894.

3. _____: Researches on circulation time and on the influences which affect it. IV. The output of the heart. J. Physiol. 22, 159, 1897.

4. _____: The pulmonary circulation time, the quantity of blood in the lungs and the output of the heart. Am. J. Physiol., 58, 20, 1921.

5. _____: Researches on the circulation time in organs and on the influences which affect it. V. The circulation time of the spleen, kidney, intestine, heart (coronary circulation) and retina, with some further observations on the time of the lesser circulation. Am. J. Physiol., 58, 278, 1921-22.

6. Blumgart, H.L., and Weiss, S.: Studies on the velocity of blood flow. VII. The pulmonary circulation time in normal resting individuals. J. Clin. Invest., 4, 399, 1927.

7. Kinsman, J.M., Moore, J.W., and Hamilton, W.F.: Studies on circulation. I. Injection method, physical and mathematical considerations. Am. J. Physiol., 89, 322, 1929.

8. Moore, J.W., Kinsman, J.M., Hamilton, W.F., and Spurling, R.G.: Studies on the circulation. II. Cardiac output determinations, comparison of the injections with direct Fick procedure. Am. J. Physiol., 89, 331, 1929.

9. Hamilton, W.F., Moore, J.W., Kinsman, J.M., and Spurling, R.G.: Blood flow and intrathoracic blood volume as determined by the injection method and checked by direct measurement in perfusion experiments. Am. J. Physiol., 93, 654, 1930.

10. _____: Further analysis of the injection method and of changes in hemodynamics under physiological and pathological conditions. Am. J. Physiol., 99, 534, 1932.

11. Meier, P., and Zierler, K.L.: On the theory of the indicator dilution method for measurement of blood flow and volume. J. Appl. Physiol., 6, 731, 1954.

12. Cournand, A., and Ranges, H.A.: Catheterization of the right auricle in man. Proc. Soc. Exp. Biol., & Med. 46, 462, 1941.

13. Cournand, A., Riley, R.L., Breed, E.S., Baldwin, E., de F., and Richards, D.W.: Measurement of cardiac output in man using the technique of catheterization of the right auricle or ventricle. J. Clin. Invest., 24, 106 1945.

14. Hamilton, W.F., Riley, R.L. Attyah, A.M., Cournand, A., Fowell, D.M., Himmelstein, A., Noble, R.P., Remington, J.W., Richards, D.W., Wheeler, N.C., and Witham, A.C.: Comparison of the Fick and dye injection methods of measuring the cardiac output in man. Am. J. Physiol., 153, 321, 1948.

15. Werkö, L., Lagerlöf, H., Bucht, H., Wehle, B., and Holmgren, A.: Comparison of the Fick and Hamilton methods for the determination of cardiac output in man. Scand. J. Clin. Lab. Invest., 1, 109, 1949.

16. Kopelman, H., and Lee, G. de J.: The intrathoracic blood volume in mitral stenosis and left ventricular failure. Clin. Sci., 10, 383, 1951.

17. Johnson, S.R.: The effect of some anaesthetic agents on the circulation in man. Acta Chir. Scand. Suppl. 158, 1951.

18. Doyle, J.T., Wilson, J.S., Lepine, C., and Warren, J.V.: An evaluation of the measurement of cardiac output and the so-called pulmonary blood volume by the dye dilution method. J. Lab. & Clin. Med., 41, 29, 1953.

19. Eliasch, H., Lagerlöf, H., Bucht, H., Ek, J., Eriksson, K., Bergstrom, J., and Werkö, L.: Comparison of the dye dilution and the direct Fick methods for the measurement of cardiac output in man. Scand. J. Clin. Lab. Invest., 7, Suppl. 20, 73, 1954.

20. Shepherd, J.T., Bowers, D., and Wood, E.H.: Measurement of cardiac output in man by injection of dye at a constant rate into the right ventricle or pulmonary artery. J. Appl. Physiol., 7, 629, 1955.

21. Taylor, S.H., and Shillingford, J.P.: Clinical application of coomassie blue. Brit. Heart J., 21, 497, 1959.

22. Nicholson, J.W., Burchell, H.B., and Wood, E.H.: A method for the continuous recording of Evans blue dye curves in arterial blood, and its application to the diagnosis of cardiovascular abnormalities. J. Lab. & Clin. Med., 37, 353, 1951.

23. Nicholson, J.W., and Wood, E.H.: Estimation of cardiac output and Evans blue space in man using an oximeter. J. Lab. & Clin. Med., 38, 588, 1951.

24. Wood, E.H., Swan, H.J.C., and Heimholz, H.F.: Recording and basic patterns of dilution curves: Normal and abnormal. Proc. Staff Meet., Mayo Clinic. 32, 464, 1957.

25. Swan, H.J.C., Burchell, H.B., Linder, E., Birkhead, N.C., and Wood, E.H.: Technic and

diagnostic applications of dilution curves recorded simultaneously from left and right sides of heart and arterial circulations following injections of indicator at selected sites in the cardiac chambers and great vessels. Proc. Staff Meet., Mayo Clinic, *33*, 581, 1958.

26. Korner, P.I., and Shillingford, J.P.: Quantitative estimation of valvular incompetence by dye dilution curves. Clin. Sci., *14*, 553, 1955.

27. Shillingford, J.P.: Simple method for estimating mitral regurgitation by dye dilution curves. Brit. Heart J., *20*, 229, 1958.

28. Prinzmetal, M., Corday, E., Spritzler, R.J., and Flieg, W.: Radiocardiography and its clinical applications. J.A.M.A., *139*, 617, 1949.

29. MacIntyre, W.J., Pritchard, W.H., Eckstein, R.W., and Friedell, H.L.: The determination of cardiac output by continuous recording system utilizing iodinated (I^{131}) human serum albumin. I. Animal studies. Circulation, *4*, 552, 1951.

30. Pritchard, W.H., MacIntyre, W.J., Schmidt, W.C., Brofman, B.L., and Moore, D.J.: The determination of cardiac output by a continuous recording system utilizing iodinated (I^{131}) human serum albumin. II. Clinical studies. Circulation, *6*, 572, 1952.

31. Veall, N., Pearson, J.D., Hanley, T., and Love, A.E.: A method for the determination of cardiac output (preliminary report). Proc. of Second Radioisotope Conf., Oxford, p. 183, London, Butterworth Scientific Publications, 1954.

32. Huff, R.L., Feller, D.D., Judd, O.J., and Bogardus, G.M.: Cardiac output of man and dogs measured by in vivo analysis of iodinated (I^{131}) human serum albumin. Circ. Res., *3*, 564, 1955.

33. Milnor, W.R., Talbot, S.A., McKeever, W.P., Marye, R.B., and Newman, E.V.: A photographic ear densitometer for continuously recording the arterial concentration of T-1824 in the dye dilution method. Circ. Res., *1*, 117, 1953.

34. Shadle, O.W., Ferguson, T. B., Gregg, D., and Gilford, S.R.: Evaluation of a new cuvette densitometer for determination of cardiac output. Circ. Res., *1*, 200, 1953.

35. Gilford, S.R., Gregg, D.E., Shadle, O.W., Ferguson, T.B., and Marzetta, L.A.: An improved cuvette densitometer for cardiac output determination by the dye-dilution method. Rev. Scient. Instruments, *24*, 696, 1953.

36. Fox, I.J., Sutterer, W.F., and Wood, E.H.: Dynamic response characteristics of system for continuous recording of concentration changes in a flowing fluid. J. Appl. Physiol., *11*, 390, 1957.

37. Fox, I.J., Brooker, L.G.S., Heseltine, D.W., Essex, H.E., and Wood, E.H.: A tricarbocyanine dye for continuous recording of dilution curves in whole blood independent of variations in blood oxygen saturation. Proc. Staff Meet., Mayo Clinic, *32*, 478, 1957.

38. Fox, I.J., and Wood, E.H.: Indocyanine green: Physical and physiologic properties. Proc. Staff Meet., Mayo Clinic, *35*, 732, 1960.

39. Fox, I.J.: Indicators and detectors for circulatory dilution studies and their application to organ or regional blood-flow determination. Circ. Res., *10*, 447, 1962.

40. Woodward, E., Jr., Swan, H.J.C., and Wood, E.H.: Evaluation of a method for detection of mitral regurgitation from indicator dilution curves recorded from the left atrium. Proc. Staff Meet., Mayo Clinic, *32*, 525, 1957.

41. Braunwald, E., Tanenbaum, H.L., and Morrow, A.G.: A method for detection and estimation of aortic regurgitant flow in man. Circulation, *17*, 505, 1958.

42. Lange, R.L., and Hecht, H.H.: Quantitation of valvular regurgitation from multiple indicator dilution curves. Circulation, *18*, 623, 1958.

43. Sanders, R.J.: Use of radioactive gas (Kr^{85}) in the diagnosis of cardiac shunts. Proc. Soc. Exp. Biol. & Med., *97*, 1, 1958.

44. Morrow, A.G., Sanders, R.J., and Braunwald, E.: The nitrous oxide test: An improved method for the detection of left and right shunts. Circulation, *17*, 284, 1958.

45. Case, R.B., Horley, H.W., Keating, R., Keating, P., Sachs, H.L., and Loeffler, E.E.: Detection of circulatory shunts by use of radioactive gas. Proc. Soc. Exp. Biol. & Med., *97*, 4, 1958.

46. Clark, L.C., and Bargeson, L.M.: Left to right shunt detection by an intravascular electrode with hydrogen as an indicator. Science, *130*, 709, 1959.

47. Clark, L.C., Bargeson, L.M., Lyons, C., Bradley, M.N., and McArthur, K.T.: Detection of right to left shunts with an arterial potentiometric electrode. Circulation, *22*, 949, 1960.

48. Pfaff, W.W., Frommer, P., and Morrow, A.G.: Ascorbic acid dilution curves in cardiovascular diagnosis. Surg. Forum, *11*, 147, 1960.

49. Hyman, A.L., Hyman, E.S., Ouiroz, A.C., and Gantt, J.R.: Hydrogen platinum electrode system in detection of intravascular shunts. Am. Heart J., *61*, 53, 1961.

50. Wood, E. H.: Diagnostic applications of indicator-dilution techniques in congenital heart disease. Circ. Res., *10*, 531, 1962.

51. Newman, E.V., Merrell, M., Genecin, A., Minge, C., Milnor, W.R., and McKeever, W.P.: The dye dilution method for describing the central circulation. Circulation, *4*, 735, 1951.

52. Sheppard, C.W.: Mathematical considerations of indicator-dilution techniques. Minnesota Med., *37*, 93, 1954.

53. Lacy, W.W., Emanuel, R.W., and Newman, E.V.: Effect of the sampling system on the shape of indicator-dilution curves. Circ. Res., *5*, 586, 1957.

54. Pritchard, W.H., MacIntyre, W.J., and Moir, T.W.: The determination of cardiac output by the dilution method without arterial sampling. II. Validation of precordial recording. Circulation, *18*, 1147, 1958.

55. Milnor, W.R., and Jose, A.D.: Distortion of indicator-dilution curves by sampling systems. J. Appl. Physiol., *15*, 177, 1960.

56. Grodins, F.S.: Basic concepts in the determination of vascular volumes by indicator-dilution methods. Circ. Res., *10*, 429, 1962.

57. Dyson, N.A., Hugh-Jones, P., Newberry, G.R., Sinclair, J.D., and West, J.B.: Studies of regional lung function using radioactive oxygen. Brit. Med. J., *1*, 231, 1960.

58. West, J.B., and Dollery, C.T.: Distribution of blood flow and ventilation-perfusion ratio in the lung, measured with radioactive CO_2. J. Appl. Physiol., *15*, 405, 1961.

59. Ball, W.C., Stewart. P.B., Neusham, L.G.S., and Bates, D.V.: Regional pulmonary function studied with xenon,[133] J. Clin. Invest., *41*, 519, 1962.

60. Kunieda, R.: Evaluation of pulmonary blood volume in mitral valve disease by T-1824 method. Respiration and Circulation (Kokyu to Junkan), *3*, 510. 1955.

61. Milnor, W.R., Jose, A.D., and McGaff, C.J.: Pulmonary vascular volume, resistance and compliance in man. Circulation, *22*, 130, 1960.

62. Dock, D.S., Kraus, W.L., McQuire, L.B., Hyland, J.W., Haynes, F.W., and Dexter, L.: The pulmonary blood volume in man. J. Clin. Invest., *40*, 317, 1961.

63. Donato, L.: Selective quantitative radiocardiography. Prog. Cardiovasc. Dis., *5*, 1, 1962.

64. Holt, J.P.: Estimation of the residual volume of the ventricle of the dog's heart by two indicator-dilution techniques. Circ. Res., *4*, 187, 1956.

65. Thorpe, C.R., and Grodins, F.S.: Estimation of left ventricular volumes from thermodilution curves. Fed. Proc., *19*, 117, 1960.

66. Folse, R., and Braunwald, E.: Determination of fraction of left ventricular volume ejected per beat and of ventricular end-diastolic and residual volumes. Experimental and clinical observation with a precordial dilution technic. Circulation, *25*, 674, 1962.

67. Rapaport, E., Wiegand, B.D., and Bristow, J.D.: Estimation of left ventricular residual volume in the dog by a thermodilution method. Circ. Res., *11*, 803, 1962.

68. Bristow, J.D., Crislip, R.L., Farrehi, C., Harris, W.E., Lewis, R.P., Sutherland, D.W., and Griswold, H.E.: Left ventricular volume measurements in man by thermodilution. J. Clin. Invest., *43*, 1015, 1964.

69. Kuno, Y.: On the amount of blood in the lungs. J. Physiol., *51*, 154, 1917.

70. Ebert, R.V., Borden, C.W., Wells, H.S., and Wilson, R.H.: Studies of the pulmonary circulation. I. The circulation time from the pulmonary artery to the femoral artery and the quantity of blood in the lungs in normal individuals. J.Clin. Invest., *28*, 1134, 1949.

71. Borden, C.W., Ebert, R.V., Wilson, R.H., and Wells, H.S.: Studies of pulmonary circulation. II. The circulation time from pulmonary artery to the femoral artery and the quantity of blood in the lungs in patients with mitral stenosis and in patients with left ventricular failure. J. Clin. Invest., *28*, 1138, 1949.

72. Witham, A.C., and Fleming, J.W.: The effect of epinephrine on the pulmonary circulation in man. J. Clin. Invest., *30*, 707, 1951.

73. Witham, A.C., Fleming, J.W., and Bloom, W.L.: The effect of intravenous administration of dextran on cardiac output and other circulatory dynamics. J. Clin. Invest., *30*, 897, 1951.

74. Doyle, J.T., Wilson, J.S., and Warren, J.V.: The pulmonary vascular responses to short-term hypoxia in human subjects. Circulation, *5*, 263, 1952.

75. Hetzel, P.S., Swan, H.J.C., and Wood, E.H.: Influence of injection site on arterial dilution curves of T-1824. J. Appl. Physiol., *7*, 66, 1954.

76. Rapaport, E., Kuida, H., Haynes, F.W., and Dexter, L.: The pulmonary blood volume in mitral stenosis. J. Clin. Invest., *35*, 1393, 1956.

77. Lammerant, J.: *Le volume sanguin des poumons chez l'homme.* Bruxelles, Editions Arsica, 1957.

78. Pietila, K.A., and Hakkila, J.: Studies of cardiac output and pulmonary and intra-

thoracic blood volume. Cardiologia, *36*, 97, 1960.

79. Yu, P.N., Finlayson, J.K., Luria, M.N., Stanfield, C.A., Schreiner, B.F., and Lovejoy, F.W.: Indicator-dilution curves in valvular heart disease; after injection of indicators into the pulmonary artery and the left ventricle. Am. Heart J., *60*, 503, 1960.

80. Eich, R.H., Chaffee, W.R., and Chodos, R.B.: Measurement of central blood volume by external monitoring. Circ. Res., *9*, 629, 1961.

81. Moir, T.W., and Gott, F.S.: The central circulating blood volume in normal subjects and patients with mitral stenosis. Am. Heart J., *61*, 740, 1961.

82. Levinson, G.E., Frank, M.J., Palman, R.S., Landy, E.N., and Behar, A.: Effect of exercise on the blood volume of the lung and left heart in man. Circulation, *24*, 981, 1961.

83. Love, W.D., O'Meallie, L.P., and Burch, G.E.: Clinical evaluation of the volumes of blood in the right heart, left heart and lungs by use of I^{131} albumin. Am. Heart J., *61*, 397, 1961.

84. Chaffee, W.R., Smulyan, H., Kreighley, J.F., and Eich, R.H.: The effect of exercise on pulmonary blood volume. Am. Heart J., *66*, 657, 1963.

85. McIntosh, H.D., Gleason, W.L., Miller, D.E., and Bacos, J.M.: A major pitfall in the interpretation of "central blood volume." Circ. Res., *9*, 1223, 1961.

86. Marshall, R.J., and Shepherd, J.T.: Interpretation of changes in "central" blood volume and slope volume during exercise in man. J. Clin. Invest., *40*, 375, 1961.

87. Dow, P.: Estimations of cardiac output and central blood volume by dye dilution. Physiol. Rev., *36*, 77, 1956.

88. Ross, J.: Catheterization of the left heart through the interatrial septum: A new technique and its experimental evaluation. Surg. Forum, *9*, 297, 1958.

89. Ross, J., Braunwald, E., and Morrow, A.G.: Left heart catheterization by the transseptal route: A description of the technic and its applications. Circulation, *22*, 927, 1960.

90. Brockenbrough, E.C., Braunwald, E., and Ross, J.: Transseptal left heart catheterization: A review of 450 studies and description of an improved technique. Circulation, *25*, 15, 1962.

91. Fujimoto, K., Kunieda, R., and Shiba, T.: Lung blood volume in acquired valvular diseases. Jap. Heart J., *1*, 442, 1960.

92. Levinson, G.E., Frank, M.J., and Hellems, H.K.: The pulmonary vascular volume in man. Measurement from atrial dilution curves. Am. Heart J., *67*, 734, 1964.

93. Freitas, F.M., de, Faraco, E.Z., Nedel, N., Azevedo, D.F., de, and Zaduchliver, J.: Determination of pulmonary blood volume by single intravenous injection of one indicator in patients with normal and high pulmonary vascular resistance. Circulation, *30*, 370, 1964.

94. Oakley, C., Glick, G., Luria, M.N., Schreiner, B.F., and Yu, P.N.: Some regulatory mechanisms of human pulmonary vascular bed. Circulation, *26*, 917, 1962.

95. Freitas, F.M., de, Faraco, E.Z., Azevedo, D.F., de, Zaduchliver, J., and Lewin, I.: Behavior of normal pulmonary circulation during changes of total blood volume in man. J. Clin. Invest., *44*, 366, 1963.

96. McGaff, C.J., Roveti, G.C., Glassman, E., and Milnor, W.R.: The pulmonary blood volume in rheumatic heart disease and its alteration by isoproterenol. Circulation, *27*, 77, 1963.

97. Yu, P.N., Glick, G., Schreiner, B.F., and Murphy, G.W.: Effects of acute hypoxia on the pulmonary vascular bed of patients with acquired heart disease. With special reference to the demonstration of active vasomotion. Circulation, *27*, 541, 1963.

98. Schreiner, B.F., Murphy, G.W., Glick, G., and Yu, P.N.: Effect of exercise on the pulmonary blood volume in patients with acquired heart disease. Circulation, *27*, 559, 1963.

99. Glick, G., Schreiner, B.F., Murphy, G.W., and Yu, P.N.: Effects of inhalation of 100 per cent oxygen on the pulmonary blood volume in patients with organic heart disease. Circulation, *27*, 554, 1963.

100. Roy, S.B., Singh, I., Bhatia, M.L., and Khanna, P.K.: Effect of morphine on pulmonary blood volume in convalescents from high altitude pulmonary edema. Brit. Heart J., *27*, 876, 1965.

101. Freitas, F.M., de, Faraco, E.Z., Azevedo, D.F., de, and Lewin, I.: Action of bradykinin on human pulmonary circulation: Observations in patients with mitral valvular disease. Circulation, *34*, 385, 1966.

102. Yu, P.N., Murphy, G.W., Schreiner, B.F., and James, D.H.: Distensibility characteristics of the human pulmonary vascular bed. Study of the pressure-volume response to exercise in patients with or without heart disease. Circulation, 35, 710, 1967.

103. Donato, L., Giuntini, C., Lewis, M.L., Durand, J., Rochester, D.F., Harvey, R.M., and Cournand, A.: Quantitative radiocardiog-

raphy. I. Theoretical consideration. Circulation, *26,* 174, 1962.

104. Donato, L., Rochester, D.F., Lewis, M.L., Durand, J., Parker, J.O., and Harvey, R.M.: Quantiative radiocardiography. II. Technic and analysis of curves. Circulation, *26,* 183, 1962.

105. Lewis, M.L., Giuntini, C., Donato, L., Harvey, R.M., and Cournand, A.: Quantitative radiocardiography. III. Results and validation of theory and method. Circulation, *26,* 189, 1962.

106. Giuntini, C., Lewis, M.L., Sale Luis, A., and Harvey, R.M.: A study of the pulmonary blood volume in man by quantitative radiocardiography. J. Clin. Invest., *42,* 1589, 1963.

107. Segre, G., Turco, G.L., and Ghemi, F.: Determination of the pulmonary weighting function, of the mean pulmonary transit time and of the pulmonary blood volume in man by means of radiocardiograms. Cardiologia, *46,* 295, 1965.

108. Roughton F.J.W.: The average time spent by the blood in the human lung capillary and its relation to the rates of CO uptake and elimination in man. Am. J. Physiol., *143,* 621, 1945.

109. Filley, G.F., MacIntosh, D.J., and Wright, G.W: CO uptake and pulmonary diffusing capacity in normal subjects at rest and during exercise. J. Clin. Invest., *33,* 530, 1954.

110. Forster, R.E., Roughton, F.J.W., Cander, L., Briscoe, W.A., and Kreuzer, F.: Apparent pulmonary diffusing capacity for CO at varying alveolar O_2 tensions. J. Appl. Physiol., *11,* 277, 1957.

111. Roughton, F.J.W., and Forster, R.E.: Relative importance of diffusion and chemical reaction rates in determining rate of exchange of gases in human lung, with special reference to true diffusing capacity of pulmonary membrane and volume of blood in the lung capillaries. J. Appl. Physiol., *11,* 291, 1957.

112. Forster, R.E.: Exchange of gases between alveolar air and pulmonary capillary blood: Pulmonary diffusing capacity. Physiol. Rev., *37,* 391, 1957.

113. Ogilive, C.M., Forster, R.E., Blakemore, W.S., and Morton, J.W.: A standardized breath holding technique for clinical measurement of the diffusing capacity of the lung for carbon monoxide. J. Clin. Invest., *36,* 1, 1957.

114. McNeill, R.S., Rankin, J., and Forster, R.E.: The diffusing capacity of the pulmonary membrane and the pulmonary capillary blood volume in cardiopulmonary disease. Clin. Sci., *17,* 465, 1958.

CHAPTER 2

Functional Anatomy of the Human Pulmonary Vascular Bed

A detailed description of the morphology and structure of the human pulmonary vascular bed is beyond the scope of this monograph. The reader is referred to the excellent books or monographs written by many authors.[1-9]

The functioning lung involves the three basic components of tissue, blood, and air. The tissue is relatively stationary, but blood and air move into and out of the lung rapidly and constantly. The tissue framework consists of the bronchopulmonary tree and the pulmonary vascular bed, including the alveolo-capillary interface.

In the mature lung the bronchopulmonary tree and pulmonary blood vessels have a characteristic relationship to each other. The pulmonary arteries closely accompany the bronchopulmonary tree, and the pulmonary veins are located between the branches of the tree.

The bronchial arteries are nutrient arteries which deliver oxygenated blood to the walls of tracheobronchopulmonary tree, and to the tissues of pulmonary arteries and veins. Most of the bronchial venous blood enters the azygous veins, but a small portion drains into the pulmonary veins. The bronchial arterial blood flow in normal man is too small to be measured by the indirect techniques now available.[10,11] It probably is of the order of less than 100 ml/min.[12,13] The pulmonary circulation extends from the pulmonary valve to the orifices of the pulmonary veins in the wall of the left atrium. The three segments of the pulmonary vascular bed are arteries, capillaries, and veins. From the most distal point where pulmonary arterioles can be recognized to the point where pulmonary venules can be distinguished, 25 or more capillary networks can usually be identified.[6]

The pulmonary arteries are end arteries and consist of (a) a pulmonary trunk, which is about 5 cm long and 3 cm in diameter; (b) main arteries, either elastic (exceeding 1 cm in diameter) or muscular (from 0.1 to 1 cm in diameter); and (c) pulmonary arterioles (less than 0.1 cm in diameter).[5]

Histologically, the media of the pulmonary trunk and the elastic pulmonary arteries consists predominantly of elastic fibrils with some smooth muscle fibers, collagen substance and acid mucopolysaccharide. Both the intima and adventitia are fibrous tissue. The media of the muscular arteries consist of smooth muscle fibers lined by internal and external elastic laminae. The larger pulmonary arteries are distensible structures and are able to hold over one third of each right ventricular systolic volume at normal pulmonary arterial pressure.[14-16]

The anatomic characteristics of the small muscular pulmonary arteries suggest they are best suited for vasomotor activity manifested by active change in caliber and altered resistance to perfusion. These vessels are not really muscular in the sense that they resemble the thick-walled muscular arteries in the systemic circulation.[5] The pulmonary arterioles lie between muscular pulmonary arteries and capillaries. They do not have a heavy coat of circular smooth muscle, and their wall consists of an endothelial lining and a single elastic lamina. They have no muscular media or adventitia. In contrast to the systemic circulation, sphincteric precapillary vessels are absent in the low-pressure pulmonary circulation.

Since the pulmonary arteries closely accompany the bronchopulmonary tree and are in the same connective tissue as the bronchi, they are subjected to the same external forces. Normally the pressure around the pulmonary arteries is subatmospheric. During inspiration, however, the tissue pressure becomes more negative, while the transmural pressure becomes more positive. Thus, there is a tendency for the vessels to become dilated.[3,17-19]

The volume of the pulmonary arteries was estimated by Smith and Dexter in 26 patients at post-mortem examination.[20,21] The patients were considered to have normal lungs by gross and microscopic criteria, and their ages ranged from sixteen to ninety-one years. The pulmonary arterial tree was injected with modified Schlesinger mass, the volume of injectate required to fill the arterial system was recorded, and subsequent arteriograms of the lungs were made. The pulmonary arterial volume of the right lung in 12 patients ranged between 56 and 67 ml/M[2] with a mean ± S.D. of 62 ± 3.3 ml/M[2], while the arterial volume of the left lung in 14 patients ranged between 50 and 64 ml/M[2] with a mean ± S.D. of 55 ± 4.0 ml/M[2].

The pulmonary capillaries form a dense network which is enclosed in the alveolar wall. The capillary network is like a large vascular sheet with a surface of approximately 40-80 M[2] extending throughout the major part of the lungs.[6] The capillary networks in different portions of the lung vary in length, caliber, size, and number of vessels. Hayek and Weibel respectively estimated 300 million as the average number of alveoli in each of five human lungs.[3,6] By electron microscopy the thinnest portion of the alveolo-capillary tissue barrier separating blood and air has been measured to be around 0.4 μ.[6]

The capillaries do not appear to have smooth muscle in the wall or contractile cells surrounding them. Therefore, change in the caliber of the capillaries is probably achieved by mechanical means such as alteration in alveolar pressure, movement of adjacent structures, and the pressure of perivascular fluid.

The total capillary surface and capillary volume in five normal human lungs measured by Weibel[6] are listed in Table 2-1. Both total capillary surface and capillary volume were directly proportional to the size of the lung, and the capillary bed and its surface were dependent on the degree of blood filling. If values of 7 to 9 μ are accepted as the average normal range of variation for capillary diameter, the capillary blood volume of the adult lung may be calculated to vary between 100 and 200 ml, depending upon the size of the lung

Table 2-1   Pulmonary Capillary Surface and Volume (After Weibel)

| Subject | Capillary Surface (M^2) | | Capillary Volume (ml) | |
	Total	Internal*	Total	Estimated Blood Volume**
1	43.5	40.2	87	75
2	48.0	44.0	124	108
3	70.5	65.1	192	166
4	73.0	67.7	195	168
5	82.5	76.5	244	212

*about 92% of total capillary surface
**about 85% of total capillary volume

and the degree of capillary filling.[6]

The pulmonary capillary blood volume determined *in vivo* by carbon monoxide diffusing capacity in normal subjects at rest in general is lower than that estimated by the morphometric method.[22-31] The values reported varied from 57 to 143 ml in the sitting position and from 86 to 112 ml in the supine position. The lower values estimated by physiologic methods may be due to the fact that the pulmonary capillary blood volume at rest determined by the physiologic method is an "instantaneous" and not an "anatomic" volume. However, according to Johnson and associates,[32] during peak exercise or at peak work load, the maximum pulmonary capillary blood volume in normal subjects as well as in patients with mitral stenosis agrees closely with the maximal capacity of the pulmonary capillary bed estimated by Weibel. Several workers have shown that the pulmonary vascular flow, including the capillary blood flow, is pulsatile and intermittent.[33-36] It is likely that at a given moment only part of the capillary network is filled with blood.

Thus, the distinct possibility is recognized that at rest not all of the capillary networks are patent. During heavy exercise, however, the pulmonary capillary blood volume may increase considerably. This increase has been attributed to the opening of some previously closed capillaries as well as dilatation of some already patent capillaries.

The four pulmonary veins are end veins and enter the upper posterior left atrium. Their media contains more collagenous fibers and their musculo-elastic fibers are less regularly and distinctly arranged than in the corresponding counterparts in the pulmonary arteries. In animals the blood volume in the pulmonary veins may be as much as 53% of the total pulmonary blood volume,[37] but no information is available concerning the pulmonary venous blood volume in man. Because of the relative deficiency in smooth muscle and elastic fibers, the pulmonary veins are much less vasoactive than the corresponding arteries.[5,9]

Heath has presented convincing evidence that human pulmonary vasculature undergoes profound structural changes with increasing age.[38] In fetal life the pulmonary vessels are similar to systemic vessels with thick muscular walls, and pulmonary arterial pressure is correspondingly high. In adult life the pulmonary vessels are thin walled and highly distensible with low resistance to blood flow. In old age the pulmonary vascular tree becomes progressively arteriosclerotic, more fibrous, and less elastic. It was his contention that circumferential extensibility of the pulmonary trunk and the distensibility of the pulmonary vascular bed decrease with increasing age. Recent observations by several workers have indicated that the elasticity or static retractive force of the lung decreases progressively with age.[39-41] These mechanical changes may reflect irreversible alteration in the deposition of fibrous tissue or in the loss of lung tissue.

On the other hand, by means of hemodynamic and post-mortem radiographic studies, Dexter and co-workers[21] found no relationship between age and the following parameters: pulmonary arterial pressure, pulmonary vascular resistance, pulmonary arterial volume, and gross appearance or cross sectional area of the pulmonary vasculature. It is indeed very difficult to determine whether the structural changes in the pulmonary vessels are sufficient to interfere with what is called "normal" function.

Larsell and Dow[42] have described the distribution of the nerves and their endings within the human lungs, the innervation of which arises from the vagi and the sympathetic nerves. The pulmonary plexuses which communicate with the cardiac, aortic and esophageal plexuses consist of larger vagal and smaller sympathetic contributions. The vagal pulmonary branches contain both preganglionic and afferent fibers. The sympathetic pulmonary fibers are derived from the second to the fifth or sixth thoracic ganglia. Intensive studies of the pulmonary vasomotor nerves (vasoconstrictors and vasodilators) in animals have been carried out by Daly and Daly.[43-45] These fibers have been identified both in the vagus nerves and in the upper sympathetic chain. The caliber of the pulmonary vessels does change after these nerves are stimulated. In isolated experiments, pulmonary vasoconstrictor fibers were demonstrated to run primarily through the sympathetic system. However, in many instances,

because of the overlapping and intertwining of the nerve fibers, it was not possible to distinguish whether sympathetic or vagal effect was predominant in specific instances.[9] The recent demonstrations of both baroreceptor and chemoreceptor-like tissue in the wall of pulmonary trunk and the physiologic study of the nature of chemoreceptors will undoubtedly throw new light toward our understanding of the regulatory mechanisms of pulmonary vessels.[46-50]

The study of whole lung and its blood vessels in the normally inflated state has been a recent advance of major interest in cardiopulmonary investigation.[51] The new information has been derived from (a) the examination of whole lung slices;[52] (b) study of air-dried or fixed inflated whole lung;[53-55] (c) instantaneous rapid freezing of the lung tissue;[56,57] (d) injection or angiographic study of the pulmonary vasculature and parenchyma;[58-62] (e) electron microscopic studies of the fine structures of the lungs;[63,64] and (f) in vivo study of the movement of the lung segments and pulmonary vessels.[65,66] Emphasis on the pulmonary surface tension in relation to pulmonary function has been another important aspect of recent advances in cardiopulmonary physiology.[67,68]

Recently, the need has been emphasized for in vivo studies of pulmonary anatomy and physiology in four dimensions—length, width, depth and time.[69] Increasing awareness of the importance of four dimensional studies is evident in recent articles on four-dimensional anatomy, four-dimensional histopathology, and four-dimensional microscopy.[70-72] Krahl states "Closed chest techniques for in vivo microscopy of the lung afford the best opportunity to obtain reliable information on pulmonary structure and function."[69] He further elicited the following important information obtained by observation and cinemicrography of living lungs through the thoracic window: (*a*) There was no movement in a lateral area of lung lying opposite the second rib (dog) and the third rib (rabbit) during inspiration. (*b*) Pulmonary arterioles of rabbits' lung underwent both passive and dynamic changes in length and diameter at rest as well as under various experimental conditions. (*c*) Evidence was presented of relative ischemia due to periodic and localized constrictions of peripheral pulmonary arterioles which regulate blood flow to discrete groups of alveoli. (*d*) Marked differences were shown in the vascular perfusion of secondary pulmonary lobules throughout the lung at a given time. (*e*) Marked constriction of the vessels could be produced by electrical stimulation of ipsilateral vagus nerve.

Opportunities for further investigation along this line are virtually unlimited, particularly in relation to the pharmacodynamics of the pulmonary circulation, neural and chemical regulation of pulmonary and bronchial circulation, and response of the pulmonary vessels to unusual gas mixtures.

REFERENCES

1. Miller, W.S.: *The Lung*, 2nd ed., Springfield, Charles C Thomas, 1947.

2. Mitchell, G.A.G.: *Cardiovascular Innervation*, Edinburgh, E. & S. Livingstone Ltd., 1956.

3. Hayek, H. Von: *The Human Lung* (translated by Krahl, V.E.), New York, Hafner Publishing Company, 1960.

4. Engel, S.: *Lung Structure*, Springfield, Charles C Thomas, 1962.

5. Harris, P., and Heath, D.: *Human Pulmonary Circulation*, Baltimore, Williams and Wilkins Co, 1962.

6. Weibel, E.R.: *Morphometry of the Human Lung*, New York, Academic Press, Inc., 1963.

7. Burton, A.C.: Relation of structure to function of the tissues of the wall of blood vessels. Physiol. Rev., *34*, 619, 1954.

8. Krahl, V.E.: The mammalian lung. In *Handbook of Physiology*. Section 3, Respiration, Vol. 1, Chapter 6, p. 213, Washington, D.C., American Physiological Society, 1963.

9. Fishman, A.P.: Dynamics of the pulmonary circulation. In *Handbook of Physiology*. Section 2, Circulation, Vol. 2, Chapter 48, p. 1667, Washington, D.C., American Physiological Society, 1963.

10. Fishman, A.P., Turino, G.M., Brandfonbrenner, M., and Himmelstein, A.: The effective pulmonary collateral blood flow in man. J. Clin. Invest., *37*, 1071, 1958.

11. Fritts, H.W., Jr., Harris, P., Chidsey, C.A., Clauss, R.H., and Cournand, A.: Validation of a method for measuring the output of the right ventricle in man by inscription of dye dilution curves from the pulmonary artery. J. Appl. Physiol., *11*, 362, 1957.

12. Fritts, H.W., Hardewig, A., Rochester, D.F., Durand, J., and Cournand, A.: Estimation of pulmonary arteriovenous shunts flow using intravenous injections of T 1824 dye and Kr.[85] J. Clin. Invest., *39*, 1841, 1960.

13. Cudkowics, L., Abelman, W.H., Levinson, G.E., Katznelson, G., and Jreissaty, R.M.: Bronchial arterial blood flow. Clin. Sci., *19*, 1, 1960.

14. Meyer, W.W., and Schollmeyer, P.: Die Volumendehnbarkeit und die Druch-Amfang-Beziehungen des Lungenschlagader-Windkessels in Abhangigkeit vom alter und pulmonalen Hochdruck. Klin. Wochenschrit, *35*, 1070, 1957.

15. Patel, D.J., Freitus, F.M., de, and Mallos, A.J.: Mechanical function of main pulmonary artery. J. Appl. Physiol., *17*, 205, 1962.

16. Staub, N.C.: The interdependence of pulmonary structure and function. Anesthesiology, *24*, 831, 1963.

17. Macklin, C.C.: Evidence of increase in the capacity of the pulmonary arteries and veins of dogs, cats and rabbits during inflation of the freshly excised lung. Rev. Canad. Biol., *5*, 199, 1946.

18. Altmann, K.: Experimentell-morphologische unter Suchungen über die Beziehungen zwischen der Lungen capillar weite und dem Lungendehnungs grad. Z. Exp. Med., *122*, 516, 1954.

19. Howell, J.B.L. Permutt, S., Proctor, D.F. and Riley, R.L.: Effect of inflation of the, lung on different parts of pulmonary vascular bed. J. Appl. Physiol., *16*, 71, 1961.

20. Dexter, L., and Smith, G.T.: Quantitative studies of pulmonary embolism. Am. J. Med. Sci., *247*, 37, 1964.

21. Dexter, L., Haynes, F.W., and Smith, G.T.: Physiologic changes in the pulmonary circulation with age. *In* L. Cander and J.H. Moyer (eds), *Aging of the Lung*, p, 194, New York, Grune and Stratton, 1964.

22. Roughton, F.J.W., and Forster, R.E.: Relative importance of diffusion and chemical reaction rates in determining rate of exchange of gases in the human lung. With special reference to true diffusing capacity of pulmonary membrane and volume of blood in the lung capillaries. J. Appl. Physiol., *11*, 290, 1957.

23. McNeill, R.S., Rankin, J., and Forster, R.E.: The diffusing capacity of the pulmonary membrane and the pulmonary capillary blood volume in cardiopulmonary disease. Clin. Sci., *17*, 465, 1958.

24. Lewis, B.M., Lin, T.H., Noe, F.E., and Kamisaruk, R.: The measurement of pulmonary capillary blood volume and pulmonary membrane diffusing capacity in normal subjects; the effects of exercise and position. J. Clin. Invest., *37*, 1061, 1958.

25. Bates, D.V., Varvis, C.J., Donevan, R.E., and Christie, R.V.: Variations in the pulmonary capillary blood volume and membrane diffusion component in health and disease. J. Clin. Invest., *39*, 1401, 1960.

26. Johnson, R.L., Spicer, W.S., Bishop, J.M., and Forster, R.E.: Pulmonary capillary blood volume, flow and diffusing capacity during exercise. J. Appl. Physiol., *15*, 893, 1960.

27. Flatley, F.J., Constantine, H., McCredie, R. M., and Yu, P.N.: Pulmonary diffusing capacity and pulmonary capillary volume in normal subjects and in cardiac patients. Am. Heart J., *64*, 159, 1962.

28. Daly, W.J., Ross, J.C., and Behnke, R.H.: The effect of changes in the pulmonary vascular bed produced by atropine, pulmonary engorgement and positive pressure breathing on diffusing and mechanical properties of the lung. J. Clin. Invest., *42*, 1083, 1963.

29. McCredie, R.M.: The diffusing characteristics and pressure-volume relationships of the pulmonary capillary bed in mitral valve disease. J. Clin. Invest., *43*, 2279, 1964.

30. Daly, WJ., Giammocia, S.T., Ross, J.C., and Feigenbaum, H.: Effects of pulmonary vascular congestion on postural changes in the perfusion and filling of the pulmonary vascular bed. J. Clin. Invest., *43*, 68, 1964.

31. McCredie, R.M., Lovejoy, F.W., and Yu, P.N.: Pulmonary diffusing capacity and pulmonary capillary blood volume in patients with intracardiac shunts. J. Lab. & Clin. Med., *63*, 914, 1964.

32. Johnson, R.L., Taylor, H.F., and Lawson, W.H.: Maximal diffusing capacity of the lung for carbon monoxide. J. Clin. Invest., *44*, 349, 1965.

33. Lee, G., de J., and DuBois, A.B.: Pulmonary capillary flow in man. J. Clin. Invest., *34*, 1380, 1955.

34. Bosman, R., Honour, A.J., Lee, G. de J., Marshall, R.M., and Stott, F.D.: Instantaneous pulmonary blood flow measurement in man. J. Physiol., *159*, 15, 1961.

35. Wasserman, K., and Comroe, J.H.: A method for estimating instantaneous pulmonary capillary blood flow in man. J. Clin. Invest., *41*, 400, 1962.

36. Chrispin, A.R., and Steiner, R.E.: Pulsatile flow in the pulmonary circulation: A cinefluoroscopic study. Brit. Heart J., *26*, 592, 1964.

37. Landis, E.M., and Hortenstine, J.C.: Functional significance of venous blood pressure. Physiol. Rev., *30*, 1, 1950.

38. Heath, D.: Structural changes in the pulmonary vasculature associated with aging. *In* L. Cander and J.H. Moyer (eds), *Aging of the Lung,* p. 70, New York, Grune & Stratton, 1964.

39. Pierce, J.A., and Ebert, R.V.: The elastic properties of the lungs in the aged. J. Lab. & Clin. Med. *51*, 63, 1958.

40. Wright, R.R.: Elastic tissue of normal and emphysematous lungs. Am. J. Path., *39*, 355, 1961.

41. Radford, E.P.: Static mechanical properties of lungs in relation to age. *In* L. Cander and J.H. Moyer (eds), *Aging of the Lung*, p. 152, New York, Grune and Stratton, 1964.

42. Larsell, O., and Dow, R.S.: The innervation of the human lung. Am. J. Anat., *52*, 125, 1933.

43. Daly, I. de B. and Daly, M. de B.: The effects of stimulation of the carotid chemoreceptors on pulmonary vascular resistance in the dog. J. Physiol., *137*, 436, 1957.

44. Daly, I. de B.: Intrinsic mechanisms of the lung. Quart. J. Exp. Physiol., *43*, 2, 1958.

45. Daly, I. de B., and Daly, M. de B.: The nervous control of the pulmonary circulation. *In* A.V.S. de Reuck and M. O'Connor (eds),

Ciba Foundation Symposium on Problems of Pulmonary Circulation, p. 44, London, J. and A. Churchill Ltd.; Boston, Little, Brown and Co, 1960.

46. Krahl, V.E.: The glomus pulmonale; its location and microscopic anatomy. *In* A.V.S. de Reuck and M. O'Connor (eds), *Ciba Foundation Symposium on Pulmonary Structure and Function*, p. 53, London, J. and A. Churchill Ltd.; Boston, Little, Brown and Co, 1962.

47. Verity, M.A., and Bevan, J.A.: Distribution of nerve endings in the pulmonary artery of the cat. Science, *135*, 785, 1962.

48. Bevan, J.A., and Verity, M.A.: Nerve supply of the pulmonary bifurcation baroreceptor area and its significance. Nature, *194*, 151, 1962.

49. Duke, H.N., Green, J.H., and Heffron, P.F.: Pulmonary artery chemoreceptors. J. Physiol., *164*, 8, 1962.

50. Duke, H.N., Green, J.H., Heffron, P.F., and Stubbens, V.W.: Pulmonary chemoreceptors. Quart. J. Exp. Physiol., *48*, 164, 1963.

51. Comroe, J.H., Rahn, H., Rankin, J., and Richards, D.W.: Respiratory function and pulmonary disease. *In* Andrus, E.C. (ed), *The Heart and Circulation*. Second National Conference on Cardiovascular Diseases, p. 469, Washington, D.C., Vol. 1 / Research, 1964.

52. Gough, J., and Wentworth, J.C.: Thin sections of entire organ mounted on paper. J. Roy. Microscop. Soc., *69*, 231, 1949.

53. Tobin, C.E.: Methods of preparing and studying human lungs expanded and dried with compressed air. Anat. Rec., *114*, 453, 1952.

54. Blumenthal, B.J., and Boren, H.G.: Lung structure in three dimensions after inflation and fume fixation. Am. Rev. Tuber., *79*, 764, 1959.

55. Boren, H.G.: Alveolar fenestrae: Relationship to the pathology and pathogenesis of pulmonary emphysema. Am. Rev. Resp. Dis., *85*, 328, 1962.

56. Staub, N.C.: Microcirculation of the lung utilizing very rapid freezing. Angiology, *12*, 469, 1961.

57. Staub, N.C., and Storey, W.F.: Relation between morphological and physiological events in lung studied by rapid freezing. J. Appl. Physiol., *17*, 381, 1962.

58. Steinberg, I.: Angiocardiography in pulmonary disease. Am. J. Surg., *89*, 215, 1955.

59. Doyle, A.E., Goodwin, J.F., Harrison, C.V., and Steiner, R.E.: Pulmonary vascular patterns in pulmonary hypertension. Brit. Heart J., *19*, 353, 1957.

60. Steiner, R.E.: Radiological appearances of the pulmonary vessels in pulmonary hypertension. Brit. J. Radiol., *31*, 188, 1958.

61. Dotter, C.T.: Congenital abnormalities of the pulmonary arteries and acquired abnormalities of the pulmonary arteries. *In* Abrams, H.L. (ed), *Angiography*, p. 319, Boston, Little, Brown and Co, 1961.

62. Alexander, J.K., Gonzalez, D.A., and Fred, H.L.: Angiographic studies in cardiorespiratory diseases. J.A.M.A., *198*, 575, 1966.

63. Low, F.N.: The pulmonary alveolar epithelium of laboratory mammals and man. Anat. Rec., *117*, 241, 1953.

64. Karrer, H.E.: The fine structure of connective tissue in the tunica propria of bronchioles. J. Ultrastruct. Res., *2*, 96, 1958.

65. Alva, W.E. de, Rainer, W.G., and Filley, G.F.: A method for high speed *in vivo* pulmonary microcinematography under physiologic conditions. Anat. Rec., *142*, 349, 1962 (abstract).

66. Krahl, V.E., Alva, W.E. de, Rainer, W.G., and Filley, G.F.: A method of studying the living lung in the closed thorax and some preliminary observations. Angiology, *14*, 149, 1963.

67. Clements, J.A., Brown, E.S., and Johnson, R.P.: Pulmonary surface tension and the mucous lining of the lungs: Some theoretical considerations. J. Appl. Physiol., *12*, 262, 1958.

68. Clements, J.A.: Sixth Bowditch Lecture. Surface phenomena in relation to pulmonary function. Physiologist, *5*, 11-28, 1962.

69. Krahl, V.E.: Living pulmonary histology. *In* L. Cander and J.H. Moyer (eds), *Aging of the Lung*, p. 55, New York, Grune and Stratton, 1964.

70. Lazarow, A.: The fourth dimension of anatomy. Lancet, *82*, 135, 1962.

71. Pinkus, H.: Four-dimensional histopathology. Arch. Derm., *82*, 681, 1960.

72. Krahl, V.E.: Four-dimensional microscopy applied to the study of the lung. Turtox News, *39*, 13, 1961.

CHAPTER 3

Measurement of Pulmonary Blood Flow and Pulmonary Vascular Pressures

Several excellent books and monographs should be consulted for detailed technical consideration regarding the measurement of pulmonary blood flow and pulmonary vascular pressure.[1-6] Only a summary of the pertinent information is included in this monograph.

Measurement of Pulmonary Blood Flow

In the absence of an intracardiac shunt or severe cardiopulmonary disease, the pulmonary blood flow may be considered approximately identical to the systemic blood flow. The small flow contributed by the bronchial and thebesian vessels probably does not materially influence the calculation.

The Direct Fick Method

In 1870 Fick[7] proposed that the cardiac output can be calculated from the following formula:

$$\text{Cardiac output} \ (\text{L/min}) = \frac{\text{oxygen uptake (ml/min)}}{\text{A-V oxygen difference (ml/L)}}$$

The A-V oxygen difference is the difference in oxygen content between arterial and mixed venous blood.

The validity of the principle depends upon the assumption that the lungs themselves do not extract oxygen and that truly mixed venous blood samples can be obtained for analysis.

Support for the first assumption has been the demonstration that the metabolism of lung tissue utilizes a negligible amount of oxygen. The second assumption is valid when blood is sampled directly from the right heart or pulmonary artery during right heart catheterization. Arterial blood may be drawn from an arterial needle or from a catheter inserted into a brachial, femoral, or radial artery.

Theoretically, the determination of pulmonary blood flow would be more accurate if oxygen consumption were divided by the difference in oxygen content between pulmonary venous and pulmonary arterial blood. A pulmonary venous blood sample can be obtained readily by transseptal left atrial catheterization, and a pulmonary arterial blood sample by routine right heart catheterization. This can be done if both right and transseptal left heart catheterizations are routinely performed. In practice, however, arterial blood is usually used, since the difference in oxygen content between the arterial and pulmonary venous (left atrial) blood samples withdrawn simultaneously is small enough not to affect the interpretation of the result.

The oxygen uptake is calculated by multiplying the volume of the expired air by the fraction which is oxygen. The latter is the difference between the oxygen content in the inspired air and that in the expired air. The calculation should take into account the respiratory exchange ratio of the expired gas, and the value should be converted to conditions of standard temperature and pressure.

Samples of expired air are analyzed by standard laboratory methods or read directly from a reliable oxygen analyzer. Samples of blood are analyzed by the Van Slyke manometric method, a spectrophotometric technique, or by an oxygen tension meter.

Accurate determination of cardiac output by the Fick procedure depends upon the achievement of a steady state—a state in which apparent oxygen consumption mirrors tissue oxygen utilization. Absence of a steady state may be manifested by tachycardia, increased and variable minute ventilation, and high respiratory exchange ratio in the expired gas.[8]

The reproducibility of this method has been tested by various groups of investigators, and the average variation between duplicate determinations has been about 10%.[2]

The Fick principle has recently been used with radioactive krypton (^{85}Kr) for the determination of cardiac output.[9,10] This chemically inert and poorly soluble gas may be dissolved in normal saline solution and infused continuously into the right atrium. When the gas reaches the pulmonary capillaries, most of it is excreted from the alveoli into the expired air. If blood is sampled simultaneously from the pulmonary artery and from a systemic artery and the concentrations of ^{85}Kr are measured, the cardiac output can be estimated according to the Fick principle. This method is rapid and permits many determinations within a short period, regardless of the steady state; but its technical complexity, particularly in handling blood samples and in recording radioactivity, has deterred its use in many centers.

The potential errors in the conventional application of Fick principle for the determination of cardiac output have been emphasized by various workers.[2-6,11]

Indicator-Dilution Methods

Varieties of Indicators Available. As outlined by Fox,[12] an ideal intravenous liquid indicator should possess the following attributes: (a) water solubility, (b) lack of toxicity, (c) suitability for sterilization, (d) freedom from disturbing effects on cardiac or respiratory function, (e) ability to be measured precisely in whole blood or plasma, (f) absence of metabolic degradation during its first circulation from injection to sampling sites, (g) complete retention in the blood stream during its initial circulation through the heart and lungs, and (h) rapid loss from the blood stream preferably complete after its first circulation (except when an indicator is used for determination of blood or plasma volume).

Various indicators have been used to measure rate of blood flow or cardiac output, to estimate total or regional blood volumes, and to detect intracardiac shunts or valvular regurgitation. They may be divided into three groups.

The first group consists of substances that change physical or chemical properties of flowing blood in a manner permitting their detection and measurement in the whole blood or plasma because of one of the following three characteristics: (a) absorption of light in a particular spectral region, (b) emission of light, or (c) emission of ionizing radiation. The most commonly used indicators under this category are indocyanine green (Cardiogreen) and radioactive iodinated human serum albumin (RISA).[13-15] Other dyes include Coomassie blue,[16] Evans blue,[17] methylene blue,[18] indigo carmine,[19] and bromsulphalein.[20] Other radioisotopes and radioactive foreign gases include ^{85}Kr,[9,10] and methyl iodide or ethyl iodide containing ^{131}I.[21,22]

A second group of indicators include reducing substances which increase current flow at a positively charged platinum polarographic electrode or induce a change in potential at a potentiometric electrode. Hydrogen gas and ascorbic acid belong to this group.[23,24]

A third group of indicators consist of warmed or cooled isotonic aqueous solutions. The resulting temperature change produced in the blood can be detected and measured. In this manner, normal saline has been used to estimate cardiac output and left ventricular residual volume.[25-28]

Principles and Procedures.[29-33] The principles of the method may be summarized as follows. In a closed system of circulation (human body), if an indicator is injected into a proximal site (pulmonary artery), it mixes with the fluid in the system, traverses the various alternate pathways and is carried to a distal site (brachial artery). There the indicator may be sampled through a needle or tube, and its concentration in the circulation may be recorded as a function of time following injection. When recirculation of indicator occurs before sampling of the first circulation is completed, a second rise in concentration is recorded.

The cardiac output is calculated from the formula:

$$\text{Cardiac output} \atop (\text{L/min}) = \frac{I \times 60}{C \times t}$$

Where I = the amount of dye injected (mg)
C = average concentration of the dye during the primary circulation (mg/L)
t = time interval of the primary circulation (sec)

The theoretical and mathematical validity of the method has been well established.[34-36] Before densitometer and electronic recording systems were developed, arterial blood samples were usually collected and analyzed in a series of mechanically timed test tube specimens. A time-concentration curve was then plotted semilogarithmically, and the early (straight line) portion of the downslope was extrapolated in order to separate the primary circulation from recirculation. The area under the primary circulation curve, replotted linearly and measured by a planimeter, is the product of time (sec) and average concentration (mg/L). The concentration of the dye was determined by standard methods after blood samples were diluted and calibrated against a set of samples containing known concentrations of dye. The procedure was tedious and cumbersome; and, accordingly, the indicator-dilution technique was not widely adopted for the determination of cardiac output.

With the introduction of the cuvette densitometer and convenient recording instruments, however, blood from a distal site could be sampled continuously and the concentration of the indicator inscribed instantaneously. Instruments are available which make the semilogarithmic extrapolation electronically and provide a numerical read-out of cardiac output. These technical improvements considerably simplified the procedure and facilitated the widespread use of indicator-dilution techniques in cardiovascular diagnosis and research in many institutions. The number of curves that can be recorded with indocyanine green is virtually unlimited. More than 90 curves were recorded in animal experiments during a single study without technical difficulties or apparent ill effects on the dogs.[12] During one period of two hours we have inscribed more than 20 curves with the same dye in a patient and encountered no difficulty.

Figure 3-1 illustrates a set of typical curves recorded in a normal subject after the injection of indocyanine green into various sites in the right heart and pulmonary circulation and sampling of blood from a systemic artery.

Using an earpiece cuvette and Coomassie blue dye, cardiac output may be estimated with fair accuracy in man.[16] The method has the advantage of simplicity and can be used conveniently at the patient's bedside, but more extensive trials are necessary before it can be widely adopted for clinical use.

The time-concentration curve of a radioactive indicator may be also recorded after the injection of the indicator into a peripheral vein using a scintillation counter over the precordium. Prinzmetal and co-workers[37] first reported the feasibility of estimating cardiac output from precordial dilution curves recorded by a relatively unshielded Geiger tube after a

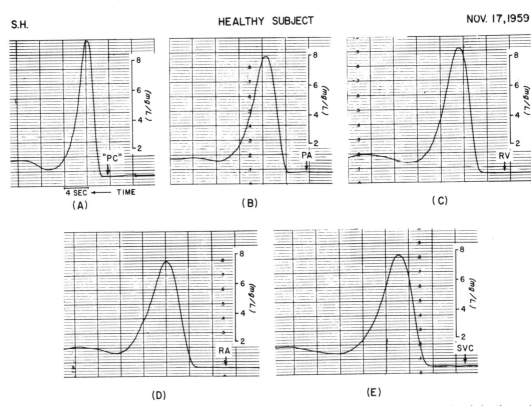

S.H.   HEALTHY SUBJECT   NOV. 17, 1959

Figure 3-1. A set of indicator-dilution curves in a normal subject after the injection of indocyanine green into various sites in the right heart and pulmonary circulation and sampling of blood from a systemic artery. "PC" = pulmonary wedge position, PA = pulmonary artery, RV = right ventricle, RA = right atrium and SVC = superior vena cava.

single intravenous injection of ^{24}Na. Work of a more sophisticated nature was described shortly thereafter by MacIntyre, Pritchard and associates.[14,15] Subsequent studies by Shipley and co-workers[38] with modern scintillation equipment and wide angle counting of RISA yielded estimates of rate of blood flow approximately twice those obtained by conventional methods. Veall, Huff, MacIntyre, Pritchard and their respective associates[39-42] refined the technique by improving collimation of the detector head and positioning the detector near the aorta. Their estimates of flow approximated those obtained by direct arterial sampling and by the Fick procedure.

This external counting method gained popularity because cardiac catheterization and arterial sampling are unnecessary. Some workers have confirmed in patients that measurements of cardiac output by the external counting method correspond very well with those determined by the Fick principle or by any dye injection and arterial sampling.[43,44] Others, however, have found an overestimate of about 12% with the external counting method.[45] The position of the scintillation counter over the precordium is critical in this method, and the use of a narrow collimeter may reduce the error appreciably. Safety and technical considerations, however, establish a limit to the number of curves that can be inscribed at one time using radioisotope. Ordinarily, only 5 or 6 curves may be recorded if a total dose of 300 μc of radioisotope (RISA) is used.

Comparison of Direct Fick and Indicator-Dilution Methods

Wade and Bishop compared and tabulated measurements of cardiac output or cardiac index by the direct Fick principle with simultaneous determinations by indicator-dilution methods as reported from twelve centers.[2] The Fick and indicator-dilution methods failed to agree in one quarter of all reported cases, but little systematic error was found between the results of the two methods.

The same authors have also reported an extensive search for data concerning the resting cardiac output in normal subjects, determined by either the Fick or indicator-dilution method. Up to 1961 they found 45 reports with 510 measurements (247 by the Fick procedure and 263 by indicator-dilution methods; 431 in men and 79 in women). They constructed a freqency distribution table of the means and standard deviations of the data reported by various authors and found that the most frequently reported mean values for resting cardiac index for both methods lie between 3.2 and 3.8 L/min/M^2. These authors enumerated various factors which may influence cardiac output at rest. These include body size, sex, age, posture, emotion, temperature, pregnancy, and oxygen tension. For detailed information, the reader is referred to their monograph.

Other Methods of Measuring Cardiac Output or Pulmonary Blood Flow

Foreign Gas Method. These indirect methods involve breathing from a bag a foreign gas which is soluble in plasma but does not combine with hemoglobin. Knowing the solubility coefficient of the gas in plasma and the amount of gas removed from the bag in a given time, one can estimate the rate of blood flow through the lungs.

Acetylene Method. This method

was originally developed by Grollman.[46] The procedure consists "in rebreathing a mixture of acetylene in air from a bag until a homogeneous mixture of acetylene is obtained in the lung-bag system. A sample of the gas, which is in equilibrium with the blood traversing the lungs, is analyzed for its oxygen, nitrogen and acetylene contents." The percentages of these gases may be designated as $(O_2)_I$, $(N_2)_I$ and $(C_2H_2)_I$, respectively. After an interval of t (usually 12 seconds), during which the subject continues to breath, a second sample of gas is withdrawn and analyzed. The percentages of oxygen, nitrogen, and acetylene in the second sample may be respectively represented by $(O_2)_{II}$, $(N_2)_{II}$, and $(C_2H_2)_{II}$. Cardiac output or pulmonary blood flow is calculated by the following formula:

$$C.O. = \frac{(\dot{V}_{O_2}) \cdot (C_2H_2)\,diff.}{(O_2)\,diff. \cdot (C_2H_2)\,av. \cdot (B-48.1) \cdot (0.00974)}$$

Where
  C.O. = cardiac output in L/min
  $\dot{V}_{O_2}$ = oxygen uptake in ml/min
  (C_2H_2) diff.= (C_2H_2) cor. $- (C_2H_2)_{II}$

  (C_2H_2) cor. = $(C_2H_2)_I \times \dfrac{(N_2)_{II}}{(N_2)_I}$

  (O_2) diff.= (O_2) cor. $- (O_2)_{II}$

  (O_2) cor.= $(O_2)_I \times \dfrac{(N_2)_{II}}{(N_1)_I}$

  (C_2H_2) av.= $\dfrac{(C_2H_2)_I + (C_2H_2)_{II}}{2}$

  B = barometric pressure in mm Hg
  48.1 = water vapor pressure in mm Hg
  0.00974 = solubility coefficient of acetylene

Although this method was used by many workers for a relatively short period, its estimates of cardiac output were considered to be inaccurate because samples were being taken after recirculation had occurred. Compared with the results obtained by cardiac catheterization, the cardiac output estimated by the acetylene method in its original form was far too low.[47,48]

Recent work by Cander and

Forster,[49] however, indicates that the acetylene method may be useful in the determination of cardiac output if rebreathing is eliminated and the error due to recirculation can be avoided.

Nitrous Oxide Method. In 1912 Krogh and Lindhard[50] used nitrous oxide to measure pulmonary blood flow in man by spirometry. The method aroused little general interest, however, because of its practical technical difficulties and because the direct Fick and indicator-dilution techniques were widely used in the determination of cardiac output. In 1955, Lee and Du-Bois[51] reported substitution of the body plethysmograph for the spirometer in measuring the uptake of nitrous oxide. These two workers were able to measure both mean and instantaneous pulmonary capillary blood flow. Later, modified plethysmographic techniques were developed for more convenient measurement of instantaneous pulmonary capillary blood flow.[52]

In 1962, DuBois and associates[53] published data comparing the cardiac output estimated by the Fick procedure with mean pulmonary capillary blood flow measured by the plethysmographic nitrous oxide absorption method. No significant statistical difference was observed. They further compared the pulsatile pulmonary capillary blood flow curves with pulmonary artery-pulmonary wedge pressure gradient curves. The general features of these curves were remarkably similar.

The basic equation for calculating the pulmonary capillary blood flow from the plethysmographic nitrous oxide absorption method is as follows:

$$\dot{Q}_C = \frac{\dot{V}_{N_2O}}{F_{A_{N_2O}} \times \alpha_{N_2O}}$$

Where
  $\dot{Q}_C$ = pulmonary capillary blood flow per minute
  $\dot{V}_{N_2O}$ = volume of nitrous oxide absorbed per minute (BTPS)

$F_{A_{N_2O}}$ = fraction of alveolar nitrous oxide (BTPS)

$\propto_{N_2O}$ = coefficient of solubility of nitrous oxide in whole blood at 37° C.

Although this technique has not been widely used for routine determination of pulmonary blood flow, it has its distinct value in research.

Angiocardiographic Methods. Left ventricular volume has been measured by angiocardiography after injection of radiopaque media. Recently, special formulae have been used for the measurement of the left ventricular volume by either biplane or single plane angiocardiography.[54-59] The end-diastolic and end-systolic volumes are measured and the difference between the two during each cycle is the stroke volume. Cardiac output per minute can be obtained by the product of the stroke volume and the heart rate per minute. The stroke volume so measured agrees well with that determined by the Fick procedure and by indicator-dilution technique.[56-61]

Electrical Impedance Plethysmography.* Plethysmography is the process of recording internal fluid flow by measuring changes in external volume. If the recording is based on measurements of electrical impedance instead of volume, the term electrical impedance plethysmography (EIP) is used. Several workers have reported the application of EIP to the estimation of pulmonary blood flow or cardiac output.[62,63]

In our laboratory a plethysmograph was constructed for application to the human thorax. It consists of four circumferential electrodes—two for placement around the neck and two around the abdomen—a 100 kHz

---

*I am indebted to Dr. Edwin Kinnen, Associate Professor of Electrical Engineering, University of Rochester School of Medicine, for the material in this section.

constant current source and a voltage balance circuit. Thoracic impedance fluctuations appear as voltage variations across the inner electrodes, possibly resulting from changes in the blood volume of the pulmonary vascular bed. Impedance records are taken during the cardiac catheterization, either before or after determinations of cardiac output by the Fick procedure or indicator-dilution technique. A phonocardiogram and an electrocardiogram are recorded simultaneously with the impedance variations.

The stroke volume is calculated according to the following formula:

$$S.V. = \frac{Pb l^2 \triangle R}{R^2}$$

Where   Pb = resistivity of blood (150 ohm cm)

l = distance between the lower cervical and upper abdominal electrodes in cm

$\triangle R$ = magnitude of resistance (or impedance) change measured from extrapolated slopes of the recorded waveform during the period of systole

R^2 = average balance resistance of the basically resistive body impedance

An example of the construction used to obtain R is shown in Figure 3-2 for a typical waveform. The negative slope is always clearly indicated during the rapid ejection phase of systole. The positive slope is estimated from the waveform during the portion of the second heart sound associated with the pulmonary valve closure. The distance from the peak of the impedance wave during the first heart sound to the middle point between the vertical distance projecting from the intersection of the positive and negative slopes and the second sounds is taken as $\triangle R$.

We have completed a study correlating cardiac output determined by the indicator-dilution technique and the Fick procedure with corresponding

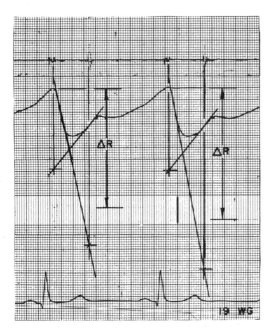

Figure 3-2. An example of a typical electrical impedance plethysmographic (EIP) waveform recorded in a patient with patent ductus arteriosus. The top line shows the first and second heart sounds. The EIP waveform is recorded in the middle. The negative slope is clearly indicated during the early systolic ejection, while the positive slope is estimated from the waveform during the portion of second sound. The distance from the peak of the impedance wave during the first heart sound to the middle point between the vertical distance projecting from the intersection of the positive and negative slopes and the second sound is taken as △ R.

values estimated from the impedance plethysmograph in a group of cardiac patients. The correlation of the data is excellent if it is limited to values derived from patients in sinus rhythm with typical impedance waveforms. From our previous work we have postulated that the impedance estimates of cardiac output are based on right ventricular stroke volume as reflected by changes in pulmonary blood volume over a heart cycle.

Studies have been undertaken to estimate pulmonary arterial and venous flow in dogs with chronically implanted electromagnetic flow probes.

Our approach has been similar to that reported by other workers.[64a,65b] In addition, pulmonary arterial and venous signals were combined electronically to allow us to record the integral of their difference. Preliminary observations have demonstrated that over each cycle the waveforms derived from the integrated flow difference varied with characteristics in common with the impedance plethysmographic waveforms recorded from human subjects.

Regional Pulmonary Blood Flow

A variety of techniques are now available for the estimation of regional pulmonary blood flow. These include angiography of the pulmonary vessels,[65-67] differential bronchospirometry,[68] external detection of either inhaled or injected radioactive bases,[69-72] and external radioisotope scanning.[73-75]

The earlier method for the measurement of regional lung function is differential bronchospirometry. In skillful hands, this technique provides reliable information; but the procedure is time consuming, tedious, and uncomfortable for the patient. Furthermore, the measurements are made under somewhat unphysiologic conditions and differences within one lung cannot be reliably assessed.

Using gases such as $C^{15}O$, $C^{15}O_2$, and xenon[133], the blood flow and ventilation of small regions of the lung can be measured by placement of multiple probes on the chest under normal physiologic conditions and without discomfort to the patient.[69-72]

In the normal human lung, with the patient upright, blood flow is much less at the apices than at the dependent zones of the lungs; and the high ventilation-perfusion ratio at the apices gradually converts to low values as the base of lung is approached. When the subject lies supine, the blood flow to the upper zone increases until it becomes virtually equal to that in the lower zone.[69,71,75] The differences in regional lung perfusion in the erect position have been attributed to effects of gravity.

On moderate exercise in the upright position, blood flow in the upper zone increases proportionately more than that in the dependent zone so that the distribution of blood flow becomes more uniform. Pulmonary hypertension not associated with an increased pulmonary blood flow also results in a more even distribution of flow. Patients with moderate mitral stenosis show a uniform distribution of blood flow at the apices and base of the lung.[70,72,75] In patients with severe or advanced mitral stenosis, an inversion of the normal pattern may be observed so that the apical blood flow exceeds basal flow.

West and associates found that the distribution of blood flow in an isolated dog lung preparation is influenced by changes in both pulmonary vascular and alveolar pressures.[76,77] Increase in pulmonary arterial pressure resulted in a more uniform flow while decrease in pulmonary arterial pressure caused under-perfusion of the apex. Increase in pulmonary venous pressure also caused a more even distribution of blood flow. The apex of the lung became unperfused when alveolar pressure was increased. Based on the observation on regional pulmonary blood flow in man and in isolated dog lungs, the human lung may be divided into three zones, blood flow through which is influenced by the factors summarized in Table 3-1.

Utilizing external scintillation scanning technique following the intravenous administration of macroaggregates of ^{131}I labeled human serum

TABLE 3-1   (After West)

Zone	Pressure Relationship*	Conditions of Flow
Top	$P_A > Pa > Pv$	Virtually no flow due to collapsible vessels (capillaries?) directly exposed to P_A
Middle	$Pa > P_A > Pv$	The vessels behave like Starling resistors and flow is determined by the difference between Pa which is higher than at the apex down the lung and P_A which is constant
Bottom	$Pa > Pv > P_A$	Flow is determined by the pressure difference between Pa and Pv. Both Pa and Pv are higher in this region than at the apex. Flow increases further because the transmural pressure of the vessels is larger so that the vessels have a larger caliber

*P_A = alveolar pressure
Pa = pulmonary arterial pressure
Pv = pulmonary venous pressure

albumin (^{131}I MAA), the pattern of distribution of pulmonary arterial blood flow also can be delineated.[73-75] This technique is simpler than that employing radioactive gases. There is a small, though systematic, difference in the results reported by these two techniques. In the erect position, the radioactive gas technique yields lower values for the ratio of blood flow per unit of tissue in the upper and lower thirds of the lung (U/L) than those obtained by ^{131}I MAA technique. This may be due to the fact that maximum inspiratory position required for the radioactive gas method exaggerates the relative decrease in blood flow at the apices. In a series of patients with mitral valve disease, Friedman and Braunwald[75] found a close correlation between the U/L and the mean left atrial pressure. Thus, in these patients the extent of the abnormality of distribution of the pulmonary arterial blood flow may be indeed an index of the hemodynamic severity of the disease.

Measurement of Pulmonary Vascular Pressures

Pressure in the pulmonary vascular bed may be measured via a catheter by means of right heart catheterization.[78,79] The catheter, filled with heparinized saline or 5% dextrose in water, is connected to a strain gauge with a rigid chamber and a flexible diaphragm. The gauge is filled with sodium citrate or saline solution and connected to a carrier amplifier and an electronic recorder. In some instances a built-in manometer is mounted at the tip of the catheter. Pressure alterations in the pulmonary artery are transmitted through the solution and cause mechanical movements of the metal diaphragm in the gauge. These mechanical movements are converted into electrical signals which are amplified and recorded on a direct-writing or photographic electronic recorder.

The catheter-manometer systems do have their limitations, however, particularly when they are required to record pressure which is changing rapidly from moment to moment. The most frequent artifacts are those produced by movements of the catheter with heart beat.

For the measurement of absolute intravascular pressure in the lungs the zero or reference level for the externally placed manometer is usually taken at a level 5 to 6 cm below the angle of Louis or 10 to 12 cm above the table top. This point is presumed to be the center of the right atrium. It is obvious that different reference levels may be adopted by different laboratories. Reliable consecutive measurements under various conditions may be made with a fixed reference to any reasonable level.

Pulmonary Arterial Pressure

The pulmonary arterial pressure was first measured in man when right heart catheterization was introduced. The contour of the pulmonary arterial pressure pulse generally resembles that of the ascending aorta with a systolic peak, a dicrotic incisura or notch, and a decline to the diastolic level. In a patient with normal pulmonary arterial pressure the configuration of the pressure curve may be so distorted by artifacts that identification of its various components requires critical damping (Figure 3-3). On the other hand, satisfactory pulmonary arterial pressure curves are usual in patients with moderately severe or severe pulmonary hypertension in whom the distorting artifacts are much less frequently encountered (Figure 3-4).

In general, the normal pulmonary arterial systolic pressure is less than 30 mm Hg, the diastolic pressure less than 12 mm Hg, and the mean pressure less than 20 mm Hg. In a series of 52 normal subjects the average systolic pressure was found to be about 22 mm Hg and the diastolic pressure 10 mm Hg.[80] The mean pressure has been obtained heretofore by planimetric measurement of the pressure curves. Now, mean pressure may be reliably approximated electronically. The measurement of pressure should take into account the respiratory variations, since intrathoracic pressure is higher in expiration than in inspiration. Thus, it is routine to average pressure over at least two respiratory cycles.

In many patients apprehension or anxiety may cause temporary elevation of the pulmonary arterial pressure during the initial phase of cardiac catheterization. A gradual decline of the pressure is not uncommon later in the course of the procedure. As previously reported, a difference as large as 8 mm Hg was found between duplicate determinations of pulmonary arterial mean pressure in a subject at rest over a period of an hour.[81] Because of such pressure variations the effects of physiologic or pharmacologic interventions on the pulmonary circulation may not necessarily be interpret-

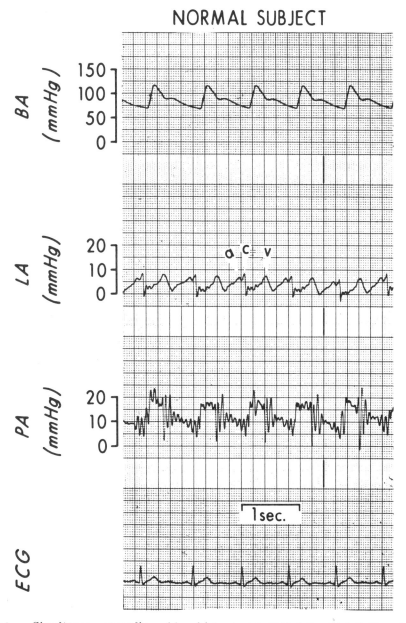

Figure 3-3. Simultaneous recording of brachial arterial (BA), left atrial (LA) and pulmonary arterial (PA) pressures and electrocardiogram (ECG) in a normal subject. Note a, c, and v waves in the left atrial tracings and marked distortion of the configuration of the pulmonary arterial pressure curve by artifacts.

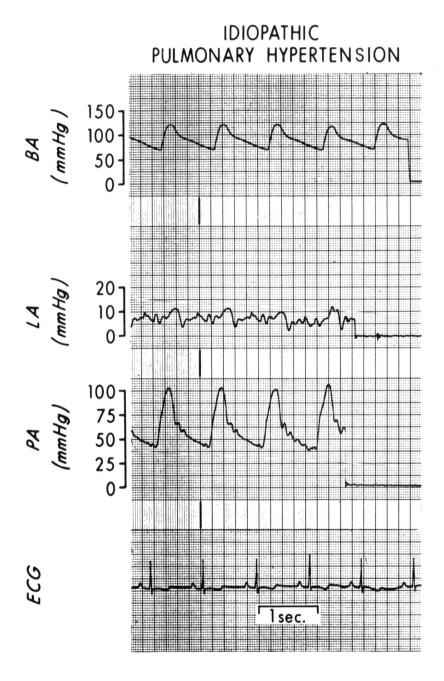

IDIOPATHIC PULMONARY HYPERTENSION

Figure 3-4.   Simultaneous recording of brachial arterial (BA), left atrial (LA) and pulmonary arterial (PA) pressures and electrocardiogram (ECG) in a patient with idiopathic pulmonary hypertension. Both the brachial arterial and the left atrial pressures are normal, but the pulmonary arterial pressure is markedly elevated. In this patient the pulmonary arterial pressure curve is satisfactory without distorting artifacts although there is slight delay in the upstroke of the curve.

ed with confidence at face value. Hence, in any physiologic or pharmacologic study the pressure taken immediately prior to an experimental maneuver should be used as the control pressure. This general precaution, of course, applies to hemodynamic studies all pressures in the pulmonary vasular bed.

Pulmonary Arterial Wedge Pressure

By advancing a cardiac catheter to a terminal branch of the pulmonary artery, one may record the so-called pulmonary arterial wedge pressure or pulmonary wedge pressure.[82,83] This measurement was originally called pulmonary "capillary" pressure because it was assumed that it measured pressure in the pulmonary capillary bed. It has since been demonstrated that the pulmonary wedge pressure closely approximates pressure in the pulmonary veins and in the left atrium Figure 3-5). *

Pulmonary wedge and left atrial pressures have been recorded simultaneously in many patients with normal pulmonary arterial pressure and in others with pulmonary hypertension.[85-93] A clearly pulsatile tracing with two distinct waves is found in only about half of patients with normal pulmonary arterial pressure, but such a tracing is found in nearly all patients with pulmonary venous hypertension. The contour of the pulmonary wedge and left atrial pressures may show phasic differences, but the mean values are virtually identical in most cases (Figure 3-5). The mean wedge pressure may be several mm Hg higher in a few.[93]

Several criteria have been proposed to ensure that the catheter occupies the wedge position. These include (a) a characteristic left atrial pressure pattern with a, c, and v waves on the wedge pressure recording and normal respiratory variation; (b) a lower wedge mean pressure than the pulmonary arterial mean pressure; (c) the withdrawal of fully oxygenated pulmonary capillary blood from the wedged catheter; (d) a sudden snap of the catheter and change in the pressure pattern as the catheter is withdrawn from the wedge position to the proximal portion of the pulmonary artery. Often, however, even when a satisfactory wedge pressure is recorded, blood cannot be withdrawn from the wedged catheter. In other instances, when the catheter is impacted near the diaphragm, the pressure recorded may be simply an undulating line without discernible individual waves. In patients with marked pulmonary hypertension, wedging of a catheter in the terminal portion of a pulmonary artery is often impossible. Notwithstanding the limitations, the pulmonary wedge pressure has been generally accepted as an estimate of pulmonary venous or left atrial pressure. When left heart catheterization is not successful or not feasible, a recording of the wedge pressure does provide pertinent information about the magnitude of pulmonary venous or left atrial pressure. It also helps to distinguish so-called precapillary from postcapillary pulmonary hypertension.[94] The former group includes patients with idiopathic or thromboembolic pulmonary hypertension, those with chronic pulmonary disease, and many patients with congenital heart

---

*In a recent paper, Brody and associates described a new method for measuring pulmonary capillary pressure in isolated lung lobes of dogs.[84] The average mid-capillary pressure was found to be 13.3 cm H_2O, while pulmonary arterial pressure averaged 20.4 cm H_2O, and pulmonary venous pressure averaged 9.2 cm H_2O.

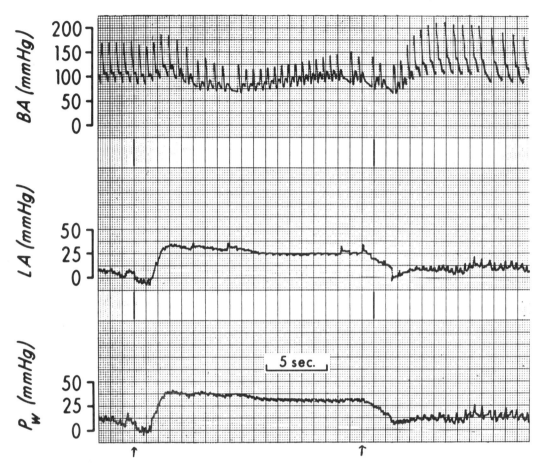

Figure 3-5. Brachial arterial (BA), left atrial (LA) and pulmonary wedge (P_w) pressures simultaneously recorded in a normal subject before, during and after Valsalva maneuver. Note the normal response of the brachial arterial pressure and the close approximation of the changes of both left atrial and pulmonary wedge pressures.

disease. The latter group consists of patients with left ventricular decompensation and the majority of patients with disease of the mitral or aortic valves. In normal subjects the mean pulmonary wedge pressure is less than 12 mm Hg and usually is 5 to 9 mm Hg.[83]

Pulmonary Venous and Left Atrial Pressures

In the past, pulmonary venous and left atrial pressures were recorded after fortuitous passage of a cardiac catheter through an atrial septal defect;[95] or the left atrial pressure was measured by various approaches including punctures during operation,[96,97] through the posterior chest wall,[90] through a bronchus,[98,99] or by suprasternal puncture.[100]

With the introduction of the transseptal technique,[101-103] the left atrial and pulmonary venous pressures could be measured with relative ease and a catheter might be left *in situ* for several hours without undue discomfort to patients. This technique has enabled many studies of pulmonary hemodynamics when prolonged periods are required for measuring pulmonary blood flow, pressure and volume.

In animal studies, significant differences have been found between pulmonary wedge and left atrial pressures, especially during acute hypoxia, indicating constriction of the pulmonary veins.[104,105] Experimental study of the volume-pressure relationship of the pulmonary vein-left heart vascular segment also suggested the presence of valve-like closure in the pulmonary vein.[106] Findings of a similar nature have also been demonstrated in man by histologic examination.[107] We have previously reported almost identical pulmonary wedge and left atrial pressures in five patients during periods of acute hypoxia.[108] For practical purposes, the left atrial pressure is almost the same as the pulmonary venous pressure in single subjects, and the two pressures may be considered interchangeable in studies of pulmonary hemodynamics in man.

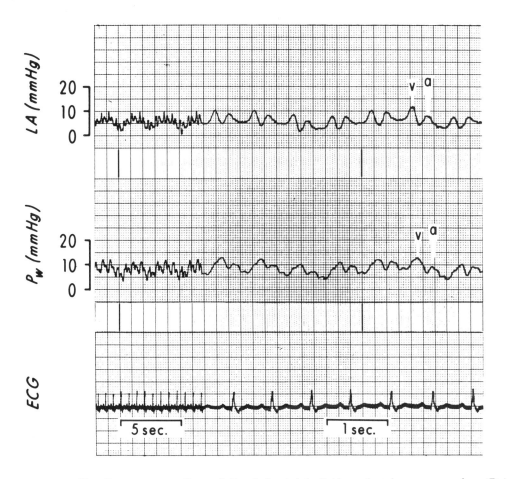

Figure 3-6. Simultaneous recording of the left atrial (LA) and pulmonary wedge (P_w) pressures and electrocardiogram (ECG) in a normal subject. The a and v waves are clearly recorded in both pressure curves. The mean values of the two pressures are almost identical although there are phasic differences.

The contour of the left atrial pressure pulse (Figure 3-6) during transseptal left heart catheterization has been fully described.[109,110] In normal subjects the values of the various components of the left atrial pressure pulse have been reported by Braunwald and associates[109] and by Samet and co-workers[110] as follows:

	Range		Average	
	Braunwald	Samet	Braunwald	Samet
LAm	2-12	5-12	7.9	9
LAm-RAm	1-7	–	3.9	6
"a" onset	1-12	–	7.1	–
"a" peak	4-16	7-16	10.4	11
"a" wave pulse pressure	1-7	–	3.4	–
"z" point	1-13	6-14	7.6	10
"v" peak	6-21	9-18	12.8	14

Definition of Three Kinds of Pressure[111,112]

Three kinds of pressure may be considered in the vascular system. (a) *Intravascular pressure* is the actual blood pressure measured in the lumen of a vessel at any point, relative to atmospheric pressure. (b) *Driving pressure* is the difference between the intravascular pressure at one proximal point and at another distal point in a vessel. This pressure is responsible for the flow of blood between two points. For the total pulmonary circulation the driving pressure is the difference between pressure in the pulmonary artery and that in the pulmonary vein or left atrium. (c) *Transmural or distending pressure* is the difference between the intravascular pressure and the tissue pressure around the vessel. The tissue pressure around the pulmonary arteries and veins is the intrathoracic pressure. The pressure around the pulmonary arterioles, capillaries, and venules is probably intermediate between alveolar and intrapleural pressure. Transmural pressure is the pressure which tends to distend the vessel. In the pulmonary circulation the approximate overall transmural pressure can be estimated by subtracting the intrathoracic pressure from the average of pulmonary arterial and venous pressures. In this monograph, the pulmonary vascular distending pressure is approximated by averaging pulmonary arterial and venous pressure. Intrathoracic pressure is not taken into account.

REFERENCES

1. Adams, W.R., and Veith, I. (eds): *Pulmonary Circulation*, New York, Grune and Stratton, 1959.

2. Wade, O.L., and Bishop, J.M.: *Cardiac Output and Regional Blood Flow*, Oxford, Blackwell Scientific Publications, 1962.

3. Harris, P., and Heath, D.: *Human Pulmonary Circulation*, Baltimore, Williams & Wilkins Co, 1962.

4. Hamilton, W.F.: Measurement of the cardiac output. *In* W.F. Hamilton and P. Dow (eds), *Handbook of Physiology*. Section 2, Vol. 1, p. 551, Washington, D.C., American Physiological Society, 1962.

5. Guyton, A.C.: *Circulatory Physiology: Cardiac Output and Its Regulation,* Philadelphia, W.B. Saunders Co, 1963.

6. Fishman, A.P.: Dynamics of the pulmonary circulation. In *Handbook of Physiology.* Section 2, Circulation, Vol. 2, p. 1681, Washington, D.C., American Physiological Society, 1963.

7. Fick, A.: Über die messung des Blutquatums in den Herzventrikeln. Verhandl d. physical med. gesellsch Z Wurzburg, *2*, 16, 1870.

8. Fishman, A.P., McClement, J., Himmelstein, A., and Cournand, A.: Effects of acute anoxia on the circulation and respiration in patients with chronic pulmonary disease studied during the "steady state." J. Clin. Invest., *31*, 770, 1952.

9. Chidsey, C.A., Fritts, H.W., Hardewig, A., Richards, D.W., and Cournand, A.: Fate of radioactive krypton (Kr[85]) introduced intravenously in man. J. Appl. Physiol., *14*, 63, 1959.

10. Rochester, D.F., Durand, J., Parker, J.O., Fritts, H.W., and Harvey, R.M.: Estimation

of right ventricular output in man using radioactive krypton (Kr85). J. Clin. Invest., *40*, 643, 1961.

11. Visscher, M.B., and Johnson,J.A.: The Fick principle: Analysis of potential errors in its conventional application. J. Appl. Physiol., *5*, 635, 1953.

12. Fox, I.J.: Indicators and detectors for circulatory dilution studies and their application to organ or regional blood flow determination. Circ. Res., *10*, 447, 1962.

13. Fox, I.J., and Wood, E.H.: Indocyanine green: Physical and physiologic properties. Proc. Staff Meet., Mayo Clinic, *35*, 732, 1960.

14. MacIntyre, W.J., Pritchard, W.H., Eckstein, R.W., and Friedell, H.L.: The determination of cardiac output by a continuous recording system utilizing iodinated(I131) human serum albumin. I. Animal studies. Circulation, *4*, 552, 1951.

15. Pritchard, W.H., MacIntyre, W.J., Schmidt, W.C., Brofman, B.L., and Moore, D.J.: The determination of cardiac output by a continuous recording system utilizing iodinated (I131) human serum albumin. II. Clinical studies. Circulation, *6*, 572, 1952.

16. Taylor, S.H., and Shillingford, J.P.: Clinical application of Coomassie blue. Brit. Heart J., *21*, 497, 1959.

17. Gibson, J.G., II, and Evans, W.A.: Clinical studies of the blood volume. I. Clinical application of a method employing the azo dye "Evans blue" and the spectrophotometer. J. Clin. Invest., *16*, 301, 1937.

18. Fox, I.J., and Wood, E.H.: Use of methylene blue as an indicator for arterial dilution curves in the study of heart disease. J. Lab. & Clin. Med., *50*, 598, 1957.

19. Lacy, W.W., Ugaz, C., and Newman, E.V.: The use of indigo carmine for dye dilution curves. Circ. Res., *3*, 570, 1955.

20. Wassen, A.: The use of bromsulphalein for determination of the cardiac output. Scand. J. Lab. & Clin. Invest., *8*, 189, 1956.

21. Amplatz, K., and Marvin, J.F.: A simple and accurate test for left-to-right cardiac shunts. Radiology, *72*, 585, 1959.

22. Case, R.B., Hurley, H.W., Keating, R.P., Keating, P., Sachs, H.L., and Loeffler, E.E.: Detection of circulatory shunts by use of a radioactive gas. Proc. Soc. Exp. Biol. & Med., *97*, 4, 1958.

23. Clark, L.C., and Bargeron, L.M.: Detection and direct recording of left-to-right shunts with hydrogen electrode catheter. Surgery, *46*, 797, 1959.

24. Pfaff, W.W., Frommer, P., and Morrow, A.G.: Ascorbic and dilution curves in cardiovascular diagnosis. Surg. Forum, *11*, 147, 1960.

25. Fegler, G.: Measurement of cardiac output in anesthetized animals by a thermodilution method. Quart. J. Exp. Physiol., *39*, 153, 1954.

26. Holt, J.P.: Estimation of the residual volume of the ventricle of the dog's heart by two indicator dilution techniques. Circ. Res., *4*, 187, 1956.

27. Evonuk, E., Imig, C.J, Greenfield, W., and Eckstein, J.W.: Cardiac output measured by thermal dilution of room temperature injectate. J. Appl. Physiol., *16*, 271, 1961.

28. Khalil, H.H.: Determination of cardiac output in man by a new method based on thermodilution. Lancet, *1*, 1352, 1963.

29. Stewart, G.N.: The pulmonary circulation time: Quantity of blood in lungs and output of heart. Am. J. Physiol., *58*, 20, 1921.

30. Hamilton, W.F., Moore, J.W., Kinsman, J.M., and Spurling, R.G.: Simultaneous determination of the pulmonary and systemic circulation times in man and of a figure related to the cardiac output. Am. J. Physiol., *84*, 338, 1928.

31. Kinsman, J.M., Moore, J.W., and Hamilton, W.F.: Studies on the circulation. I. Injection method: Physical and mathematical considerations. Am. J. Physiol., *89*, 322, 1929.

32. Hamilton, W.F., Moore, J.W., Kinsman, J.M., and Spurling, R.G.: Studies on the circulation. IV. Further analysis of the injection method, and of changes in hemodynamics under physiological and pathological conditions. Am. J. Physiol., *99*, 534, 1932.

33. Dow, P.: Estimations of cardiac output and central blood volume by dye dilution. Physiol. Rev., *38,* 77, 1956.

34. Meier, P., and Zierler, K.L.: On the theory of the indicator dilution method for the measurement of blood flow and volume. J. Appl. Physiol., *6*, 731, 1954.

35. Zierler, K.: Theoretical basis of indicator dilution methods for measuring flow and volume. Circ. Res., *10*, 393, 1962.

36. Sheppard, C.W.: Mathematical considerations of indicator dilution techniques. Minnesota Med., *37*, 93, 1954.

37. Prinzmetal, M., Corday, E., Spritzler, R.J., and Flieg, W.: Radiocardiography and its clinical application. J.A.M.A., *139*, 617, 1949.

38. Shipley, R.A., Clark, R.E., Liebowitz, D., and Krohmer, J.S.: Analysis of the radiocardiogram in heart failure. Circ. Res., *1*, 428, 1953.

39. Veall, N. Pearson, J.D., Hanley, T., and Lowes, A.E.: A method for the determination of cardiac output(preliminary report), Proc. of Second Radioisotope Conf., Oxford, p. 183, London, Butterworth Scientific Publications, 1954.

40. Huff, R.L., Feller, D.D., Judd, O.J., and Bogardus, G.M.: Cardiac output of men and dogs measured by *in vivo* analysis of iodinated(I^{131}) human serum albumin. Circ. Res., *3*, 564, 1955.

41. MacIntyre, W.J., Pritchard, W.H., and Moir, T.W.: The determination of cardiac output by the dilution method without arterial sampling. I. Analytical concepts. Circulation, *18*, 1139, 1958.

42. Pritchard, W.H., MacIntyre, W.J., and Moir, T.W.: The determination of cardiac output by the dilution method without arterial sampling. II. Validation of precordial recording. Circulation, *18*, 1147, 1958.

43. Schreiner, B.F., Lovejoy, F.W., and Yu, P.N.: Estimation of cardiac output from precordial dilution curves in patients with cardiopulmonary disease. Circ. Res., *7*, 595, 1959.

44. Pietila, K.A., and Hakkila, J.: Studies of cardiac output and of pulmonary and intrathoracic blood volume. Cardiologia, *36*, 97, 1960.

45. Van der Feer, Y., Donma, J.H., and Klip, W.: Cardiac output measurement by the injection method without arterial sampling. Am. Heart J., *56*, 642, 1958.

46. Grollman, A.: The determination of the cardiac output of man by the use of acetylene. Am. J. Physiol., *88*, 432, 1929.

47. Werkö, L., Berseus. S., and Lagerlöf, H.: A comparison of the direct Fick method and the Grollman method for determination of cardiac output in man. J. Clin. Invest., *28*, 516, 1949.

48. Chapman, C.B., Taylor, H.L., Borden, C., Ebert, R.V., Keys, A., and Carlson, W.S.: Simultaneous determination of the resting arteriovenous difference by the acetylene and direct Fick methods. J. Clin. Invest., *29*, 651, 1950.

49. Cander, L., and Forster, R.E.: Determination of pulmonary parenchymal tissue volume and pulmonary capillary blood flow in man. J. Appl. Physiol., *14*, 541, 1959.

50. Krogh, A., and Lindhard, J.: Measurements of the blood flow through the lungs of man. Scand. Arch. Physiol., *27*, 100, 1912.

51. Lee, G. de J., and DuBois, A.B.: Pulmonary capillary blood flow in man. J. Clin. Invest., *34*, 1380, 1955.

52. Wasserman, K., and Comroe, J.H.: A method for estimating instantaneous pulmonary capillary blood flow in man. J. Clin. Invest., *41*, 400, 1962.

53. Linderholm, H., Kimbel, P., Lewis, D.H., and DuBois, A.B.: Pulmonary capillary blood flow during cardiac catheterization. J. Appl. Physiol., *17*, 135, 1962.

54. Chapman, C.B., Baker, O., Reynolds, J., and Bonte, F.J.: Use of biplane cinefluorography for measurement of ventricular volume. Circulation, *18*, 1105, 1958.

55. Dodge, H.T., Hay, R.E., and Sandler, H.: An angiocardiographic method for directly determining left ventricular volume in man. Circ. Res., *11*, 739, 1962.

56. Arvedsson, H.: Angiocardiographic determination of left ventricular volume. Acta Radiol., *56*, 321, 1961.

57. Dodge, H.T., Sandler, H., Ballew, D.W., and Lord, J.D.: The use of biplane angiocardiography for the measurement of left ventricular volume in man. Am. Heart J., *60*, 762, 1962.

58. Dodge, H.T., Sandler, H., Baxley, W.A., and Hawley, R.R.: Usefulness and limitations of radiographic methods for determining left ventricular volume. Am. J. Cardiol., *18*, 10, 1966.

59. Greene, D.G., Carlisle, R., Grant, C., and Bunnell, I.L.: Estimation of left ventricular volume by one-plane cineangiography. Circulation, *35*, 61, 1967.

60. Gribbe, P.: Comparison of the angiocardiographic and the direct Fick methods in determining cardiac output. Cardiologia, *36*, 20, 1960.

61. Hallerman, F.J., Rastelli, G.C., and Swan, H.J.C.: Comparison of left ventricular volumes by dye dilution and angiocardiographic methods in the dog. Am. J. Physiol., *204*, 446, 1963.

62. Nyboer, J.: *Electrical Impedance Plethysmography*, Springfield, Charles C Thomas, 1952.

63. Kinnen, E., Kubicek, W., and Patterson, R.: Thoracic cage impedance measurements, impedance plethysmographic determination of cardiac output: A comparative study. U.S.A.F. School of Aviation Medicine, SAM-TDR-64-15, 1964.

64a. Morkin, E., Collins, J.A., Goldman, H.S., and Fishman, A.P.: The pattern of blood flow in the pulmonary veins of the dog. J. Appl. Physiol., *20*, 118, 1965.

64b. Morgan, B., Dillard, D.H., and Guntheroth, W.G.: Effect of cardiac and respiratory cycle in pulmonary vein flow, pressure and diameter. J. Appl. Physiol., *21*, 1276, 1966.

65. Davies, L.G., Goodwin, J.F., Steiner, R.E., and Van Leuven, B.D.: Clinical and radiological assessment of the pulmonary arterial pressure in mitral stenosis. Brit. Heart J., *15*, 393, 1953.

66. Doyle, A.E., Goodwin, J.F., Harrison, C.V., and Steiner, R.E.: Pulmonary vascular patterns in pulmonary hypertension. Brit. Heart J., *19*, 353, 1957.

67. Steiner, R.E.: Radiological appearance of the pulmonary vessels in pulmonary hypertension. Brit. J. Radiol., *31*, 189, 1958.

68. Mattson, S.B., and Carlens, E.: Lobar ventilation and oxygen uptake in man: Influence of body position. J. Thorac. Cardiov. Surg., *30*, 676, 1955.

69. West, J.B., and Dollery, C.T.: Distribution of blood flow and ventilation perfusion ratio in the lung, measured with radioactive CO_2. J. Appl. Physiol., *15*, 405, 1960.

70. Dollery, C.T., and West, J.B.: Regional uptake of radioactive oxygen, carbon monoxide and carbon dioxide in the lungs of patients with mitral stenosis. Circ. Res., *8*, 765, 1960.

71. Ball, W.C., Stewart, P.B., Newsham, L.G.S., and Bates, D.V.: Regional pulmonary function studied with xenon[133]. J. Clin. Invest., *41*, 519, 1962.

72. Dawson, A., Kaneko, K., and McGregor, M.: Regional lung function in patients with mitral stenosis studied with xenon[133] during air and oxygen breathing. J. Clin. Invest., *44*, 999, 1965.

73. Taplan, G.V., Johnson, D.E., Dore, E.K., and Kaplan, H.S.: Suspension of radioalbumin aggregates for photoscanning the liver, spleen, lung and other organs. J. Nucl. Med., *5*, 259, 1964.

74. Wagner, H.N., Sabiston, D.C., McAfee, J.G., Iio, M., Meyer, J.K., and Langan, J.K.: Regional pulmonary blood flow in man by radioisotope scanning. J.A.M.A., *187*, 601, 1964.

75. Friedman, W.F., and Braunwald, E.: Alterations in regional pulmonary blood flow in mitral valve disease studied by radioisotope scanning. A simple non-traumatic technique for estimation of left atrial pressure. Circulation, *34*, 363, 1966.

76. West, J.B., Dollery, C.T., and Naimark, A.: Distribution of blood flow in isolated lung; relation to vascular and alveolar pressures. J. Appl. Physiol., *19*, 713, 1964.

77. West, J.B., Dollery, C.T., and Heard, B.E.: Increased pulmonary vascular resistance in the dependent zone of the isolated dog lung caused by perivascular edema. Circ. Res., *17*, 191, 1965.

78. Cournand, A., and Ranger, H.A.: Catheterization of the right auricle in man. Proc. Soc. Exp. Biol. & Med., *46*, 462, 1941.

79. Dexter, L., Haynes, F.W., Burwell, C.S., Eppinger, E.C., Seibel, R.E., and Evans, J.M.: Studies of congenital heart disease. I. Technique of venous catheterization as a diagnostic procedure. J. Clin. Invest., *26*, 547, 1947.

80. Harris, P., and Heath, D.: *Human Pulmonary Circulation*, Baltimore, Williams & Wilkins Co, 1962.

81. Yu, P.N., Nye, R.E., Lovejoy, F.W., Schreiner, B.F., and Yim, B.J.B.: The effects of intravenous hexamethonium on pulmonary circulation in patients with mitral stenosis. J. Clin. Invest., *37*, 194, 1958.

82. Hellems, H.K., Haynes, F.W., Dexter, L., and Kinney, T.D.: Pulmonary capillary pressure in animals estimated by venous and arterial catheterization. Am. J. Physiol., *155*, 98, 1948.

83. Lagerlöf, H., and Werkö, L.: Studies on the circulation of blood in man. VI. The pulmonary capillary venous pressure pulse in man. Scand. J. Clin. Lab. Invest., *1*, 147, 1949.

84. Brody, J.S., Stemmler, E.J., and DuBois, A.B.: Longitudinal distribution of vascular resistance in the pulmonary arteries capillaries and veins. J. Clin. Invest., *47*, 783, 1968.

85. Calazel, P., Gerard, R., Daley, R., Draper, A., Foster, J., and Bing, R.J.: Physiological studies in congenital heart disease. XI. A comparison of the right and left auricular capillary and pulmonary artery pressures in nine patients with auricular septal defect. Bull. Johns Hopkins Hosp., *88*, 20, 1951.

86. Ankeney, J.L.: Interrelation of pulmonary arterial, "capillary" and left atrial pressures under experimental conditions. Am. J. Physiol., *169*, 40, 1952.

87. Epps, R.G., and Adler, R.H.: Left atrial and pulmonary capillary venous pressures in mitral stenosis. Brit. Heart J., *15*, 298, 1953.

88. Werkö, L., Vernauskas, E., Eliasch, H., Lagerlöf, H., Senning, A., and Thomasson, B.: Further evidence that the pulmonary capillary venous pressure pulse in man reflects cyclic pressure changes in the left atrium. Circ. Res., *1*, 337, 1953.

89. Wilson, R.H., McKenna, W.T., Johnson, F.E., Jenson, N.K., Mazzitello, W.F., and Dempsey, M.E.: The significance of the pulmonary arterial wedge pressure. J. Lab. & Clin. Med., *42*, 408, 1953.

90. Björk, V.D., Malmström, G., and Uggla, L.G.: Left auricular pressure measurements in man. Ann. Surg., *138*, 718, 153.

91. ⸻ : Left atrial and pulmonary "capillary" pressure curves during Valsalva's experiment. Am. Heart J., *47*, 635, 1954.

92. Connolly, P.C., Kirklin, J.W., and Wood, E.H.: The relationship between pulmonary artery wedge pressure and left atrial pressure in man. Circ. Res., *2*, 434, 1954.

93. Luchsinger, P.C., Seipp, H.W., and Patel, D.J.: Relationship of pulmonary artery wedge pressure to left atrial pressure in man. Circ. Res., *11*, 315, 1962.

94. Yu, P.N., Simpson, J.H., Lovejoy, F.W., Joos, H.A., and Nye, R.E.: Pulmonary circulatory dynamics in patients with mitral stenosis at rest. Am. Heart J., *47*, 330, 1954.

95. Cournand, A., Motley, H.L., Himmelstein, A., Dresdale, D., and Baldwin, J.S.: Recording of blood pressure from the left auricle and the pulmonary veins in human subjects with interauricular septal defects. Am. J. Physiol., *150*, 267, 1947.

96. Munnel, E.R., and Lam, C.R.: Cardiodynamic effects of mitral commissurotomy. Circulation, *4*, 321, 1951.

97. Wynn, A., Matthews, M.B., McMillan, I.K.R., and Daley, R.: Left auricular pressure pulse in normals and in mitral valve disease. Lancet, *2*, 216, 1952.

98. Facquet, J., Lemoin, J.M., Alhomme, P., and Lefeboie, J.: La mesure de la pression auriculaire gauche par voie transbronchique. Arch. mal coeur, 48, 741, 1952.

99. Allison, P.R., and Linden, R.J.: The bronchoscopic measurement of left auricular pressure. Circulation, *7*, 669, 1953.

100. Radner, S.: Suprasternal puncture of left atrium for flow studies. Acta Med. Scand., *148*, 57, 1954.

101. Ross, J., Jr.: Transseptal left heart catheterization. Ann. Surg., *149*, 395, 1959.

102. Brockenbrough, E.C., and Braunwald, E.: A new technic for left ventricular angiocardiography and transseptal left heart catheterization. Am. J. Cardiol., *6*, 1062, 1960.

103. Ross, J.: Considerations regarding the technique for transseptal left heart catheterization. Circulation, *34*, 391, 1966.

104. Rivera-Estrada, C., Saltzman, P.W., Singer, D., and Katz, L.N.: Action of hypoxia on pulmonary vasculature. Circ. Res., *6*, 10, 1958.

105. Tsagaris, T.J., Kuida, H., and Hecht, H.H.: Evidence for pulmonary venoconstriction in brisket disease. Fed. Proc., *21*, 108, 1962.

106. Little, R.C.: Volume pressure relationships of the pulmonary left heart vascular segment. Evidence for a "valve-like" closure of the pulmonary veins. Circ. Res., *8*, 594, 1960.

107. Burch, G.E., and Romney, R.B.: Functional anatomy and "throttle valve" action of the pulmonary veins. Am. Heart J., *47*, 58, 1954.

108. Yu, P.N., Glick, G., Schreiner, B.F., and Murphy, G.W.: Effects of acute hypoxia on the pulmonary vascular bed of patients with acquired heart disease. With special reference to the demonstration of active vasomotion. Circulation, *27*, 541, 1963.

109. Braunwald, E., Brockenbrough, E.C., Frahm, C.J., and Ross, J.: Left atrial and left ventricular pressures in subjects without cardiovascular disease. Circulation, *24*, 267, 1961.

110. Samet, P., Bernstein, W.H., Medow, A., and Levine, S.: Transseptal left heart dynamics in thirty-two normal subjects. Dis. Chest, *47*, 632, 1965.

111. Burton, A.C., and Patel, D.J.: Effect on pulmonary vascular resistance of inflation of rabbit lungs. J. Appl. Physiol., *12*, 239, 1958.

CHAPTER 4

Measurement of Total Blood Volume and "Central Blood Volume"

Total Blood Volume[1-4]

In recent years the measurement of total blood volume has become a routine laboratory procedure and a valuable diagnostic and research tool.

Total blood volume consists of plasma volume and red blood cell volume. The ratio of the two components of blood, cells and plasma, vary in the several components of the vascular bed. The factors responsible for differences in the ratio of red cells to plasma include the caliber of the blood vessels, the rate of flow, and the viscosity of blood. In large blood vessels, containing approximately 80% of the total blood volume, the hematocrit is fairly constant, usually about 40%. The remaining 20% of the blood volume is found in blood vessels of smaller caliber, and the hematocrit in these vessels may be as low as 23%.[3]

In the past, radiophosphorus,[5,6] radioiron,[7,8] or radiochromium tagged red blood cells[9,10] have been used for the measurement of red blood cell volume and Evans blue dye (T-1824)[11,12] or RISA[12-14] for the estimate of plasma volume. The total blood volume can be estimated by measuring either red blood cell volume or plasma volume, using an arbitrary correction factor for the difference between peripheral and total body hematocrit, or by measuring both red cell volume and plasma volume concurrently.[15-18]

In 1947 Nylin and Hedlund[19] summarized the opinions of many investigators concerning the accuracy and efficiency of the various methods of determining total blood volume. They pointed out that the dye method (T-1824) may produce falsely high values because of leakage of dye from the vascular compartment. More accurate determinations of total blood volumes are possible utilizing radioactive material. The most accurate total blood volume determinations require the plasma and red blood cell volumes to be measured independently with two appropriate tracers (*i.e.*, RISA for plasma volume and ^{51}Cr for red blood cell volume).

In our laboratory we have used only the radioisotope (RISA) dilution method for the determination of total blood volume. The principles of the method may be briefly described as follows: A known amount of radioisotope such as RISA is injected into the blood stream. It is assumed that this material remains unaltered and mixes evenly with the circulating blood and remains entirely within the vascular bed until after sampling. After an arbitrary interval (usually 10 minutes), a sample of blood is taken. The concentration of radioactivity in the sample is proportional to the dilution of RISA in the circulating blood volume. To calculate the total blood volume, the following equation is applied:

$$I = C \times V \qquad (1)$$

$$Or \quad V = \frac{I}{C} \qquad (2)$$

Where V = volume of diluent or blood volume in ml
I = amount of radioactive material administered in μc (microcuries) or CPM (counts per minute)
C = concentration of the radioactive material, after a period of equilibrium (CPM/ml)

This equation can be further expanded as follows:

Let I_1 = total dose of RISA injected into a 1000 ml flask as a standard (μc or CPM)
C_1 = concentration of RISA in the diluted standard (CPM/ml)
V_1 = 1000 ml, the dilution volume of the standard
And I_2 = total dose of RISA injected into the patient (μc or CPM)
V_2 = unknown volume or total blood volume of the patient (ml)
C_2 = concentration of RISA in the patient's blood after mixing (CPM/ml)
Then $I_1 = C_1V_1$ (3)
And $I_2 = C_2V_2$ (4)

Now if the ratio $I_2 / I_1 = R$ is known, the concentration volume products may be equated and solved for V_2.

Thus $I_2 = R\ I_1$ (5)
Or $C_2V_2 = R\ C_1V_1$ (6)
Hence $V_2 = R\ V_1 \dfrac{C_1}{C_2}$ (7)

Since concentration appears in both numerator and denominator, any unit of concentration such as CPM/ml may be used: C_1 being CPM/ml of diluted standard, or CPM_S; and C_2 being CPM/ml of patient's blood after 10 to 15 minutes of intravascular equilibration, or CPM_P. In practice, R is determined by weighing the dose in μc given to patient (D_P) and weighing the dose put into the standard solution (D_S).

Thus, $R = \dfrac{D_P.}{D_S}$ Substitution of these

values for those in equation (7), the total blood volume calculation follows:

$$TBV = \frac{D_P}{D_S} \cdot \frac{CPM_S}{CPM_P} \cdot 1000$$

Where TBV = total blood volume in ml

This equation, utilizing RISA for the determination of total blood volume, may not be precisely accurate and probably reflects overestimates of the red cell volume slightly. Thus for a hematocrit of 40%, a factor of 0.95 is used to correct for this error.[4] In clinical practice one tracer such as RISA may be used with reasonable accuracy for the determination of total blood volume.

The respective values of total, plasma, and red cell volumes in normal subjects reported by several groups of workers are presented in Table 4-1.[8,16-18,20-25] The values of TBV varied considerably in patients with valvular heart disease, but in general the mean value of TBV was higher in these patients than that in normal subjects. Many workers have found an increase in TBV in patients with cardiac failure, particularly in those with right heart failure, the value falling to normal limits after compensation was restored.[19,23,24,26-29] On the other hand, other workers have reported no significant increase in TBV in patients with cardiac failure.[30,31]

"Central Blood Volume"

Central blood volume (CBV) is usually measured by indicator-dilution technique according to the Stewart-Hamilton principle. It also has been estimated by precordial radioisotope counting.

Heretofore, CBV has been determined between a site of injection located anywhere from the antecubital vein to the pulmonary artery and site

Table 4-1   Total, Plasma and Red Cell Volumes in Normal Subjects

Authors	Sex of Subjects	No. of Subjects	Method	Ave. TBV		Ave. PV		Ave. RCV		Ref. No.
				ml/M²	ml/kg	ml/M²	ml/kg	ml/M²	ml/kg	
Gibson et al	Male	40	Fe^{55}, Fe^{59}					1151	29.8	8
	Male	49	E.B.		71.2	1620	43.1			20
	Female	41	E.B.			1151	41.5			20
Reeve and Veall		13	E.B. P^{32}				46.9		30.0	21
Gregerson and Nickerson	Male	53	E.B.	3112	82.3	1729	45.6			22
Berlin et al.	Female	16	P^{32}		64.4		37.0		27.0	23
Gray and Frank	Male	21	Chromic Chloride				39.3			16
	Male	25	Cr^{51}						31.8	
		10	Cr^{51}				41.1		30.3	
Hedlund	Male	35	P^{32}					1131	29.6	24
	Female	7	P^{32}					868	24.0	
Berson	Male	36	I^{131}				40.2			17
	Male	15	P^{32} or K^{32}						28.7	
Reilly et al	Male	89	C^{51}	2490	65.5					25
Samet et al	Male	30	E.B.			1527	41.1			18
	Male	30	P^{32}					1039	28.0	
	Female	30	E.B.			1463	40.5			
	Female	30	P^{32}					782	21.6	

Ave. TBV = Average total blood volume
Ave. PV = Average plasma volume
Ave. RCV = Average red cell volume
E.B.   = Evans blue

of sampling located variously anywhere from the root of aorta to a systemic artery. Because of the various sites of injection and sampling, it has not been possible to compare the values reported by various investigators, either at rest or during physiologic or pharmacologic interventions.

In 1949 Ebert and associates[32,33] used injections of Evans blue dye and reported (a) the circulation time from the pulmonary artery to the femoral artery and (b) the estimated CBV in normal subjects, in patients with mitral stenosis, and in patients with left ventricular failure. In the same year Lagerlöf and co-workers independently published their studies on the estimation of CBV.[34] However, the values of CBV in their series were generally higher than those reported by Ebert and associates. These studies stimulated considerable interest in the determination of CBV by many workers.[35-41] Ebert and associates actually measured the *median* circulation time instead of

the *mean* circulation time. In normal subjects the median circulation time is approximately the same or only slightly shorter than the mean circulation time. In cardiac patients with slow flow rates and asymmetrical indicator-dilution curves, however, the mean circulation time may be considerably longer than the median circulation time.[42]

For the sake of uniformity, CBV as used in this monograph is the volume measured by injecting an indicator (either a dye or a tracer) into the pulmonary artery and sampling from a systemic artery. This volume includes blood in the pulmonary vascular bed, left heart, a portion of the aorta and all arterial segments temporally equidistant to the point of sampling. The volume measured is recognized as indefinite and does not conform to any specific anatomic boundary.

The volume determined by injecting an indicator into a peripheral vein or right atrium is hereafter referred to as intrathoracic volume (ITV). The volume measured in this manner is even more indefinite because it includes the CBV, blood in the right heart, and, in some instances, a portion of the venous system.

Thus, "central" blood volume may be calculated by the following formula (Stewart-Hamilton):

$$CBV = \frac{Tm_{PA-BA}}{60} \times Qp$$

Where   CBV = "central" blood volume in ml
Tm$_{PA-BA}$ = mean transit time from the pulmonary artery to a systemic artery in seconds
Qp = pulmonary blood flow or cardiac output in ml/min

The accuracy of the measurement of "central" blood volume by the Stewart-Hamilton method has been established by various approaches: (a) perfusion experiments,[43,44] (b) model systems,[44-46] and (c) direct measurements.[47]

Estimations of CBV also have been made by a precordial radioisotope counting method, a technique which has been extended to the measurement of pulmonary blood volume.[48-54] In essence, one or two probes are placed over the precordium facing the right and left heart chambers. A dose of tracer (usually RISA) is injected into a peripheral vein and the radioactivity of the tracer is recorded externally. The peak time for each ventricle is obtained from semilogarithmic plot of the original tracing. The right ventricular downslope is extrapolated, and the extrapolated values subtracted from the left ventricular curve. Thus, the left side is corrected for the right-sided counts. The time between the right ventricular peak and the corrected left ventricular peak is used as the corrected "pulmonary circulation time" which unavoidably includes part of the "ventricular circulation time." This time multiplied by the cardiac output in ml/sec, as determined

either from the precordial or arterial dilution curve, is called the CBV or PBV. This volume includes blood in both right and left ventricles as well as that in the pulmonary vascular bed. The volume so determined is probably less than the CBV and greater than the PBV estimated by the conventional arterial sampling method.

In the reports of Ebert and associates,[32,33] the values of CBV were calculated by the formula of Stewart, using cardiac output determined by the Fick principle and median circulation time obtained by dye curves. For 13 normal subjects the CBV was 610 $\pm$ 128 ml/M^2 (mean $\pm$ S.D.), values similar to those reported by other workers who used mean circulation time for the calculation. In 10 patients with mitral stenosis and pulmonary hypertension the corresponding values were 720 $\pm$ 108 ml/M^2, and in 10 patients with aortic valve lesions and left ventricular failure the respective values were 975 $\pm$ 200 ml/M^2. CBV was within normal limits in the group of patients with mitral stenosis and pulmonary hypertension. Although CBV was elevated in patients with aortic valve disease and left ventricular failure, the authors felt that the elevated volume could be attributed to the increased volume of the left ventricle.

Kopelman and Lee[36] found no significant difference between the ITV measured in normal subjects and that in patients with mitral stenosis. They measured CBV in 5 normal patients and the values reported were 770 $\pm$ 130 ml/M^2. In 5 patients with mitral stenosis and congestive failure the mean value was 910 ml/M^2 (in only 2 patients was the CBV above the limits of normal), and in 4 of these patients during recovery from failure the mean value was 860 ml/M^2. In 4 patients with predominant left ventricular failure the mean value of CBV was significantly elevated to 1280 ml/M². A similar difference was also found in ITV between normal subjects and patients with heart failure.

Doyle and co-workers estimated CBV in many cardiac patients at rest and during certain physiologic and pharmacologic interventions.[38],[39],[55] They pointed out that a methodical error of ± 10% or a volume of about ± 100 ml may be anticipated in the measurement of CBV. They felt that a change of 20 to 30% in the CBV is required for definite significance.

Recently, utilizing the arterial indicator-dilution sampling technique, many workers reported an increase in the CBV or ITV during exercise in man.[37],[56-60] The magnitude of change depended upon the severity of exercise and the sites of injection and sampling of the indicator. By using the precordial monitoring technique, Chaffee and associates[61] also demonstrated an increase in "pulmonary" blood volume with exercise in 13 of 15 cardiac patients. On the other hand, Lammerant[48] and Moir and Gott,[52] who used the radioisotope precordial counting technique, failed to demonstrate any change in the CBV during exercise.

Some workers have postulated that CBV may be an important blood reservoir regulating the cardiac output.[1] Others have noted a decrease in CBV during general anesthesia.[35]

Gleason and co-workers[62] and Marshall and Shepherd[63] have pointed out certain pitfalls and limitations in the measurement of "central" blood volume from a peripheral arterial sampling site, particularly during any maneuver that causes redistribution of systemic blood flow. They demonstrated the importance of local reactive hyperemia affecting the flow characteristics of systemic arteries. For instance, during reactive hyperemia of the legs of normal subjects, the CBV was greater when measured from a brachial arterial sampling but was diminished when measured from the femoral artery. It was suggested that changes in either arterial volume or arterial flow distribution may alter the measured CBV. The model study by McIntosh and associates[64] demonstrated the distribution effect. These workers suggested that sampling from the aorta rather than from the peripheral artery avoids the distortion caused by altered distribution effect.

REFERENCES

1. Sjöstrand, T.: Volume and distribution of blood and their significance. in regulating the circulation. Physiol. Rev., *33*, 202, 1953.

2. _____ : Blood volume. *In* W.F. Hamilton and P. Dow (eds), *Handbook of Physiology.* Section 2, Circulation, Vol. 1, p. 51, Washington, D.C., American Physiological Society, 1962.

3. Lawson, H.C.: The volume of blood - A critical examination of methods for its measurement. *In* W.F. Hamilton and P. Dow (eds), *Handbook of Physiology.* Section 2, Circulation, Vol. 1, p. 23, Washington, D.C., American Physiological Society, 1962.

4. Albert, S.N., and Albert. C.A.: Blood volume methodology. Picker Scintillator, *9*, No. 5C, 1, 1965.

5. Hahn, L., and Hevesy, G.: A method of blood volume determination. Acta Physiol. Scand., *1*, 3, 1940.

6. Nylin, G.: Blood volume determination with radioactive phosphorus. Brit. Heart J., *7*, 81, 1945.

7. Hahn, P.F., Balfour, W.M., Ross, J.F., Bale, W.F., and Whipple, G.H.: Red cell volume circulating and total as determined by radioiron. Science, *93*, 87, 1941.

8. Gibson, J.G., Peacock, W.C., Segilman, A.M., and Sack, T.: Circulating red cell volume measured simultaneously by radioactive iron and dye methods. J. Clin. Invest., *25*, 838, 1946.

9. Gray, S.J., and Sterling, K.: The determination of the red cell volume by radioactive chromium. Science, *112*, 179, 1950.

10. Sterling, K., and Gray, S.G.: Determination of the circulating red cell volume in man by radioactive chromium. J. Clin. Invest., *29*, 1614, 1950.

11. Gibson, J.G., and Evans, W.A.: Clinical studies of the blood volume. I. Clinical application of a method employing the azo dye "Evans blue" and the spectrophotometer. J. Clin. Invest., *16*, 301, 1937.

12. Schultz, A.L., Hammarsten, J.F., Heller, B.I., and Ebert, R.V.: A critical comparison of T-1824 dye and iodinated albumin methods for plasma volume measurement. J. Clin. Invest., *32*, 107, 1953.

13. Fine, J., and Seligman, A.M.: Traumatic shock. IV. A study of the problem of the "lost plasma" in hemorrhagic shock by the use of radioactive plasma protein. J. Clin. Invest., *22*, 285, 1943.

14. Crispell, K.R., Porter, B., and Nieset, R.T.: Studies of plasma volume using human serum albumin tagged with radioactive iodine[131]. J. Clin. Invest., *29*, 513, 1950.

15. Gregerson, M.I.: Blood volume. Ann. Rev. Physiol., *13*, 397, 1951.

16. Gray, S.J., and Frank, H.: The simultaneous determination of red cell mass and plasma volume in man with radioactive sodium chromate and chronic chloride. J. Clin. Invest., *32*, 1000, 1953.

17. Berson, S.A.: Blood volume in health and disease. Bull. N.Y. Acad. Med., *30*, 750, 1954.

18. Samet, P., Fritts, H.W., Fishman, A.P., and Cournand, A.: The blood volume in heart disease. Medicine, *36*, 211, 1957.

19. Nylin, G., and Hedlund, S.: Weight of the red blood corpuscles in heart failure determined with labelled erythrocytes during and after decompensation. Am. Heart J., *33*, 770, 1947.

20. Gibson, J.G., and Evans, W.A.: Clinical studies of blood volume. II. The relation of plasma and total blood volume to venous pressure, blood velocity rate, physical measurements, age and sex in ninety normal humans. J. Clin. Invest., *16*, 317, 1937.

21. Reeve, E.B., and Veall, N.A.: A simplified method for the determination of circulating red-cell volume with radioactive phosphorus. J. Physiol., *108*, 2, 1949.

22. Gregersen, J.I., and Nickerson, J.L.: Relation of blood volume and cardiac output to body type. J. Appl. Physiol., *3*, 329, 1950.

23. Berlin, N.I., Hyde, G.M., Parsons, R.J., Lawrence, J.H., and Port, S.: Blood volume of the normal female as determined with P[32] labelled red blood cells. Proc. Soc. Exp. Biol. & Med., *76*, 831, 1951.

24. Hedlund, S.: Studies on erythropoiesis and total red cell volume in congestive heart failure. Suppl. 284, Acta Med. Scand., 1953.

25. Reilly, W.A., French, R.M., Lan, F.Y.K., Scott, K.G., and White, W.E.: Whole blood volume determined by radiochromium-tagged red cells. Comparative studies on normal and congestive heart failure patients. Circulation, *9*, 571, 1954.

26. Gibson, J.G., and Evans, W.A.: Clinical studies of blood volume. III. Changes in blood volume, venous pressure, and blood velocity rate in chronic congestive heart failure. J. Clin. Invest., *16*, 851, 1937.

27. Waller, J.V., Blumgart, H.L., and Volk, M.C.: Studies of the blood in congestive heart failure with particular reference to reticulocytosis, erythrocyte fragility, bilirubinemia, urobilinogen excretion and changes in blood volume. Arch. Int. Med., *66*, 1230, 1940.

28. Meneely, G.R., and Kaltreider, N.L.: Study of volume of blood in congestive heart failure and relation to other measurements in 15 patients. J. Clin. Invest., *22*, 521, 1943.

29. Seymour, W.B., Pritchard, W.H., Longley, L.P., and Hayman, J.M.: Cardiac output, blood and interstitial fluid volumes, total circulating serum protein, and kidney function during cardiac failure and after improvement. J. Clin. Invest., *21*, 229, 1942.

30. Prentice, T.C., Berlin, N.I., Hyde, G.M., Parsons, R.J., Lawrence J.H., and Port, S.: Total red cell volume, plasma volume and sodium space in congestive heart failure. J. Clin. Invest., *30*, 1471, 1951.

31. Ross, J.F., Chodos, R.B., Baker, W.H., and Freis, E.D.: The blood volume in congestive heart failure. Trans. Ass. Am. Physicians, *66*, 75, 1952.

32. Ebert, R.V., Borden, C.W., Wells, H.S., and Wilson, R.H.: Studies of the pulmonary circulation. The circulation time from the pulmonary artery to the femoral artery and the quantity of blood in the lungs in normal individuals. J. Clin. Invest., *28*, 1134, 1949.

33. Borden, C.W., Ebert, R.V., Wilson, R.H., and Wells, H.S., Studies of the pulmonary circulation. The circulation time from the pulmonary artery to the femoral artery and the

quantity of blood in the lungs in patients with mitral stenosis and in patients with left ventricular failure. J. Clin. Invest., *28*, 1138, 1949.

34. Lagerlöf, H., Werkö, L., Bucht, H., and Holmgren, A.: Separate determination of the blood volume of the right and left heart and the lungs in man with the aid of the dye injection method. Scand. J. Clin. & Lab. Invest., *1*, 114, 1949.

35. Johnson, S.R.: The effect of some anesthetic agents on the circulation in man: With special reference to the significance of pulmonary blood volume for circulatory regulation. Acta Chir. Scand., Suppl. 158, 1951.

36. Kopelman, H., and Lee, G. de J.: The intrathoracic blood volume in mitral stenosis and left ventricular failure. Clin. Sci., *10*, 383, 1951.

37. Ball, J.D., Kopelman, H., and Witham, A.C.: Circulatory changes in mitral stenosis at rest and on exercise. Brit. Heart J., *14*, 363, 1952.

38. Doyle, J.T., Lee, R.A., and Kelley, E.B.: Observations on the elasticity of the pulmonary vasculature in man. Am. Heart J., *44*, 565, 1952.

39. Doyle, J.S, Wilson, J.S. Lépine, C., and Warren, J.V.: An evaluation of the measurement of the cardiac output and of the so-called pulmonary blood volume by the dye dilution method. J. Lab. & Clin. Med., *41*, 29, 1953.

40. Rapaport, E., Kuida, H., Haynes, F.W., and Dexter, L.: The pulmonary blood volume in mitral stenosis. J. Clin. Invest., *35*, 1393, 1956.

41. Yu, P.N., Finlayson, J.K., Luria, M.N., Stanfield, C.A., Schreiner, B.F., and Lovejoy, F.W.: Indicator-dilution curves in valvular heart disease: After injection of indicator into the pulmonary artery and left ventricle. Am. Heart J., *60*, 503, 1960.

42. Hamilton, W.F.: The physiology of cardiac output. Circulation, *8*, 527, 1953.

43. Kinsman, J.M., Moore, J.W., and Hamilton, W.F.: Studies on the circulation. I. Injection method: Physical and mathematical considerations. Am. J. Physiol., *89*, 322, 1929.

44. Sheppard, C.W., Cough, B.L., and Crowder, B.L.: Dye dilution in canine heart-lung preparations. Circ. Res., *8*, 837, 1960.

45. Hamilton, W.F., Moore, J.W., Kinsman, J.M., and Spurling R.G.: Studies on the circulation. IV. Further analysis of the injection method and of changes in hemodynamics under physiological and pathological conditions. Am. J. Physiol., *99*, 534, 1931.

46. Crane, M.G., Adams, R., and Woodward, I.: Cardiac output measured by the injection method with use of radioactive material and continuous recording. J. Lab. & Clin. Med., *47*, 802, 1956.

47. Schlant, R.C., Novack, P., Kraus, W.L., Moore, C.B., Haynes, F.W., and Dexter, L.: The determination of central blood volume. Comparison of Stewart-Hamilton method with direct measurements in dogs. Am. J. Physiol., *196*, 499, 1959.

48. Lammerant, J.: *Le volume sanguin des poumons chez l'homme*. Bruxelles, Editions Arsica, 1957.

49. Weissler, A.M., McCraw, B.H., and Warren, J.V.: Pulmonary blood volume determined by a radioactive tracer technique. J. Appl. Physiol., *14*, 531, 1959.

50. Pietila, K.A., and Hakkila, J.: Studies of cardiac output and of pulmonary and intrathoracic blood volume. Cardiologia, *36*, 97, 1960.

51. Eich, R.H., Chaffee, W.R., and Chodos, R.B.: Measurement of central blood volume by external monitoring. Circ. Res., *9*, 626, 1961.

52. Moir, T.W., and Gott, F.S.: The central circulating blood volume in normal subjects and patients with mitral stenosis. Am. Heart J., *61*, 740, 1961.

53. Love, W.D., O'Meallie, L.P., and Burch, G.E.: Clinical estimation of the volumes of blood in the right heart, left heart, and lungs by use of I[131] albumin. Am. Heart J., *61*, 397, 1961.

54. Kashemsant, U., Smulyan, H., and Eich, R.H.: The pulmonary blood volume. Measurement in patients with rheumatic heart disease. Am. J. Med. Sci., *249*, 667, 1965.

55. Doyle, J.T., Wilson, J.S., and Warren, J.V.: The pulmonary vascular responses to short-term hypoxia in human subjects. Circulation, *2*, 263, 1952.

56. Mankin, H.T., and Swan, H.J.C.: Arterial dilution curves of 1824 during rest and exercise. Fed. Proc., *12*, 93, 1953.

57. Mitchell, J.H., Sproule, B.J., and Chapman, C.B.: The physiological meaning of the maximal oxygen intake test. J. Clin. Invest., *37*, 539, 1958.

58. Mitchell, J.H., Sproule, B.J., and Chapman, C.B.: Factors influencing respiration during heavy exercise. J. Clin. Invest., *37*, 1693, 1958.

59. Thompson, H.K., Berry, J.N., and McIntosh, H.D.: Comparison of the cardiac output responses to hyperventilation and exercise. Clin. Res., *7*, *136*, 1959.

60. Braunwald, E., and Kelly, E.R.: The effects of exercise on central blood volume in man. J. Clin. Invest., *39*, 413, 1960.

61. Chaffee, W.R., Smulyan, H., Keighley, J.F., and Eich, R.H.: The effect of exercise on pulmonary blood volume. Am. Heart J., *66*, 657, 1963.

62. Gleason, W.L., Bacos, J.M., Miller, E., and McIntosh, H.D.: A major pitfall in the inter-pretation of the central blood volume. Clin. Res., *7*, 227, 1959.

63. Marshall, R.J., and Shepherd. J.T.: Inter-pretation of changes in "central" blood vol-ume and slope volume during exercise in man. J. Clin. Invest., *40*, 375, 1961.

64. McIntosh, H.D., Gleason, W.L., Miller, D.E., and Bacos, J.M.: A major pitfall in the inter-pretation of "central blood volume." Circ. Res., *9*, 1223, 1961.

CHAPTER 5

Interrelationships—Pulmonary Vascular Pressure, Flow and Volume

Understanding the hemodynamic interrelationships in the pulmonary vascular bed requires appreciation of several physical laws and the conventional formulae which express them quantitatively.[1-8]

Pressure, Flow and Resistance

The rate of flow of a newtonian fluid through a rigid tube may be calculated according to the Poiseuille's law, expressed in the following equation, which relates flow, pressure, size of the tube, and viscosity of the fluid under stream-line conditions.

$$\dot{Q} = \frac{\triangle P \pi r^4}{8 \eta 1}$$

$$Or \quad \triangle P = \frac{\dot{Q} \cdot 8 \cdot 1 \eta}{\pi r^4}$$

Where $\dot{Q}$ = rate of flow of a fluid in ml/sec
P = pressure differential required to drive the fluid through the tube in mm Hg or dynes/cm²
r = radius of the tube in cm
l = length of the tube in cm
η = coefficient of viscosity of the fluid in poises

This equation is analogous to Ohm's law for electrical circuits, which states "The ratio of the voltage (E) between the ends of a conductor to the current (I) flowing in it is always constant, provided the physical condition of the conductor remains constant." This is expressed as follows:

$$I = \frac{E}{R}$$

$$Or \quad R = \frac{E}{I}$$

Where I = current flowing through the conductor in amperes
E = voltage across the length of the conductor in volts
R = resistance in ohms

The vascular resistance may be considered analogous to the resistance of a conductor, blood flow through the vascular bed to the current flowing through the conductor, and the pressure differential to the voltage across the conductor. Thus,

$$R = \frac{\triangle P}{\dot{Q}}$$

Where R = vascular resistance in mm Hg/ml/ sec
$\triangle P$ = pressure differential in mm Hg
$\dot{Q}$ = rate of blood flow in ml/sec

Pulmonary vascular resistance (PVR) is defined as the ratio of the mean pressure differential across the pulmonary vascular bed to the mean blood flow through it, expressed in the following equation:

$$PVR = \frac{PAm - LAm}{\dot{Q}p}$$

$$Or \quad PVR = \frac{PAm - Pw}{\dot{Q}p}$$

Where PVR = pulmonary vascular resistance
PAm = pulmonary arterial mean pressure
LAm = left atrial mean pressure
Pw = pulmonary wedge mean pressure
$\dot{Q}p$ = pulmonary blood flow

To express the pulmonary vascular resistance in fundamental units of the metric centimeter-gram-second (cgs) system, the following calculation is made:

a. Pressure = density of the fluid (gm/cm³)
       × acceleration due to gravity
          (approx. 980 cm/sec²)
       × height of fluid column (cm)
    Thus, 1 mm Hg pressure
       = 13.6 gm/cm³ × 980 cm/sec² × 0.1 cm
       $= 1332 \dfrac{gm \cdot cm \cdot cm}{cm^3 \cdot sec^2}$ Or
       $1332 \left(\dfrac{gm \cdot cm}{sec^2} \right) \dfrac{1}{cm^2}$
    By definition, 1 dyne $= 1 \dfrac{gm \cdot cm}{sec^2}$
    Therefore, 1 mm Hg pressure = 1332 dynes /cm²
b. Blood ($\dot{Q}p$) is expressed as the cardiac output in ml or cm³ per second
c. Therefore, in cgs units, the pulmonary vascular resistance (PVR) may be expressed as
       $\dfrac{dynes/cm^2}{cm^3/sec}$ Or dynes sec/cm⁵
    Some workers express the PVR in arbitrary numerical units, i.e.:
       $PVR = \dfrac{20 \text{ mm Hg}}{4 \text{ L/min}} = 5 \text{ units}$

To convert this arbitrary unit to cgs units, a factor of 80 is used. This factor is derived as follows:
$$\frac{1.36 \times 980 \times 60}{1000} = 80$$
Where 1.36 = conversion factor from mm Hg to cm H₂O
       980 = gravity acceleration factor
       60   = 60 seconds
       1000 = 1000 ml

Thus, the PVR of 5 units as previously calculated is equivalent to 5 × 80 or 400 dynes · sec/cm⁵.

It should be pointed out that in many instances, particularly under certain stressful conditions, such as exercise and acute hypoxia, accuracy in the measurements of pulmonary blood flow and pressures may be greatly influenced by the exaggerated respiratory excursions. Thus, under these circumstances, the change of the calculated pulmonary vascular resistance should be interpreted with caution.[6]

Furthermore, Permutt and associates have recently stressed that in any condition in which the alveolar pressure is greater than the pulmonary venous pressure, by interrupting a continuity in pressure between the pulmonary capillaries and veins, the pulmonary venous pressure cannot reliably be used for the calculation of pulmonary vascular resistance.[9,10]

Poiseuille's equation assumes that the viscosity of the flowing fluid remains constant, that the tube is relatively rigid, and that flow occurs at a steady state. The pressure-flow relationship in a rigid tube differs considerably from that in a distensible tube. When flow is increased in a rigid tube, the pressure differential along the tube increases proportionately. If the flow remains streamlined, the relation between these two parameters is linear and the resistance remains constant regardless of the rate of flow.

However, an increase in flow through a distensible tube causes it to dilate because of increased transmural pressure. As the tube dilates, it offers less resistance to flow. Thus, the pressure-flow relationship becomes curvilinear, the increase in pressure differential along the tube is proportionately less marked than the increase in flow, and the resistance to flow tends to diminish as flow increases.

The pulmonary blood vessels are distensible, pulmonary blood flow is pulsatile, and the blood flow through the system is nonhomogeneous. Thus, the application of the Poiseuille principle to the calculation of pulmonary vascular resistance in animal or man may be liable to considerable error. Further, when the pulmonary arterial pressure is low or the difference between the pulmonary arterial and left atrial pressure is small, a slight error in the measurement of pressure may result in a large error in the calculation of pulmonary vascular resistance.[11] The effects of various interventions on the pulmonary vascular resistance have sometimes been confusing and inconsistent. Burton and Patel[12] pointed out two possible reasons. (a) Pulmonary arterial pressure is inaccurate as a measure of driving pressure in the pulmonary circulation, driving pressure in fact being the difference in pressure between the pulmonary artery and the pulmonary vein. (b) Pressure passively distending pulmonary vessels has been assumed to be the intravascular pressure, rather than the transmural pressure which is the difference between the intravascular pressure and surrounding tissue pressure. Simmons and co-workers[13] mentioned a third possible source of confusion in the evaluation of pulmonary vascular resistance, namely, variation in lung volume from one study to another, the effect of which is discussed briefly later in this chapter.

Interpretation of changes in pulmonary vascular resistance is further complicated by uncertainty regarding active or passive changes in the caliber of the pulmonary vessels.[5,6,14] Active or vasomotor changes denote alterations in the intrinsic "tone" of vessels and are considered "primary," while passive or mechanical changes in caliber result simply from transmural pressure variation and are "secondary" in nature. The calculated vascular resistance may be affected either by vasomotor or mechanical effects or both.

Changes in "tone" of the pulmonary vessels may indicate either stiffening or relaxation of the vessel walls. Stiffening of a vessel wall means increase in "tone" and causes vasoconstriction. Under this condition a de-creased volume in the vessel is associated with an elevation in transmural pressure. Relaxation indicates reduction in "tone" and permits vasodilatation, manifested by an increase in pulmonary vascular volume and a reduction in transmural pressure. Both active vasoconstriction and vasodilatation are accompanied by a *discordant* change in pulmonary vascular pressure-volume relationships and may be elicited by local, neurohumoral, or chemical factors.[5,6,15]

"Distention" and "collapse" of a pulmonary vessel are passive, depending largely if not solely on the transmural pressure. "Distention" is caused by an increase in transmural pressure and is accompanied by an increase in vascular volume. "Collapse" is accompanied by a reduction in volume and a decrease in transmural pressure. Thus, passive mechanisms are reflected by *concordant* changes in pulmonary vascular volume and transmural pressure.[5,6,15]

The two important groups of factors which may be involved in a change in pulmonary vascular resistance have been well summarized by Fishman.[6] Passive mechanical factors include (a) cardiocirculatory effects such as change in left atrial or pulmonary blood flow, change in pulmonary blood volume, and change in the state of the bronchial circulation; and (b) respiratory effects such as change in alveolar pressure, change in intrathoracic pressure, change in the state of interstitial muscle, and the presence or absence of interstitial edema. On the other hand, the factors affecting vasomotor activity of the pulmonary vessels may originate from without or within the lungs. The former include effects of the autonomic nervous system and influences of catecholamines; the latter include "critical" closure of small vessels, intravascular chemoreceptors, chemical stimuli affecting vascular muscle, and local reflexes. In general, vasomotion in pulmonary vessels is greatest in the pulmonary arteries which are rich in smooth muscle and elastic tissue in comparison with pulmonary capillaries and veins.

Passive cardiocirculatory and respiratory effects have been further elaborated in animal studies.[9-13,16-22] An elevation of either pulmonary arterial or left atrial pressure is followed by passive dilatation of the vessels, a decrease in pulmonary vascular pressure gradient, and a decline in pulmonary vascular resistance. Conversely, pulmonary vascular resistance may rise if pulmonary arterial or left atrial pressure is reduced. Furthermore, at low pulmonary arterial and left atrial pressures, small changes in either pressure have a pronounced influence on pulmonary vascular resistance. On the other hand, small changes in resistance occur with large changes of pulmonary arterial or left atrial pressure in the high ranges.

Pulmonary vascular resistance is increased in intact animals when lung volume is either increased or decreased. The increase in pulmonary vascular resistance at increased lung volume probably results from a decrease in the caliber of the small vessels of the lung because of a reduction in their effective distending pressure. On the other hand, the rise in pulmonary vascular resistance associated with a decreased lung volume is attributed to change in the geometry of the arterioles (arteriolar "snarliness") and collapse of large pulmonary arteries. The various aspects of active vasomotion in animals have been studied by many workers.[5-7,14,23]

In human subjects, however, the precise relationships of pressure and flow in the pulmonary circulation have not been conclusively elucidated.[6,24,25] For more than two decades many investigators have demonstrated relatively normal or slightly elevated pulmonary arterial pressure under conditions which are associated with a 2 or 3 fold increase in pulmonary blood flow. Such conditions included (a) patients with large atrial septal defects,[26-28] (b) patients who had previously undergone pneumonectomy,[29] and (c) normal subjects during moderate exercise.[30-35] Such observations may suggest a decrease in pulmonary vascular resistance, but the data cannot be interpreted to represent the acute and uncomplicated effects on pressure-flow relationships. Under conditions (a) and (b) the distensibility of the pulmonary vessels may have occurred over periods of months or years. Under condition (c) many complex factors may be influencing pulmonary circulation.

Harris and Heath[5,36,37] have analyzed the reported data on physiologic effects of occluding one pulmonary artery in man and plotted the changes in pulmonary arterial pressure and flow before and after unilateral occlusion. This maneuver was considered to provide the most direct information available concerning the effects of acutely altered arterial pressure-flow relationship in the human pulmonary circulation. In 5 subjects the average mean pulmonary arterial pressure rose from 15.4 to 20.8 mm Hg, while the averaged pulmonary blood flow through one lung increased from 3.8 to 8.0 L/min. Thus, there is an average pressure rise of approximately 1.3 mm Hg for an increase in flow of 1 L/min through one lung. Since pulmonary wedge or left atrial pressure was not measured in these cases, it is indeed difficult to interpret the precise flow-pressure relationship. However, if a hypothetical normal value for the pulmonary wedge pressure, which is assumed to be the mean pulmonary arterial pressure at zero flow, was plotted on the diagram, the line between this point and the average values for the other two points (pressure and flow before and after occlusion) gives a possible indication of the slight curvilinearity of the relation between flow and pressure. This curvilinear relationship is similar to that observed in a distensible tube and in anesthetized dogs. The effects of unilateral occlusion of the pulmonary artery in patients with cardiac or chronic pulmonary disease will be discussed in Chapter 11.

A passive increase in pulmonary blood volume following blood transfusion or infusion of isotonic solution may increase or decrease the pulmonary vascular resistance but the change is small.[38-40]

Pressure-Volume Relationship and the Effects of Compliance and Distensibility

In a distensible system at low transmural pressures, the caliber of vessels is minimal and some of the vessels may be closed completely. As mentioned earlier, an elevation in transmural pressure increases the caliber of the vessel and its resistance to flow decreases in proportion to the fourth power of change in the radius. When the increasing caliber of the vessel nears its limit of acute distensibility, the volume-pressure relationships of the vessel behave like a more rigid system, a small increase in volume causing a large rise in pressure. Thus, at high levels of pressure and volume, the pressure-volume relationship becomes curvilinear instead of linear. In the linear region of the

pulmonary pressure-volume relationship, the approximate pulmonary vascular compliance may be expressed by the following formula:[5-7,41]

$$C = \frac{\triangle V}{\triangle Pd}$$

Where   C = pulmonary vascular compliance in ml/mm Hg

$\triangle V$ = change in pulmonary blood volume in ml

$\triangle Pd$ = change in pulmonary distending or transmural pressure in mm Hg

The pulmonary vascular compliance under static conditions may be calculated as the ratio of pulmonary blood volume to the pulmonary distending pressure. Alteration of the pulmonary vascular pressure-volume relationship in an animal or human subject requires physiological or pharmacological intervention. The classical examples in animal studies were reported by Sarnoff and Berglund[42] and Lanari and Agrest.[43] A more detailed discussion in human subjects will be included in Chapter 17.

In a pulsatile system such as the pulmonary vascular bed, the volume distensibility of the large vessels depends upon their storage capacity or capacitance. Distensibility may be expressed as increase in volume per unit increase in pressure. The "coefficient of distensibility" is defined by the following equation:[5-7,44]

$$D = \frac{1}{V} \cdot \frac{\triangle V}{\triangle Pd}$$

Where   D = coefficient of distensibility

V = original pulmonary blood volume in ml

$\triangle V$ = increase in pulmonary blood volume in ml

$\triangle Pd$ = increase in distending pressure in mm Hg

As pointed out by Fishman,[6] the term "pulmonary vascular distensibility" is a composite one. It is influenced by (*a*) the elastic properties of the walls of the pulmonary vessels, (*b*) the tone of the smooth muscle, (*c*) the perivascular pressures, (d) the effects of alveolar surface tension, (e) the presence of excessive interstitial fluid, and (f) the mechanical distortion from the adjacent pulmonary tissues.

Since the pulmonary vascular bed is not fixed and since a number of the relevant factors listed are unknown, the calculated coefficient of distensibility represents an oversimplification of a complex physiologic situation. Furthermore, the coefficient of distensibility cannot be used with reference to any particular segment of the vasculature until reliable and simple techniques are available for the measurement of pressures and volume in the three components of the pulmonary vessels. Interpretation of the coefficient of distensibility may be further limited and uncertain when changes in volume and distending pressure are small or insignificant.

REFERENCES

1. Green, H.D.: Circulatory system: Physical principles. In Glasser, O. (ed), Medical Physics, Vol. 2, p. 228, Chicago, Year Book Medical Publishers, Inc., 1950.

2. Burton, A.C.: The relation between pressure and flow in the pulmonary bed. In W. Adams and I. Veith (eds), Pulmonary Circulation, p. 26, New York, Grune & Stratton, 1959.

3. Fritts, H.W., and Cournand, A.: Physiological factors regulating pressure, flow and distribution of blood in the pulmonary circuit. In W. Adams and I. Veith (eds), Pulmonary Circulation, p. 62, New York, Grune & Stratton, 1959.

4. Randall, J.E.: Elements of Biophysics, 2nd ed., Chicago, Year Book Medical Publishers, Inc., 1962.

5. Harris, P., and Heath, D.: The Human Pulmonary Circulation, Baltimore, Williams & Wilkins Co., 1962.

6. Fishman, A.P.: Dynamics of the pulmonary circulation. In Handbook of Physiology, Section 2, Circulation, Vol. 2, p. 1695, Washington, D.C., American Physiological Society, 1963.

7. Burton, A.C.: Physiology and Biophysics of Circulation, Chicago, Year Book Medical Publishers, Inc., 1965.

8. Hill, D.W.: Principles of Electronics in Medical Research, p. 34, Washington, Butterworth, 1965.

9. Permutt, S., Howell, J.B.L., Proctor, D.F., and Riley, R.L.: Effect of lung inflation on static pressure-volume characteristic of pulmonary vessels. J. Appl. Physiol., 16, 64, 1961.

10. Howell, J.B.L., Permutt, S., Proctor, D.F., and Riley, R.L.: Effect of inflation of lung on different parts of pulmonary vascular bed. J. Appl. Physiol., 16, 71, 1961.

11. Borst, H.G., McGregor, M., Whittenberger, J.L., and Berglund, E.: Influence of pulmonary arterial and left atrial pressures on pulmonary vascular resistance. Circ. Res., 4, 393, 1956.

12. Burton, A.D., and Patel, D.J.: Effect on pulmonary vascular resistance of inflation of rabbit lungs. J. Appl. Physiol., 12, 239, 1958.

13. Simmons, D.H., Linde, L.M,. Miller, J.H., and O'Reilly, R.J.: Relation between lung volume and pulmonary vascular resistance. Circ. Res., 9, 465, 1961.

14. Feeley, J.W., Lee, T.D., and Milnor, W.R.: Active and passive components of pulmonary vascular response to vasoactive drugs in the dog. Am. J. Physiol., 205, 1193, 1963.

15. Oakley, C., Glick, G., Luria, M.N., Schreiner, B.F., and Yu, P.N.: Some regulatory mechanisms of the human pulmonary vascular bed. Circulation, 26, 917, 1962.

16. Haddy, F.J., and Campbell, G.S.: Pulmonary vascular resistance in anesthetized dogs. Am. J. Physiol., 172, 747, 1953.

17. Whittenberger, J.L., McGregor, M., Berglund, E., and Borst, H.G.: Influence of state of inflation of lung on pulmonary vascular resistance. J. Appl. Physiol., 15, 878, 1960.

18. Harasawa, M., and Rodbard, S.: Ventilatory air pressure and pulmonary vascular resistance. Am. Heart J., 60, 73, 1960.

19. Lenfant, C., and Howell, B.: Cardiovascular adjustments in dogs during continuous pressure breathing. J. Appl. Physiol., 15, 425, 1960.

20. Thomas, L.J., Griffo, Z.J., and Roos, A.: Effect of negative-pressure inflation of the lung on pulmonary vascular resistance. J. Appl. Physiol., 16, 451,1961.

21. Patel, D.J., Mallos, A.J., and Freitas, F.M. de: Importance of transmural pressure and lung volume in evaluating effect on pulmonary vascular tone. Circ. Res., *9*, 1217, 1961.

22. Roos, A., Thomas, L.J., Negel, E.L., and Prommas, D.C.: Pulmonary vascular resistance as determined by lung inflation and vascular pressures. J. Appl. Physiol., *16*, 77, 1961.

23. Rudolph, A.M., and Scarpelli, E.M.: Drug action on pulmonary circulation of unanesthetized dogs. Am. J. Physiol., *206*, 1201, 1964.

24. Cournand, A.: Some aspects of the pulmonary circulation in normal man and in chronic cardiopulmonary disease. Circulation, *2*, 641, 1950.

25. Daley, R., Goodwin, J.F., and Steiner, R.E.: *Clinical Disorders of the Pulmonary Circulation*. Boston, Little, Brown & Co., 1960.

26. Dow, J.W., and Dexter, L.: Circulatory dynamics in atrial septal defects. J. Clin. Invest., *29*, 809, 1950.

27. Dexter, L.: Atrial septal defect. Brit. Heart J., *18*, 209, 1956.

28. Weidman, W.H., Swan, H.J.C., DuShane, J.W., and Wood, E.H.: A hemodynamic study of atrial septal defect and associated anomalies involving the atrial septum. J. Lab. & Clin. Med., *50*, 165, 1957.

29a. Cournand, A., Himmelstein, A., Riley, R.L., and Lester, C.W.: A follow-up study of cardiopulmonary function in four young individuals after pneumonectomy. J. Thor. Surg., *16*, 30, 1947.

29b. Mendelsohn, H.J., Zimmerman, B.A., and Adelman, A.: A study of pulmonary hemodynamics during pulmonary resection. J. Thor. Surg., *20*, 366, 1950.

30. Hickam, J.B., and Cargill, W.H.: Effect of exercise on cardiac output and pulmonary arterial pressure in normal persons and in patients with cardiovascular disease and pulmonary emphysema. J. Clin. Invest, *27*, 10, 1948.

31. Riley, R.L., Himmelstein, A., Motley, H.L., Weiner, H.M., and Cournand, A.: Studies of the pulmonary circulation at rest and during exercise in normal individuals and in patients with chronic pulmonary disease. Am. J. Physiol., *152*, 372, 1948.

32. Dexter, L., Whittenberger, J.L., Haynes, F.W., Goodale, W.T., Gorlin, R., and Sawyer, C.G.: Effect of exercise on circulatory dynamics of normal individuals. J. Appl. Physiol., *3*, 439, 1951.

33. Slonim, N.B., Ravin, A., Balchum, O.J., and Dressler, S.H.: The effect of mild exercise in the supine position on the pulmonary arterial pressure of five normal human subjects. J. Clin. Invest. *33*, 1022, 1954.

34. Donald, K.W., Bishop, J.M., Cumming, G., and Wade, O.L.: The effect of exercise on the cardiac output and circulatory dynamics of normal subjects. Clin. Sci., *14*, 37, 1955.

35. Sancetta, S.M., and Rakita, L.: Response of pulmonary artery pressure and total pulmonary resistance of untrained convalescent man to prolonged mild steady-state exercise. J. Clin. Invest., *36*, 1138, 1957.

36. Brofman, B.L., Charms, B.L., Kohn, P.M., Elder, J., Newman, R., and Rizika, M.: Unilateral pulmonary artery occlusion in man. Control studies. J. Thor. Surg., *34*, 206, 1957.

37. Soderholm, B.: The hemodynamics of the lesser circulation in pulmonary tuberculosis. Effect of exercise, temporary unilateral pulmonary occlusion, and operation. Scand. J. Clin. & Lab. Invest., *9*, Suppl. 26, 1957.

38. Doyle, J.T., Wilson, J.S., Estes, E.H., and Warren, J.V.: The effect of intravenous infusions of physiological saline solution on the pulmonary arterial and pulmonary capillary pressure in man. J. Clin. Invest., *30*, 345, 1951.

39. Witham, A.C., Fleming, J.W., and Bloom, W.L.: The effect of the intravenous administration of dextran on cardiac output and other circulatory dynamics. J. Clin. Invest., *30*, 897, 1951.

40. Freitas, F.M. de, Faraco, E.Z., Azevedo, D. F. de, Zaduchliver, J., and Lewin, I.: Behavior of normal pulmonary circulation during changes of total blood volume in man. J. Clin. Invest., *44*, 366, 1965.

41. Milnor, W.R., Jose, A.D., and McGaff, C.J.: Pulmonary vascular volume, resistance and compliance in man. Circulation, *12*, 130, 1960.

42. Sarnoff, S.J., and Berglund, E.: Pressure-volume characteristics and stress relaxation in the pulmonary vascular bed of the dog. Am. J. Physiol., *171*, 238, 1952.

43. Lanari, A., and Agrest, A.: Pressure-volume relationship in the pulmonary vascular bed. Acta Physiol. Latinam, *4*, 116, 1954.

44. Yu, P.N., Murphy, G.W., Schreiner, B.F., and James, D.H.: Distensibility characteristics of the human pulmonary vascular bed. Study of pressure-volume response to exercise in patients with and without heart disease. Circulation, *35*, 710, 1967.

Section II

CHAPTER 6

Estimate of Pulmonary Blood Volume in Animals

Direct Method

The earliest direct measurements of the quantity of blood in animals' lungs were based upon washing blood out of the lungs.[1-5] The amount of blood in the lungs of various species was found to approximate 7 to 9% of the total blood volume.

Heger and Spehl[1] measured the volume of blood in rabbit lungs after ligation of blood vessels to and from the lungs. They found that the ratio of pulmonary blood volume (PBV) to total blood volume (TBV) varied from 0.06 to 0.10. Plumier[2] made similar studies in anesthetized dogs. The mean PBV/TBV was 0.11 during inspiration and 0.09 during expiration.

In 1917 Kuno[3] reported studies of blood volume in a dog heart-lung preparation under various conditions. The quantity of the blood in the lungs was estimated by Welcker's method. This method required (a) mincing and grinding of the lung tissues, (b) repeated washing and extraction of the tissue with distilled water until complete discoloration, and (c) comparison of the color of the resultant distilled water with a standard solution of blood diluted 200 times with distilled water. With this technique Kuno found that the amount of blood in the lungs varied from 6.15 to 13.8 ml/kg of the body weight or from 8.8 to 19.4% of the total blood volume, which was assumed to be 7% of body weight. In 10 preparations the average amount of the blood in the right lung was about 150% of that in the left lung.

Kuno further found the amount of blood in the lungs to be increased when the blood circulation became more vigorous. If the lungs were made edematous, the amount of blood in both lungs might be as much as one fourth of the total blood volume. He realized, however, that his results were not unequivocal and that the experimental conditions might not be analogous to the pulmonary edema which occurred under pathophysiologic circumstances.

Indirect Methods

Pulmonary blood volume was measured indirectly in animals by employing dye or radioisotope dilution curves. These techniques made possible several consecutive determinations of pulmonary blood volume in a single animal. A few examples are cited below.

Stewart-Hamilton Method

Pulmonary blood volume has been measured in dogs by indicator-dilution technique after injection of a dye sequentially into the pulmonary artery and the left atrium and sampling blood from a systemic artery, according to the Stewart-Hamilton principle.[6],[7]

$$PBV = Tm_{(PA - BA)} - Tm_{(LA - BA)} \times C.O.$$

Where   PBV = pulmonary blood volume in ml

$Tm_{(PA - BA)}$ = mean transit time from the pulmonary artery to a systemic artery in seconds

$Tm_{(LA - BA)}$ = mean transit time from the left atrium to a systemic artery in seconds

C.O. = cardiac output in ml/sec

Feeley, Lee, and Milnor[7] found the average PBV of 10.9 ml/kg in a series of 31 closed-chest dogs and of 10.6 ml/kg in a series of 20 open-chest dogs using this method. It is likely that an unknown portion of the left atrial blood volume is included in the calculated PBV.

Employing indicator-dilution methods, Marshall and co-workers[8] measured the components of the "central" blood volume in 7 intact anesthetized dogs. The mean blood volume between the pulmonary artery and the femoral artery was 22.6 ml/kg, of which half or less was in the lungs. Measurements made before and during occlusion of the right pulmonary artery indicated that the right lung contained about a third of the total blood volume in the lungs and left side of the heart. Assuming that the left heart blood volume remains stable, they felt that measurements of volume between the pulmonary and aortic valves might indicate the quantity of blood in the vessels of the lungs.

Ether Method (Feisal, Soni and DuBois)

Feisal, Soni, and DuBois[9] developed a method for estimating the blood volume in the part of the pulmonary arteries in dogs which does not participate in gas exchange. This method is based upon the measurement of the circulation time in the pulmonary arterial tree multiplied by the pulmonary blood flow. The circulation time is measured by a rise in plethysmographic pressure caused by the entry of gaseous ether into the alveoli after the injection of a small amount of ether in alcohol into the main pulmonary artery.

The pulmonary arterial circulation time was measured in 12 dogs. In order to estimate the pulmonary blood volume from the pulmonary flow and circulation time through the total pulmonary vascular bed, indocyanine green dilution curves also were recorded from the femoral artery in 5 dogs, after sequential injections of the dye into the pulmonary artery and the left atrium.

In the total series of 12 dogs the pulmonary arterial circulation time ranged from 0.4 sec to 2.8 sec. In the 5 dogs with pulmonary blood flow studies, the pulmonary arterial circulation times varied from 0.7 to 1.5 sec (average 1.1 sec), while the circulation times from the pulmonary artery to the left atrium ranged from 2.8 to 6.2 sec (average 4.1 sec).

The average pulmonary arterial volume was estimated to be 51 ml (range from 35 to 83 ml), and the average total pulmonary blood volume was 190 ml (range from 102 to 262 ml).

The ratio of pulmonary arterial circulation time to total pulmonary circulation time averaged 0.28 (range from 0.15 to 0.41), while the ratio of pulmonary arterial volume to total pulmonary blood volume averaged 0.29 (range from 0.15 to 0.47).

The authors discussed in great detail the limitations and sources of error in this method. They also pointed out its possible application in studies of pulmonary circulatory dynamics, regional ventilation, pulmonary arterial compliance and gas exchange kinetics. Further, the combination of this method, the indicator-dilution technique for determining total pulmonary blood volume, and the carbon monoxide method for estimating the pulmonary capillary blood volume, will make possible the subdivision of the blood volume in the three compartments of pulmonary vascular bed (arteries, capillaries, and veins).

It should be recognized that this method requires measurement of the earliest appearance time of ether rather than its mean circulation time. The circulation time measured by the method therefore may be actually shorter than the mean circulation time, and the measured pulmonary arterial volume may be accordingly smaller.

Radioisotope Method (Lindsay and Guyton)

By detecting RISA in the blood from a circumscribed portion of lung field, Lindsay and Guyton[10] devised a method for continuously recording pulmonary blood volume in intact dogs. The counts per minute (CPM) from the chest wall after removing from the lung at the end of the experiment were subtracted from the recorded CPM throughout the experiment. Since the CPM from the chest wall were found to be stable, it was concluded that the changes in total CPM were caused by changes in pulmonary blood volume in the segment examined.

These authors produced respectively left ventricular failure by gradually constricting the ascending aorta and right ventricular failure by gradually constricting the pulmonary artery with loops of plastic tubing previously placed around the aorta or the pulmonary artery. When the ascending aorta was constricted, pulmonary blood volume increased an average of 79.5%, systemic arterial pressure decreased, and both left atrial and pulmonary arterial pressures increased. On the other hand, when the pulmonary artery was constricted, both the pulmonary arterial pressure distal to the constriction and the systemic arterial pressures decreased, and the pulmonary blood volume decreased an average of 38%.

Equilibration Method (Bradley)[11]

When a non-diffusible indicator is injected into the pulmonary artery the amount of the indicator entering the pulmonary vascular bed during the equilibration period is equal to the product of the pulmonary blood flow and the mean concentration of the indicator in the pulmonary arteries during that period. The amount of indicator leaving the pulmonary vascular bed during this period is the same as the pulmonary blood flow multiplied by the mean concentration of the indicator in the pulmonary veins. The difference between these two values is the amount of indicator remaining in the pulmonary vascular bed at equilibrium.

Equilibration of the indicator within the pulmonary vascular bed may be considered complete when the concentration of the indicator becomes identical in both the pulmonary arteries and the pulmonary veins (left atrium or a systemic artery). At this time it is assumed that the concentration of the indicator within the pulmonary vascular bed is identical with that entering and leaving the bed. The pulmonary blood volume is determined by dividing the calculated amount of the indicator remaining in the system at equilibrium by the concentration of the indicator at equilibrium.

$$PBV = \frac{C.O. \cdot t \cdot (PAct - PVct)}{CEq}$$

Where   PBV = circulating blood volume within the pulmonary vascular bed in ml

C.O. = cardiac output in ml/sec

t = time in seconds required for equilibration of the indicator

PAct = mean concentration of indicator in the pulmonary arteries during the time t in mg/ml

PVct = mean concentration of indicator in the pulmonary veins during the time t in mg/ml

If left atrial blood is sampled, the calculated blood volume will include a portion of or total left atrial volume. If systemic arterial blood is used, the calculated blood volume will include that in the left heart chambers, aorta, and arteries temporally equidistant.

CEq = concentration of indicator at equilibrium in mg/ml

The applicability and limitations of this method will be discussed in Chapter 7.

Partition of Pulmonary Blood Volume

Estimate of pulmonary blood volume in animals has been made by various authors. Table 6-1 lists the approximate proportions in the three segments of the lung (arteries, capillaries and veins) estimated by various workers. It would appear that in animals the combined capacity of pulmonary arteries and capillaries is approximately the same as that of pulmonary veins.

Table 6-1   Partition of Pulmonary Blood Volume in Animals

Authors	Per Cent of PBV			Ref. No.
	Arteries	*Capillaries*	*Veins*	
Landis and Hortenstine	26	21	53	12
Green	38.0	14.5	47.5	13
Engelberg and DuBois	25	15	60	14

REFERENCES

1. Heger, P., and Spehl, E.: Recherches sur la fistule peri-cardique chez le lapin. Arch. Biol. (Liege), *2*, 154, 1881.

2. Plumier, L.: La circulation pulmonarire chez le chien. Arch. Internat. Physiol., *1*, 176, 1904.

3. Kuno, Y.J.F.: On the amount of blood in the lungs. J. Physiol., *51*, 154, 1917.

4. Stewart, G.N.: The pulmonary circulation time, the quantity of blood in the lungs and the cardiac output of the heart. Am. J. Physiol., *58*, 20, 1921.

5. Lindsey, A.W., Banahan, B.F., Cannon, R.H., and Guyton, A.C.: Pulmonary blood volume of the dog and its changes in acute heart failure. Am. J. Physiol., *190*, 45, 1957.

6. McGaff, C.J., and Milnor, W.R., Effects of serotonin on pulmonary blood volume in the dog. Am. J. Physiol., *202*, 957, 1962.

7. Feeley, J.W., Lee, T.D., and Milnor, W.R.: Active and passive components of pulmonary vascular response to vasoactive drug in the dog. Am. J. Physiol., *205*, 1193, 1963.

8. Marshall, R.J., Wang, Y., and Shepherd, J.T.: Components of the "central" blood volume in the dog. Circ. Res., *8*, 93, 1960.

9. Feisal, K.A., Soni, J., and DuBois, A.B.: Pulmonary arterial circulation time, pulmonary arterial blood volume and the ratio of gas to tissue volume in the lungs of dogs. J. Clin. Invest., *41*, 390, 1962.

10. Lindsey, A.W., and Guyton, A.C.: Continuous recording of pulmonary blood volume: Pulmonary pressure and volume changes. Am. J. Physiol., *197*, 959, 1959.

11. Rabinowitz, M., and Rapaport, E.: Determination of circulating pulmonary blood volume in dogs by an arteriovenous dye equilibrium method. Circ. Res., *2*, 525, 1954.

12. Landis, E.M., and Hortenstine, J.C.: Functional significance of venous blood pressure. Physiol. Rev., *30*, 1, 1950.

13. Green, H.D.: Circulation system: Physical principles. *In* Glasser, O.(ed), *Medical Physics*, Vol. 2, p. 228, Chicago, Year Book Medical Publishers, Inc, 1950.

14. Engelberg, J., and DuBois, A.B.: Mechanics of pulmonary circulation in isolated rabbit lungs. Am. J. Physiol., *196*, 401, 1959.

CHAPTER 7

Measurement of Pulmonary Blood Volume in Man

General Principles

Indicator-dilution techniques measure only the circulating portion of the pulmonary blood volume. Any stagnant blood not in direct contact with the indicator and not equally diluted during transit through the pulmonary vascular bed will not be included in the estimated volume. Stagnant pools of blood could not be demonstrated in canine lungs,[1] however; and no evidence exists to suggest any such pools in the human pulmonary vascular bed.[2-4]

The bronchial circulation contributes only small amounts to the pulmonary blood volume in normal subjects or in patients with minor cardiovascular disease. In patients with severe cardiopulmonary disease, however, the measurement of pulmonary blood volume may be appreciably distorted by a larger number of bronchopulmonary anastomoses and increased flow.[5-8]

Major Approaches

Use of Dyes (Stewart-Hamilton)

Double Injection and Single Sampling. Routine right heart catheterization (Cournand) and percutaneous left atrial puncture (Björk) were employed in the first measurements of pulmonary blood volume (PBV) by

Kunieda and associates, utilizing both single and double injection techniques.[9,10] Their studies were divided into two parts. The first part of the study consisted of sequential injections of Evans blue dye into the pulmonary artery (PA) and left atrium (LA) followed by sampling of blood from a brachial artery (BA) every two seconds. In the second part, the dye was injected into the main PA and blood sampled from the LA every two seconds.

The PBV was calculated according to the conventional formula:

$$PBV = \frac{C.O. \times Tm_{(PA - LA)}}{60}$$

The authors used the median circulation time instead of the mean circulation time for calculation. The results in patients with various types of valvular heart disease are listed in Table 7-1.

In 1959-61 Dock and associates[11,12] and Milnor and co-workers[13,14] independently reported their studies of PBV in 64 patients. Both groups employed the combined technique of right heart catheterization and percutaneous or transbronchial left atrial puncture. The right heart catheter was positioned in the main PA and a polyethylene or polyvinyl tubing was advanced through a needle into the LA. Blood was sampled from the BA, and the procedure

Table 7-1.   Pulmonary Blood Volume Determined by Double Injection and Single Sampling Method

Year	Authors	LA Cath	PA & LA Injections	Arterial Sampling	Indicators used	Diagnosis	No.	Mean ± SE	Range	Ref. No.
1955	Kunieda	PC	Sequential	Q2S	E.B.	MS	16	361	299–419	9, 10
						MR	7	399	329–487	
						AR	2	434	417–451	
						Total	25	375	299–487	
1959 61	Dock et al.	PC	Simultaneous	Q2S	E.B.	"Normal"	4	246	219–269	11, 12
						MS	15	335	193–634	
						MR	13	358	172–521	
						AS	7	303	185–423	
						AR	3	368	177–401	
						Combined lesions	3	298	190–359	
						Total	45	322	172–634	
1959–60	Milnor et al.	PC or TB	Sequential	Continuous	I.G.	Mostly valvular Lesions	19			13, 14
						Normal PVR		372	126–598	
						High PVR		357	222–493	
1961	Fermoso et al.	TS	Sequential	Q2S	E.B.	MS	11	461	283–642	15
1962	Oakley et al.	TS	Sequential	Continuous	I.G.	MS	32	280 ± 12.7	175–435	16
						AS	4	268	152–307	
1963	McGaff et al.	PC	Sequential	Continuous	I.G.	"Normal"	5	230 ± 13.6		17
						MS	5	229 ± 34.3		
						MS & AS	25	359 ± 23.7		
						MR	4	308 ± 89.9		
						ASHD	3	153 ± 11.8		
1963	Yu, Schreiner Glick and Murphy	TS	Sequential	Continuous	I.G.	MS and MR	12	277 ± 16.7	215–388	18–20
						AS and AR	14	320 ± 24.1	169–546	
						Other Lesions	3	239	202–286	
1964	Forsberg and Varnauskas	TS	Simultaneous	Q1S	I.G. and BSP	Mostly valvular Lesions				21, 22
						Old series	33	311	126–451	
						New series	36	343	206–469	
						Total	69	328	126–469	
1965	Samet et al.	TS	Sequential	Continuous	I.G.	Normal subjects	32	231	140–302	23
1965	Roy et al.	TS	Sequential	Continuous	I.G.	Normal	15	211	145–310	24
						MR	4	266	242–296	
						MS					
						I	5	370	215–451	
						II	11	420	294–584	
						III	13	473	232–592	
						Total	29	419	215–592	
1966	Samet et al.	TS	Sequential	Continuous	I.G.	Mostly valvular Lesions	96	262 ± 7.2	156–685	25
1966	Schreiner et al.	TS	Sequential	Continuous	I.G.	"Normal"	12	271 ± 10		26
						CHF				
						MS	6	238 ± 26.3		
						Other	7	292 ± 21.4		

LA Cath	= Left atrial catheterization	MR	= Mitral regurgitation
PC	= Percutaneous	AR	= Aortic regurgitation
TB	= Transbronchial	AS	= Aortic stenosis
TS	= Transseptal	ASHD	= Ischemic heart disease
Q2S or Q1S	= Intermittent sampling every two seconds or every second	PVR	= Pulmonary vascular resistance
		I, II, & III	= Classification according to functional capacity
Continuous	= Through a cuvette densitometer		
E.B.	= Evans blue	CHF	= Congestive heart failure
I.G.	= Indocyanine green	PBV	= Pulmonary blood volume in ml.
BSP	= Bromsulphalein	Ref. No.	= Reference number
I.C.	= Indigo-carmine		
MS	= Mitral stenosis		

was similar to the double-injection method described by Kunieda and associates.

Dock and associates[12] injected Evans blue dye into the PA, and RISA into the LA simultaneously, while Milnor and co-workers[14] used sequential injections of indocyanine green. Most of the patients studied had valvular heart disease and data from only a few "normal" subjects were included.

Dock and associates used the average of the two cardiac output determinations calculated from the Evans blue and RISA curves for nearly all of the volume calculations. The mean PBV for 45 patients was 322 ml/M², ranging from 172 to 634 ml/M². The mean PBV for those with predominant mitral valvular disease was 335 ml/M²; for those with predominant aortic valvular disease, 323 ml/M²; for those with combined mitral and aortic disease, 298 ml/M²; and for 4 patients with no recognized hemodynamic disturbance, 246 ml/M².

In the study of Milnor and co-workers, the interval between the sequential injections into PA and LA was usually less than 5 minutes. For unknown reasons cardiac output calculated from the LA injection was consistently higher than that calculated from the PA injection. The mean difference was 0.37 L/min and was statistically significant. The authors used only cardiac output measured from PA injection for the calculation of PBV. In 19 patients, most of whom had valvular heart disease, the PBV ranged from 147 to 598 ml/M² with a mean value of 365 ml/M.

With improvements in the methodology and technique of instantaneous inscription of the indicator-dilution curves and with the introduction of transseptal left heart catheterization, multiple determinations of PBV in a patient may be made with ease at rest as well as during various physiologic or pharmacologic interventions. The technique of double injection and single sampling has been used most widely. Values reported from various sources are listed in Table 7-1.[15-26]

Single Injection and Double Sampling. Freitas and associates measured PBV by a single injection of indocyanine green into the upper inferior vena cava with simultaneous sampling from PA and LA, the latter catheterized by transseptal technique.

Two groups of patients were studied. The first group consisted of 12

Table 7-2 Pulmonary Blood Volume Estimated by Single Injection and Double Sampling
Method

Year	Authors	LA Cath	Site of Injection	Site of Sampling	Indicator Used	Patients Diagnosis	No.	PBV/M² Mean ± S.E.	Range	Ref.
1964	Freitas et al.	T.S.	IVC	PA and LA	I.G.	Pulmonary hypertension (M.S.) Normal pulmonary arterial pressure	12 (11) 12	375 ± 29 310 ± 6.4	220–525 173–385	27
1965	Freitas et al.	T.S.	IVC	PA and LA	I.G.	Normal hemodynamics	21	295 ± 16	–	28
1966	Samet et al.	T.S.	IVC	PA and LA	I.G.	Mostly V.H.D.	96	271	75–915	25
1966	Freitas et al.	T.S.	IVC	PA and LA	I.G.	M.S. with pulmonary hypertension Hypertension	15 5	337 ± 11.5	–	29

IVC = inferior vena cava
Other symbols and abbreviations are identical to those used in Table 7-1

Table 7-3   Pulmonary Blood Volume Estimated by Single Injection and Single Sampling Method

Year	Authors	LA Cath	Site of Injection	Site of Sampling	Indicator Used	Patients		PBV/M²		Ref. No.
						Diagnosis	No.	Mean	Range	
1965	Levinson et al.	T.S.	PA	LA	I.G.	V.H.D.	10	311	236–405	30
1966	Samet et al.	T.S.	PA	LA	I.G.	Mostly V.H.D.	96	427	235–1060	25
1966	Schreiner et. al.	T.S.	PA	LA	I.G.	Mostly V.H.D.	10	482	386–688	31

V.H.D. = Valvular heart disease
Other symbols and abbreviations are identical to those used in Table 7-1

patients with pulmonary hypertension, 11 of whom had mitral stenosis. The second group included 12 patients without known hemodynamic disturbances. The PBV in patients of the first group was 375 ± 97 ml/M² (mean ± S.D.). The PBV in the second group was 310 ± 21 ml/M² (Table 7-2).

Reproducibility was such that two successive determinations of PBV in a given patient under the same conditions rarely varied more than 12%. Table 7-2 also includes the values of PBV determined by a similar method reported in another three papers.[25,28,29]

Single Injection and Single Sampling. As mentioned previously, Kunieda and associates[9,10] also injected an indicator into the PA and sampled blood from LA. Subsequently, Levinson and co-workers[30] used this approach to measure PBV. PBV was determined as the product of cardiac index and mean transit time from PA to LA. In 10 patients with 15 measurements the mean PBV was 311 ml/M² with a range of 236 to 403 ml/M² (Table 7-3). In Table 7-3 are listed the data obtained by two other groups of workers using similar technique.[25,31]

Use of Radioisotopes (Lammerant)

Precordial Counting. At about the same time that Kunieda and associates published measurements of PBV based on the injection and sampling of dyes, Lammerant[32] proposed the measurement of pulmonary mean transit time and pulmonary circulating blood volume using precordial radioisotope dilution curves. Subsequently, other workers have reported determination of the estimated "PBV," derived from the precordial radioisotope curves.[33-37] All the proposed methods lead to a gross overestimation of the pulmonary mean transit time, since transit time through part of both right and left heart is invariably included.

In a different approach, Donato, Giuntini and co-workers[38-41] devised a new technique for the measurement of PBV. Immediately after injection of a calculated dose of RISA through a catheter placed in the right atrium, a precordial radioisotope curve was recorded.

The mean pulmonary circulation time ($\overline{PCT}$) is obtained from the RISA radiocardiogram by subtracting the extrapolated exponential downslope of the right heart curve from the corrected ratemeter curve in order to obtain the isolated left heart curve. The first heart cycle after injection during which the radioisotope is ejected from the right ventricle is considered as t_o. The heart cycle during which the total ratemeter tracing deviates from the right exponential downslope is taken as t_a. The heart cycle during which the left heart curve reaches its peak is t_p.

It is assumed that the mean pulmonary circulation time is (a) longer than the time measured from the first heart cycle during which the radioisotope is ejected to the time at which radioactivity appears in the left heart, and (b) shorter than the time measured from the same origin to the peak of the left heart curve. If these two values are averaged, a reasonable estimate of mean pulmonary circulation time may be made.

Thus

$$(t_a - t_o) < \overline{PCT} < (t_p - t_o)$$

and $$\overline{PCT} = (t_a - t_o) + (t_p - t_o)$$

To obtain mean pulmonary blood volume $(\overline{PBV})$, the following formula is used:

$$\overline{PBV} = SV \frac{(t_a - t_o) + (t_p - t_o)}{2}$$

Where SV = stroke volume in ml

The theory, technique, results, and validation of the method were published in a series of papers.[38-40] The original publications should be consulted for a more detailed description.

With similar reasoning, Segre and associates[42] reported a method of measuring PBV based upon a pulmonary weighting function. The pulmonary circulation is considered as a black box formed by a system of unidirectional channels of various lengths. The model designs by the authors assume the validity of the superposition principle, that is, the linearity of the system described. The input is given by the right heart and the output by the left heart. By numerical "deconvolution" between the output and input, the weighting function of the black box (the pulmonary weighting function) is determined from which the mean transit time of the black box can be calculated. The mean transit time of the model corresponds to the mean transit time from the outflow tract of the right ventricle to the end of the pulmonary vascular system in the left atrium. The method involves complex mathematical derivation and calculation, and the reader is referred to the original publication for more detail. In 14 healthy, normal subjects the pulmonary transit time was 4.0 ± 0.45 sec (mean $\pm$ S.D.) and the PBV 263 ± 63 ml/M^2. Some published values for PBV estimated by precordial counting are listed in Table 7-4.

Table 7-4 Pulmonary Blood Volume Estimated by Precordial Counting

Year	Authors	Patients Diagnosis	No.	PBV Mean ± S.E.	Range	PBV/M² Mean ± S.E.	Range	Ref. No.
1957	Lammerant	Normal	104	1240 ± 37				32
1959-61	Eich et al.	No CV disease	12			430 ± 29[1]		33
						403 ± 38		
			10			451 ± 17[2]		
						441 ± 17		
			9			403 ± 45[3]		
						442 ± 26		
1960	Love et al.	No CP disease	9			490 ± 45		34
1960	Pietila and Hakkila	Pulmonary disease	17	718 ± 44	428-1120			35
1961	Moir and Gott	Normal	25			610 ± 33		36
		M.S.	14			678 ± 51		
1965	Kashamsant et al.	M.S.	11	1182	600-1990			37
		M.R.	10	1067	747-1478			
		A.S.	7	778	355-1180			
1962	Donoato, Giutini and associates	Mostly pulmonary tbc	18	550 ± 26.2	323-721	313 ± 14	211-403	38-41
1965	Segre et al.	Normal	14	433 ± 26	293-542	263 ± 7.4	172-416	42

CV = cardiovascular, CP = cardiopulmonary, pulmonary. tbc = pulmonary tuberculosis
(1) single counter, (2) dual counters, (3) single counter with collimation
Other symbols and abbreviations are identical to those used in Table 7-1

Arterial Sampling. Utilizing radio-isotopes as an indicator, PBV may be determined by the single injection and double sampling method described earlier. In this case, two scintillators and sampling devices should be used. The simultaneous or sequential use of radioisotope and dye for respective injections into PA and LA is also feasible, followed by sampling from a peripheral artery. Because of the relatively long interval required for counting background, however, radioisotopes are not suitable for sequential injections into PA and LA.

Other Methods

Equilibration Method (Bradley).[43] This method has been described in some detail in Chapter 6.

Exponential Downslope (Newman). Newman and associates[44] analyzed the form of the indicator-dilution curves inscribed after injecting Evans blue dye into a three-chambered model flow system. They demonstrated that the volume calculated from the slope formula was equal to the largest single volume in the system. It was assumed that the three-chambered experimental model imitated roughly the right heart, lung, and left heart chamber of human subjects and that the volume calculated from the exponential downslope of the human dilution curves represented the PBV, which was the largest volume among the three "chambers."

When a "model" was constructed with three compartments, the largest having the same volume as that calculated from the human curves and with the same flow, the similarity between the "model" dilution curve and the human dilution curves was remarkable.

The "slope" formula used is as follows:

$$V = F/S$$

Where V = the largest volume or PBV
F = rate of flow or cardiac output
S = slope of the straight line downstroke of the curve

Subsequently, they injected indicator into the right atrium, pulmonary artery, a pulmonary vein, and the aorta consecutively and sampled blood from the carotid artery of dogs.[45] They found that the serial compartment analysis of dye curves was valid and the lungs were the largest volume in the series. The volume measured by the "slope" method appeared to be the PBV.

Radiologic Technique. Lagerlöf and Werkö[46] attempted to estimate the PBV in man by a combination of indicator-dilution and radiologic findings. The central blood volume was determined by injecting Evans blue dye into the pulmonary artery and sampling arterial blood with a series of tubes every 1 to 2 seconds. The blood volume of the left heart was taken as half of the total blood volume of the heart determined roentgenographically. The blood volume of the proximal arterial tree was calculated by multiplying the area of aorta determined roentgenologically by the distance from the root of the aorta to the site of the arterial puncture. The PBV was calculated by subtracting the blood volume in the left heart and that in the proximal arterial tree from the central blood volume. The estimated PBV in the lungs varied from 511 to 968 ml. Compared with recent data obtained by various workers using other methods, these values were unusually high. One reason might be the questionable reliability of the roentgenologic technique in assessing the heart, aortic, and arterial volumes.

Post-mortem Method. Hayek[47] found about 50 ml of blood in the pulmonary arteries of man at post-mortem examination. Bachmann[48] measured PBV at post-mortem examination in 7 adults with normal lungs. The blood volume in one lung (four left and three right) ranged from 259 to 367 ml with a mean of 259 ml. Multiplying these values by two, the PBV would range from 518 to 734 with a mean of 518, values which agree with those obtained by the indicator-dilution method and by the technique of Donato and Guintini.

Dexter and Smith[49] recently studied 26 patients at post-mortem examination. They found that the pulmonary arterial blood volume of the right lung ranged from 56 to 67 ml/M^2 in 12 patients, and the corresponding volume of the left lung varied from 50 to 64 ml/M^2 in 14 patients.

Evaluation of Different Methods

Dye Dilution Method

At the present time, the dye dilution methods are most widely used to determine PBV in man. Since these methods require left and right heart catheterization, the injection of one or more indicators, and the removal of a certain amount of blood, it is reasonable to consider whether any immediate hemodynamic effects are precipitated by the procedure. The various pressures and the heart rate changed little or not at all, however, after repeated determinations of PBV. In our laboratory no systematic difference was found between the cardiac output determined by injection into the pulmonary artery and by injection into the left atrium.[16,18] Similar findings have been reported by others.[12,14,21,50] Thus, shunts from the pulmonary circulation to the bronchial vessels are not likely to cause a major systematic error. Such shunts of significant volume would cause the cardiac output estimated from the pulmonary arterial curve to exceed that estimated from the left atrial curve.

The question of adequate and complete mixing of indicator injected into the left atrium deserves special comment. Should the indicator mix incompletely within the left atrium, the calculated PBV would include that portion of the left atrial volume in which no mixing occurred and would be falsely high. Theoretically, inadequate mixing might be expected to occur more frequently in patients with larger left atrium. In practice, however, no direct correlation was found between the calculated PBV and the radiologic size of the left atrium.[16] Forsberg[22] in an extensive review concluded that indicators injected into the left atrium are adequately mixed with blood during their passage through the left heart.

It should be pointed out that all three of the methods described probably include a variable amount of left atrial volume in the calculated PBV. This inevitable error would be minimized if the left atrial catheter could be placed very close to the junction of the pulmonary veins and the left atrium. Regardless of which of the three methods is used, the reproducibility of duplicate determinations of the PBV has been excellent in the experience of many workers.

The double injection and single sampling method avoids the need to place an extra catheter in the inferior vena cava, and the requirement of two simultaneous sampling systems is obviated. As discussed in Chapter 4, the reliability of peripheral arterial sampling in the determination of "central" blood volume has been questioned, particularly during exercise.[51,52] However, the double injection method, with simultaneous or sequential injections of the indicators, overcomes such objections in the estimation of PBV because distortion of the indicator-dilution curves resulting from the location of the arterial sampling site affects the curves recorded from pulmonary artery and left atrial injections equally and is eliminated in the calculation of mean transit time from PA to LA.

The single injection and double sampling method requires that a third catheter be placed in the inferior vena cava for the injection and that two sampling systems of equal sensitivity be provided to record dilution curves from PA to LA. In addition, sampling from a long cardiac catheter may compromise the reliability of the results because of flow-volume distortion in such a sampling system.

The single injection and single sampling method is the simplest of all. However, the absence of a ventricular mixing chamber between the PA and the LA and the possible inclusion of all or a major portion of the left atrial volume makes the calculated PBV significantly higher than values measured by either of the other two methods (see below).

Samet and co-workers[25] evaluated the three dye dilution methods for the determination of PBV in 96 patients, most of whom had valvular heart disease. *Method 1* consisted of double injection(PA and LA) and single sampling (BA); *method 2* included that of single injection (PA) and single sampling (LA); and *method 3* was that of single injection (right atrium) and double sampling (PA and LA). They found that method 2 consistently overestimated the PBV. This method has failed in their hands, despite its attractive technical simplicity. These authors considered the absence of a ventricular mixing chamber between the injection and sampling sites as the most important source of error in this method, resulting in incomplete mixing of the

indicator in the PA and subsequently in the LA.

On the other hand, they found little difference between method 1 and method 3, the values of PBV estimated by these two methods comparing favorably with those reported by others. The authors preferred method 1 because the standard deviation of the mean was considerably smaller in method 1 than in method 3, and method 1 did not require a third catheter in the right atrium.

Precordial Radioisotope Technique

The major advantages of this technique are (a) simplicity of application, (b) freedom from the requirement of cardiac catheterization and arterial puncture, (c) exclusion of peripheral venous and arterial circulation from the boundaries of central volume, (d) absence of effects of redistribution of arterial flow on the measured volume under experimental conditions such as exercise or after administration of drugs.

Disadvantages of the precordial radioisotope technique are (a) the invariable inclusion in the PBV of a significant and indeterminate portion of both right and left heart volumes, (b) limitations in the number of determinations which can be made because of background accumulation and the hazards of radiation, and (c) the lack of simultaneous intracardiac or intravascular pressure information unless separate cardiac catheterization is performed. The method proposed by Donato, Giuntini and their associates[38-4] is attractive and the PBV so determined approaches that estimated by pulmonary arterial and left atrial dilution curves. The authors emphasize, however, that the main theoretical limitation of the method derives from the uncertainty concerning the actual distribution of pulmonary circulation times.

Other Methods

Equilibration Method. Braunwald and associates[53] utilized an artificial circulatory model to evaluate the accuracy of the equilibration method and the mean circulation time method (Stewart-Hamilton) for the measurement of the volume of a segment of the vascular bed. They found that the Stewart-Hamilton method was accurate over a wide range of ratios of flow rate per minute to volume (0.37/1.0 to 7.75/1.0), whereas the equilibration method was accurate only with flow to volume ratios below 4.0/1.0. The equilibration method depends upon the principle that the difference between the concentration of the indicator entering and leaving a segment of the circulation varies directly as the volume of segment and inversely as rate of flow. Thus, the difference in the concentration of the indicator will be larger when the circulatory volume is large and the rate of flow is small. When the volume is small and the rate of flow is large, this difference becomes small and a small error in the determination of indicator concentration causes a larger error in the calculation of volume. Thus, the applicability of the equilibration method to the estimate of human pulmonary blood volume is questionable inasmuch as the flow-volume ratio exceeds 4/1 in most cases.

Exponential Downslope Method. The theoretical and experimental background of this method and its simplicity make it attractive. The slope volume, however, approximates the "central" blood volume more closely than the PBV as estimated by the newer methods. Others have pointed out that dye does not mix instantaneously or completely in either the heart or lungs.[54,55] Thus, the volume determined by the slope method probably does not represent a true physiologic volume.[56,57]

Limitations and Potential Errors of the Indicator-Dilution Technique

Dye Method

The utilization of the dye method is subject to many inherent limitations and potential errors. The various sources of errors may be enumerated as follows:

Timing and Rate of Injection. It is important to make sequential injections as closely together as possible. The cardiac output and mean transit time may vary significantly if sequential injections of indicator are made at an interval of more than 5 minutes, particularly when the patient's condition is unstable. The rate of injection may influence the estimate of mean transit time.

Marking or timing the injection may be done either manually or electrically. Generally, the timing mark is made in the middle of the injection. As long as the technique of timing is consistent throughout the procedure, the volume calculation is not substantially influenced in the double injection and single sampling technique or single injection and double sampling method. With the single injection and single sampling method, however, an error of one second may alter the volume calculation as much as 25%.

Cardiac Catheter.

a. The Technique of Left Heart Catheterization (Transseptal, Percutaneous or Transbronchial). The position of the left atrial catheter during injection is important. If the catheter is near the mitral valve, a major portion of the indicator may enter the left ventricle without adequate mixing in the left atrium, and the dilution curve will show a narrow base and a high peak (Figure 7-1). On the other hand, if the catheter is positioned in or near a pulmonary vein, the mean transit time from the left atrium to a systemic artery is prolonged, and the calculated PBV will be erroneously small.

b. The right heart catheter may be positioned too far into the pulmonary artery, so that the injected dye may not traverse all of the pulmonary vascular bed equally. On the other hand, if the tip of the catheter is placed too close to the pulmonic valve, the vigorous injection of dye may cause recoil of the catheter into the right ventricle, and the calculated PBV determined will be erroneously large.

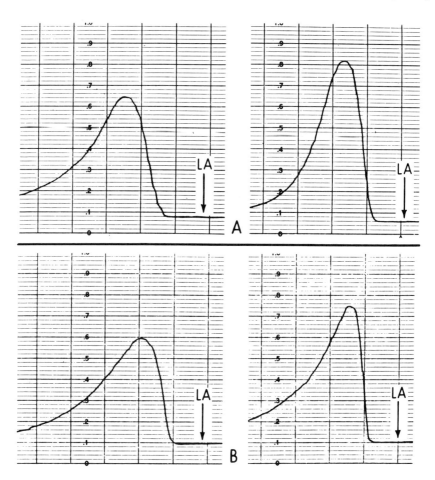

Figure 7-1.   Indicator-dilution curves recorded in two patients (A and B) after injection of indocyanine green into the left atrium and sampling of blood from a systemic artery. On the left panel the tip of the transseptal left atrial catheter was placed in the middle of the left atrium, whereas on the right panel the tip of the catheter was advanced close to the mitral valve. It is apparent that when the tip of the catheter is placed too close to the mitral valve the dilution curve shows a narrower base and higher peak. The distortion is due to the fact that a major portion of the indicator may enter the left ventricle without adequate mixing in the left atrium.

c. If the cardiac catheter is too long or its caliber too small, the time required for injection is prolonged. Even if the dead space of the catheter is accurately estimated, the calculated mean transit time may be unreliable. Injection is facilitated by using a catheter with multiple side holes rather than one with only one end hole.

Mixing Problems.

a. The mixing of indicator in the pulmonary vascular bed may be incomplete if stagnant or pooled blood is present, resulting in less indicator from the blood sampled. The possibility also exists that indicator may be lost through the pulmonary capillary-alveolar interface. Inadequate mixing of indicator is one of the criticisms of the single injection and single sampling method already discussed.[25]

b. Pulmonary regurgitation may prolong the mean transit time from the pulmonary artery to the arterial sampling site, causing the estimated PBV to be spuriously large (Figure 7-2).

c. In addition, there is the question of adequate mixing in the left atrium when the catheter lies near the pulmonary veins or the mitral valve, as

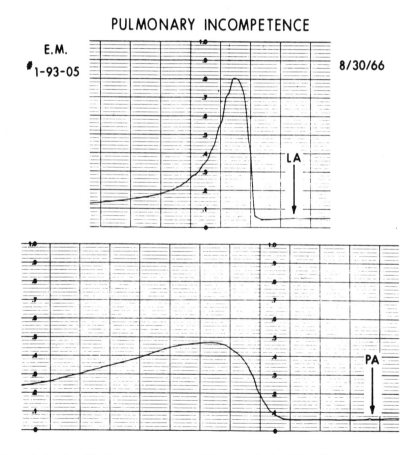

PULMONARY INCOMPETENCE

E.M.
#1-93-05   8/30/66

Figure 7-2.   Indicator-dilution curve recorded in a patient with mitral stenosis and pulmonary hypertension. There was clinical, hemodynamic and angiographic evidence of pulmonary incompetence. Note the marked distortion of the indicator-dilution curve inscribed after injection of indocyanine green into the pulmonary artery and slightly distorted dilution curve recorded after injection into the left atrium.

mentioned earlier, and injected dye may regurgitate into pulmonary veins or become sequestrated in the left atrial appendix. Finally, the timing of injection corresponding to the cardiac cycle is important. For instance, more adequate mixing would be expected if most of the indicator reaches the left atrial chamber during ventricular systole.

Sampling System.

a. The length and caliber (volume) of the sampling tubing as well as the flow rate through the sampling system may affect the time-concentration components of the indicator-dilution curve considerably. The volume/flow ratio (V/F) in the sampling system should not exceed 0.7, where V = ml and F = ml/sec.[58]

b. The dead space of collecting needle, tubing, cuvette, etc. in each study should be considered in calculating the timing of the sampling system.

c. Sampling from the ascending aorta is preferable to that from a systemic artery, since the rate of blood flow and mean transit time may be significantly influenced by local hyperemia in peripheral arteries, as discussed earlier.[51,52] This pitfall is important when "central" blood volume is measured (injection into PA and sampling from a peripheral artery). When PBV is measured with the double injection and single sampling method, however, the mean transit time through the pulmonary vascular bed is not materially affected whether the sampling is from a systemic artery or from the ascending aorta.

Status of the Indicator in the Vascular System. It is essential that the indicator remain within the vascular system during the primary circulation. When multiple dilution curves are recorded, the background concentration of the indicator should be as low as

possible for each curve. This requires that the indicator be rapidly metabolized or excreted after each injection.

Recording System. The cuvette densitometers now in general use are satisfactory and the time-concentration components of the indicator dilution may be instantaneously inscribed using any of the many available direct writing electronic recording systems.

Radioisotope Method

The limitations and potential errors of the dye method also apply to the radioisotope method, particularly if the radioisotope indicator is sampled from the left atrium, aorta, or a systemic artery. Cardiac catheterization is not required for precordial counting, but the limited depth focus of present scintillation detectors restricts their applicability. The mean transit time measured from the peak time in the right heart to the peak time in the left heart results in a falsely high PBV calculation because a portion of both right and left heart volumes is included. The techniques of radioisotope precordial counting recently developed by Donato, Guintini, Segre and their respective associates[38-42] narrow the calculated PBV to values comparable to those obtained by the dye dilution methods.

The number of radioisotope dilution curves which can be inscribed in a given subject is limited by the hazard of large doses of radioisotope and by the high background concentrations which accumulate after repeated curves.

Indirect Methods for Estimating Changes in Pulmonary Blood Volume

Change in Lung Volumes

In a normal subject the PBV is greater in the supine than in the upright position, a change which is reflected in reduction in the vital capacity in the supine position.[59-61] In patients with chronic left heart failure and pulmonary congestion, the vital capacity is usually diminished;[62-64] but the PBV may remain within normal limits[26] (see Chapter 9). Thus, the reduction in vital capacity need not necessarily reflect a significant increase in PBV. In this case, an increase in interstitial fluid in the lungs may be responsible largely for the altered lung volume.[26,62,64]

Mechanics of Breathing

Compliance is the change in lung volume in ml resulting from a change in intrapleural or esophageal pressure in cm $H_2O(\triangle V/\triangle P)$.[65,66] Compliance is significantly reduced in patients with chronic congestive heart failure,[64,66-70] an effect which has been attributed to increased PBV. Recent studies demonstrating that the PBV in these patients is not augmented[26] have supported the notion that the encroachment of the lung volume is largely due to interstitial edema resulting from inordinate increase in pulmonary venous and "capillary" pressures (see Chapter 9).

Critically Balanced Teeter Board[71-73]

This device is used to detect a shift in the center of gravity of the body when blood is displaced from one end to the other. An increase in intrathoracic blood volume causes the head portion of the teeter board to tilt downward, an effect which may represent an increase in any compartment of the intrathoracic blood volume, the pulmonary vascular bed, all four chambers of the heart, the great veins, the thoracic aorta, and more. The PBV is smaller than the volume in the heart chambers and non-pulmonary vessels, making study of PBV during physiologic or pharmacologic interventions difficult or impossible.

REFERENCES

1. Gibson, J.G., Seligman, A.M., Peacock, W.C., Aub, J.C., Fine, J., and Evans, R.D.: The distribution of red cells and plasma in large and minute vessels of the normal dog, determined by radioactive isotopes of iron and iodine. J.Clin. Invest., 25, 848, 1946.

2. Ebert, R.V., and Stead, E.A.: Demonstration that in normal man no reserves of blood are mobilized by exercise, epinephrine and hemorrhage. Am. J. Med. Sci., 201, 655, 1941.

3. Nylin, G.: The effect of heavy muscular work on the volume of circulating red corpuscles in man. Am. J. Physiol., 149, 180, 1947.

4. Holmgren, A.: Circulatory changes during muscular work in man. Scand. J. Clin. & Lab. & Invest., 8, Suppl. 24, 1956.

5. Liebow, A.A., Hales, M.R., and Bloomer, W. E: Relation of bronchial to pulmonary vascular tree. In W. Adams and I. Veith (eds), Pulmonary Circulation, p. 79, New York, Grune & Stratton, 1959.

6. Cudkowicz, L., Abelmann, W.H., Levinson, G.E., Katznelson, G., and Jreissatz, R.M.: Bronchial arterial blood flow. Clin. Sci., 19, 1, 1960.

7. Fritts, H.W., Harris, P., Chidsey, C.A., Clauss, R.H., and Cournand, A.: Estimation of flow through bronchial-pulmonary vascular anastomoses with use of T-1824 dye. Circulation, 23, 390, 1961.

8. Fishman, A.P.: The clinical significance of the pulmonary collateral circulation. Circulation, 24, 677, 1961.

9. Kunieda, R.: Evaluation of pulmonary blood volume in mitral valve disease by T-1824 method. Respiration and Circulation (Kokyu to Junkan), 3, 510, 1955.

10. Fujimoto. K., Kunieda, R., and Shiba, T.: Lung blood volume in acquired heart disease. Jap. Heart J., 1, 442, 1960.

11. Dock, D.S., Kraus, W.L., Woodward, E., Dexter, L., and Haynes, F.: Observations on pulmonary, blood volume in man. Fed. Proc., 18, 37, 1959.

12. Dock, D.S., Kraus, W.L., McQuire, L.B., Hyland, J.W., Haynes, F.W., and Dexter, L.:

The pulmonary blood volume in man. J. Clin. Invest., *40*, 317, 1961.

13. McGaff, C.J., Jose, A.D., and Milnor, W.R.: Pulmonary, left heart and arterial volume in valvular heart disease. Clin. Res., *7*, 230, 1959.

14. Milnor, W.R., Jose, A.D., and McGaff, C.J.: Pulmonary vascular volume, resistance and compliance in man. Circulation, *12*, 130, 1960.

15. Fermoso, J.D., Aramendia, P., and Taquini, A.C.: Volumen sanguineo pulmonar en la estenosis mitral. Medicina (B Air), *21*, 161, 1961.

16. Oakley, C., Glick, G., Luria, M.N., Schreiner, B.F., and Yu, P.N.: Some regulatory mechanisms of the human pulmonary vascular bed. Circulation, *26*, 917, 1962.

17. McGaff, C.J., Roveti, G.C., Glassman, E., and Milnor, W.R.: The pulmonary blood volume in rheumatic heart disease and its alteration by isoproterenol. Circulation, *27*, 77, 1963.

18. Yu, P.N., Glick, G., Schreiner, B.F., and Murphy, G.W.: Effects of acute hypoxia on the pulmonary vascular bed in patients with acquired heart disease: With special reference to the demonstration of active vasomotion. Circulation, *27*, 541, 1963.

19. Schreiner, B.F., Murphy, G.W., Glick, G., and Yu, P.N.: Effect of exercise on the pulmonary blood volume in patients with acquired heart disease. Circulation, *27*, 559, 1963.

20. Glick, G., Schreiner, B.F., Murphy, G.W., and Yu, P.N.: Effects of inhalation of 100 per cent oxygen on the pulmonary blood volume in patients with organic heart disease. Circulation, *27*, 554, 1963.

21. Varnauskas, E., Forsberg, S.A., Widimsky, J., and Paulin, S.: Pulmonary blood volume and its relation to pulmonary hemodynamics in cardiac patients. Acta Med. Scand., *173*, 529, 1963.

22. Forsberg, S.A.: Pulmonary blood volume in man. Acta Med. Scand., *175*, Suppl. 410, 1964.

23. Samet, P., Bernstein, W.H., Medow, A., and Levine, S.: Transseptal left heart dynamics in thirty-two normal subjects. Dis. Chest, *47*, 632, 1965.

24. Roy, S.B., Bhardwaj, P., and Bhatia, M.L.: Pulmonary blood volume in mitral stenosis. Brit. Med. J., *2*, 1466, 1965.

25. Samet, P., Bernstein, W.H., Lopez, A., and Levine, S.: Methodology of true pulmonary blood volume determination. Circulation, *33*, 847, 1966.

26. Schreiner, B.F., Murphy, G.W., and Yu, P.N.: Pulmonary blood volume in congestive heart failure. Circulation, *34*, 249, 1966.

27. Freitas, F.M. de, Faraco, E.Z. Nedel, N., Azevedo, D.F. de, and Zaduchliver, J.: Determination of pulmonary blood volume by single intravenous injection of one indicator in patients with normal and high pulmonary vascular pressures. Circulation, *30*, 370, 1964.

28. Freitas, F.M. de, Faraco, E.Z., Azevedo, D.F. de, Zaduchliver, J., and Lewin, I.: Behavior of normal pulmonary circulation during changes of total blood volume in man. J. Clin. Invest., *44*, 366, 1963.

29. Freitas F.M. de, Faraco, E.Z., Azevedo, D.F. de, and Lewin, I.: Action of bradykinin on human pulmonary circulation. Observations in patients with mitral valvular disease. Circulation, *34*, 385, 1966.

30. Levinson, G.E., Frank, M.J,., and Hellems, H.K.: The pulmonary vascular volume in man. Measurement from atrial dilution curves. Am. Heart J., *67*, 734, 1964,

31. Schreiner, B.F., Murphy, G.W., and Yu, P.N.: Unpublished data.

32. Lammerant, J.: *Le volume sangiune des poumons chez l'homme*. Bruxelles, Edition Arsica, 1957.

33. Eich, R.H., Chaffee, W.R., and Chodos, R.B.: Measurement of central blood volume by external monitoring. Circ. Res., *9*, 626, 1961.

34. Love, W.D., O'Meallie, L.P., and Burch, G.E.: Clinical estimation of the volumes of blood in the right heart, left heart, and lungs by use of I[131] albumin. Am. Heart J., *61*, 397, 1961.

35. Pietila, K.A., and Hakkila, J.: Studies of cardiac output and of pulmonary and intrathoracic blood volume. Cardiologia, *36*, 97, 1960.

36. Moir, T.W., and Gott, F.S.: The central circulating blood volume in normal subjects and patients with mitral stenosis. Am. Heart J., *61*, 740, 1961.

37. Kashemsant, U., Smulyan, H., and Eich, R.H.: The pulmonary blood volume measurement in patients with rheumatic heart disease. Am. J. Med. Sci., *249*, 667, 1965.

38. Donato, L., Guintini, C., Lewis, M.L., Durand, J., Rochester, D.F., Harvey, R.M., and Cournand, A.: Quantitative radiography. I. Theoretical considerations. Circulation, *26*, 174, 1962.

39. Donato, L., Rochester, D.F., Lewis, M.L., Durand, J., Parker, J.O., and Harvey, R.M.: Quantitative radiography. II. Technic and analysis of curves. Circulation, *26*, 183, 1962.

40. Lewis, R.L., Giuntini, C., Donato, L., Harvey, R.M., and Cournand, A.: Quantitative radiography. III. Results and validation of theory and method. Circulation, *26*, 189, 1962.

41. Giuntini, C., Lewis, M.L., Sales Luis, A., and Harvey, R.M.: A study of the pulmonary blood volume in man by quantitative radiocardiography. J. Clin. Invest., *42*, 1589, 1963.

42. Segre, G., Turco, G.L., and Ghemi, F.: Determination of pulmonary weighting function, of the mean pulmonary transit time, and of the pulmonary blood volume in man by means of radiocardiograms. Cardiologia, *46*, 295, 1965.

43. Rabinowitz, M., and Rapaport, E.: Determination of circulating pulmonary blood volume in dogs by an arteriovenous dye equilibrium method. Circ. Res., *2*, 525, 1954.

44. Newman, E.V., Merrell, M., Genecin, A., Monge, C., Milnor, W.R., and McKeever, W.P.: The dye dilution method for describing the central circulation. An analysis of factors shaping the time-concentration curves. Circulation, *4*, 735, 1951.

45. Pearce, M.L., McKeever, W.P., Dow, P., and Newman, E.V.: The influence of injection site upon the form of dye-dilution curves. Circ. Res., *1*, 112, 1953.

46. Lagerlöf, H., Werkö, L., Bucht, H., and Holmgren, A.: Separate determination of blood volume of the right and left heart and the lungs in man with the aid of the dye injection method. Scand. J. Clin. & Lab. Invest., *1*, 114, 1949.

47. Hayek, H. Von: *Die Menschliche Lunge*. Berlin, Springer Verlag, 1953. Translated by V.E. Krahl, New York, Hafner, 1960.

48. Backmann, R.: Blutgehalt und Blutverteilung in den Lungen Gesunder und Kranker Menschen. Beitr. Path. Anat., *125*, 222, 1961.

49. Dexter, L., and Smith, G.T.: Quantitative studies of pulmonary embolism. Am. J. Med. Sci., *247*, 37, 1964.

50. Samet, P., Bernstein, W.H., and Medow, A.: Effect of site of injection upon left ventricular indicator-dilution output. Am. Heart J., *69*, 241, 1965.

51. McIntosh, H.D., Gleason, W.L., Miller, D.E., and Bacos, J.B.: A major pitfall in the interpretation of "central blood volume." Circ. Res., *9*, 1223, 1961.

52. Marshall, R.J., and Shepherd, J.T.: Interpretation of changes in "central" blood volume and slope volume during exercise in man. J. Clin. Invest., *40*, 375, 1961.

53. Braunwald, E., Fishman, A.P., and Cournand, A.: Estimation of volume of a circulatory model by the Hamilton and the Bradley methods at varying flow volume ratios. J. Appl. Physiol., *12*, 445, 1958.

54. Howard, A.R., Hamilton, W.F., and Dow, P.: Limitations of the continuous infusion method for measuring cardiac output by dye dilution. Am. J. Physiol., *175*, 173, 1953.

55. Fishman, A.P.: Dynamics of the pulmonary circulation. In *Handbook of Physiology*, Section 2, Circulation, Vol. 2, p. 1681, Washington, D.C., American Physiological Society, 1963.

56. Wang, Y., Shepherd, J.T., and Marshall, R.J.: Evaluation of the slope volume method as an index of pulmonary blood volume. J. Clin. Invest., *39*, 466, 1960.

57. McQuire, L.B., Dock, D.S., Hyland, J.W., Harrison, D.C., Haynes, F.W., and Dexter, L.: Evaluation of slope method for measuring pulmonary blood volume in man. J. Appl. Physiol., *17*, 497, 1962.

58. Milnor, W.R., and Jose, A.D.: Distortion of indicator-dilution curves by sampling system. J. Appl. Physiol., *15*, 177, 1960.

59. McMichael, J., and McGibbon, J.P.: Postural changes in the lung volume. Clin. Sci., *4*, 175, 1939.

60. Svanberg, L.: Influence of posture on the lung volumes, ventilation and circulation in normals. Scand. J. Clin. & Lab. Invest., *9*, Suppl. 25, 1957.

61. Moreno, F., and Lyons, H.A.: Effect of body posture on lung volumes. J. Appl. Physiol., *16*, 27, 1961.

62. Kopelman, H., and Lee, G. de J.: The intrathoracic blood volume in mitral stenosis and left ventricular failure. Clin. Sci., *10*, 383, 1951.

63. Brown, C.C., Fry, D.L., and Ebert, R.V.: The mechanics of pulmonary ventilation in patients with heart disease. Am. J. Med., *17*, 438, 1954.

64. Turino, G.M., and Fishman, A.P.: Congested lung. J. Chronic Dis., *9*, 510, 1959.

65. Mead, J.: Mechanical properties of lungs. Physiol. Rev., *41*, 281, 1961.

66. Sharp, J.T.: The effect of body position change on lung compliance in normal subjects and in patients with congestive heart failure. J. Clin. Invest., *38*, 659, 1959.

67. Christie, R.V., and Menkins, J.C.: The intrapleural pressure in congestive heart failure and its clinical significance. J. Clin. Invest., *13*, 323, 1934.

68. Richards, D.W.: The nature of cardiac and of pulmonary dyspnea. Circulation, *7*, 15, 1953.

69. Brown, C.C., Fry, D.L., and Ebert, R.V.: Mechanics of pulmonary ventilation in patients with heart disease. Am. J. Med., *17*, 438, 1954.

70. Donald, K.W.: Disturbances in pulmonary function in mitral stenosis and left heart failure. Prog. Cardiovasc. Dis., *1*, 298, 1958.

71. Cotton, F.W.: Studies in center of gravity changes. Australian J. Exp. Biol. Med. Sci., *8*, 53, 1931.

72. Tenney, S.M.: Fluid volume redistribution and thoracic volume changes during recumbency. J. Appl. Physiol., *14*, 129, 1959.

73. Fritts, H.W., Jr., Odell, J.E., Harris, P., Braunwald, E., and Fishman, A.P.: Effects of acute hypoxia on the volume of blood in the thorax. Circulation, *22*, 216, 1960.

CHAPTER 8

Pulmonary Blood Volume in Man*

This chapter includes data on pulmonary blood volume obtained at rest from 15 "normal" patients and from more than 300 patients with various types of cardiopulmonary disease studied in our laboratory.

Technique and Methodology Used in Our Laboratory

As mentioned previously, the technique of estimating pulmonary blood volume in our laboratory is adapted from that described by Milnor and associates.[1] Right heart and transseptal left heart catheterizations are carried out in the usual manner, with the left heart catheter introduced by a saphenous vein cut-down or percutaneously by a femoral vein puncture.[2,3] One catheter is placed in the main pulmonary artery and another in the left atrium. A No. 18 Cournand needle or a small polyethylene catheter is introduced into a brachial or femoral artery and connected to a cuvette densitometer.** Indicator dilution curves are recorded after indocyanine green (Cardiogreen+) is injected sequentially into

the pulmonary artery (PA) and the left atrium (LA). The system is flushed with physiologic saline solution after injection of dye. The two injections are usually accomplished within 2 minutes and the order of injection is randomized. The sampling rate is 0.7 to 0.8 ml per second, and each curve is inscribed by a direct writing recorder.+ The time of the injection period is considered zero time for all measurements of transit time. Each curve is transcribed electronically on IBM data cards which are fed into a previously programmed IBM Model 1620 computer which subsequently calculates cardiac output and mean transit time. All curves with deviations from the baseline greater than 3% of full scale deflection are automatically rejected. Points are accepted for determination of the exponential downslope of the curves only if they deviate from a true exponential by less than 2% of the peak concentration value. At least five such points are used, and the best approximation is calculated by the computer.[4,5] Figure 8-1 shows that the cardiac output determined from indicator-dilution curves by the programmed method checks well with the results of the manual method without systematic error.

Blood withdrawn during inscription of the indicator dilution curves is immediately reinfused, minimizing blood loss in each patient.

All pressure measurements are re-

---

*Much of the work summarized in this chapter was done by my colleagues, Drs. Bernard F. Schreiner, and Gerald W. Murphy.

**Gilford Instrument Laboratories, Inc., Oberlin, Ohio.

+Hynson, Westcott and Dunning, Inc., Baltimore, Maryland.

+Texas Instruments, Inc., Houston, Texas.

CALCULATIONS OF DYE CURVES

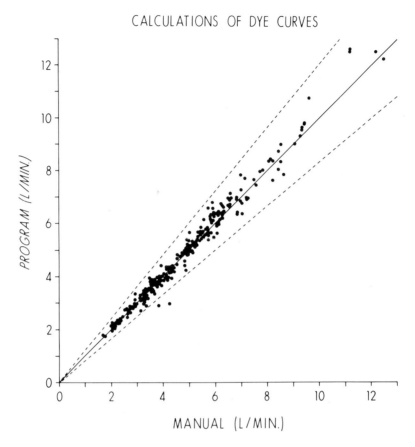

Figure 8-1.   Values for cardiac output derived from the indicator-dilution curves programmed by the IBM method are plotted against values from the same curves calculated by the manual method. The two methods checked closely without systematic error. The dotted lines indicate the range of ± 20% difference.

corded using a Statham P23 AA strain gauge and a Sanborn 350 series direct writing recorder. The gauges recording from the right and left sides of the heart are placed 6.5 and 8.5 cm below the sternal angle respectively. All pressure measurements represent mean values during at least two respiratory cycles. Left ventricular end-diastolic pressures are recorded at high gain to facilitate more accurate measurements. The pulmonary distending pressure (Pd) is the average of the pulmonary arterial and the left atrial pressures.[1]

Values of cardiac output used in the calculations of central blood volume (CBV) and pulmonary blood volume (PBV) represent the average of sequential pulmonary arterial and left atrial injections. Cardiac index (CI) is the cardiac output (CO) per M^2 of body surface area. The CBV is that volume between the main pulmonary artery and a systemic artery, including all temporally equidistant branches. It is calculated by the Stewart-Hamilton formula as follows:[6,7]

$$CBV = CI \times Tm_{(PA-BA)}$$

Where   CBV = central blood volume (ml/M^2)
CI = cardiac index (ml/sec/M^2)

$Tm_{(PA-BA)}$ = mean transit time from the pulmonary artery to a systemic artery (sec)

The PBV is that volume within the pulmonary arteries, pulmonary capillaries and pulmonary veins and an indeterminate portion of the left atrium. It is calculated by the product of cardiac index and mean transit time from the main pulmonary artery to the left atrium as follows:

$$PBV = CI \times Tm_{(PA-BA)} - Tm_{(LA-BA)}$$

Where   PBV = pulmonary blood volume (ml/M²)

$Tm_{(LA-BA)}$ = mean transit time from left atrium to a systemic artery (sec)

The blood volume in a portion of the left atrium, in the left ventricle, the aorta and its temporally equidistant tributaries is designated as left heart and aortic volume (LHV). It is the difference between CBV and PBV.

The pulmonary capillary blood volume (Vc) is the volume in the pulmonary capillary bed. It is estimated by the determination of breath-holding pulmonary diffusing capacity for carbon monoxide with ambient room air as well as with 100% O_2 as described by Ogilvie and co-workers.[8,9] The calculation of Vc is based upon the relations shown in the equation:

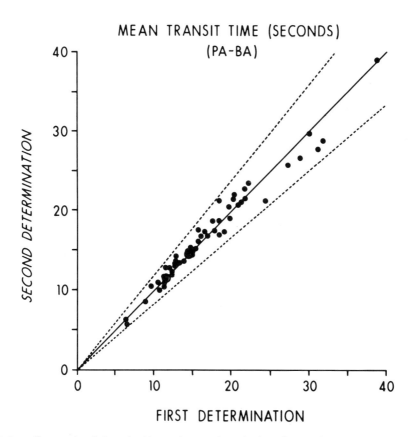

Figure 8-2.   Successive determinations of mean transit time from pulmonary artery to systemic artery. In this and subsequent figures the results of the first determination are plotted against corresponding values of the second determination. The dotted lines indicate the range of ± 20% difference.

$$1/D_L = 1/D_M + 1/\theta Vc$$

Where D_L = total pulmonary diffusing capacity for carbon monxide (ml/mm Hg/min)

D_M = membrane diffusing capacity for carbon monoxide (ml/mm Hg/min)

θ = constant related to the rate of uptake of carbon monoxide by hemoglobin at various oxygen concentrations

Vc = pulmonary capillary blood volume (ml/M^2)

Range of Variation and Reproductibility

As we have previously reported,[4,10] values of cardiac index derived from paired indicator-dilution curves following injection into the PA and the LA agreed well with each other. In paired determinations from more than 100 patients the coefficient of correlation was high ($p < 0.01$), and no systematic difference was observed.

The reproducibility of the method has been demonstrated in a series of 57 patients on whom duplicate determinations of a number of parameters were made within periods of 10 to 15 minutes. These included cardiac index (average of PA and LA curves), mean transit time from the pulmonary artery to a systemic artery (Tm_{PA-BA}) from the left atrium to a systemic artery (Tm_{LA-BA}), and from the pulmonary artery to the left artrium

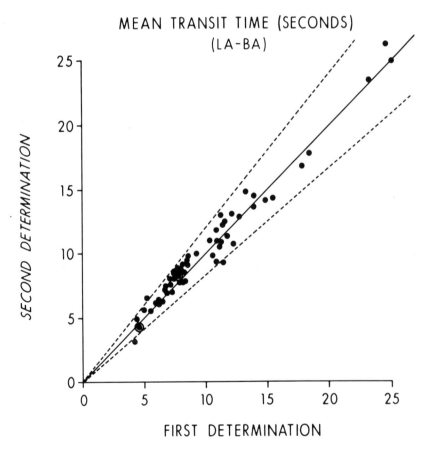

Figure 8-3.   Successive determinations of mean transit time from left atrium to systemic artery.

(Tm_{PA-LA}); central blood volume (CBV) and pulmonary blood volume (PBV). Values for the various mean transit times, CBV and PBV obtained during the first and second determinations are shown in Figures 8-2 to 8-6.

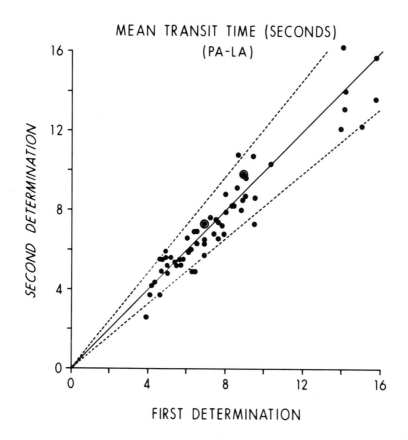

Figure 8-4. Successive determinations of mean transit time from pulmonary artery to left atrium.

TABLE 8-1 Statistical Analysis of Duplicate Determinations of Cardiac Index, Mean Transit Times, "Central" Blood Volume and Pulmonary Blood Volume

Parameters	No. of Duplicate Determinations	Standard Deviation of a Single Determination
C.I.	57	0.13 (L/min/M²)
Tm_{PA-BA}	57	0.74 (seconds)
Tm_{LA-BA}	57	0.49 (seconds)
Tm_{PA-LA}	57	0.69 (seconds)
CBV	57	26.5 (ml/M²)
PBV	57	15.6 (ml/M²)

C.I.   = Average cardiac index from PA and LA curves (L/min/M²)
Tm_{PA-BA} = Mean transit time from pulmonary artery to systemic artery (seconds)
Tm_{LA-BA} = Mean transit time form left atrium to systemic artery (seconds)
Tm_{PA-LA} = Mean transit time from pulmonary artery to left atrium (seconds)
CBV   = "Central" blood volume (ml/M²)
PBV   = Pulmonary blood volume (ml/M²)

The standard deviation of single observations for each parameter is shown in Table 8-1. For a given patient, the difference between the first and second determinations rarely exceeded 80 ml/M² for CBV and was almost always less than 45 ml/M² for PBV.

Therefore, a difference of 100 ml/M² or greater between the control and experimental values for CBV and a difference of 50 ml/M² or greater for PBV are considered significant.

The reproducibility of the method is further evident in the close agreement between the values of triplicate determinations of CBV and PBV in a series of 19 patients. The three determinations were made successively in each patient over a period of about 20 to 40 minutes with randomized injections of the indicator into the PA and the LA. The data are presented in Table 8-2. With the exception of one patient (L.N.), the CBV varied less than 100 ml/M² between any two of the three determinations. Similarly, the PBV varied less than 50 ml/M² between any two of the three determinations without exception.

Normal Subjects

The normal subjects referred to in this section were patients studied in our laboratory who had no demonstrable cardiopulmonary disease.

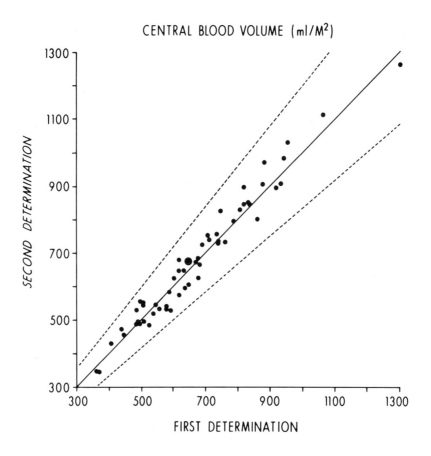

CENTRAL BLOOD VOLUME (ml/M²)

Figure 8-5.   Successive determinations of the central blood volume.

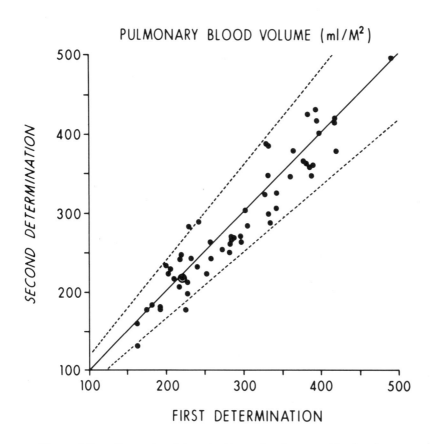

Figure 8-6. Successive determinations of pulmonary blood volume.

TABLE 8-2 Triplicate Determinations of "Central" and Pulmonary Blood Volumes

Patients	Diagnosis	F.C.	Determinations	C.I.	Tm $PA-BA$	$LA-BA$	$PA-LA$	CBV	PBV
J.S.	M.S.	III	1	1.85	21.1	11.8	9.3	649	287
			2	1.84	20.6	10.3	10.3	633	317
			3	1.66	21.8	11.7	10.1	602	279
F.T.	M.S.	III	1	2.34	25.8	16.2	9.6	1010	374
	E.H.		2	2.43	23.9	15.3	8.6	968	348
			3	2.28	26.5	16.1	10.4	1005	396
D.R.	M.S.	III	1	2.75	20.3	11.7	8.6	930	394
	M.R.		2	2.46	22.1	11.3	10.8	904	430
			3	2.30	23.4	12.6	10.8	898	415
G.B.	M.S.	III	1	1.67	17.8	10.9	6.9	496	192
	A.R.		2	1.90	17.5	11.8	5.7	554	180
			3	1.68	18.7	12.0	6.7	523	188
F.C.	M.S.	III	1	3.32	11.4	7.2	4.2	632	233
			2	3.47	11.2	7.0	4.2	649	243
			3	3.60	11.5	7.0	4.5	690	270

TABLE 8-2 Triplicate Determinations of "Central" and Pulmonary Blood Volumes (cont.)

Patients	Diagnosis	F.C.	Determinations	C.I.	Tm			CBV	PBV
					PA−BA	LA−BA	PA−LA		
E.K.	M.S.	IV	1	1.12	28.9	13.9	15.0	545	282
	T.R.		2	1.22	26.7	14.5	12.2	545	250
			3	1.24	26.8	13.5	13.3	555	276
C.B.	M.S.	IV	1	1.53	22.9	13.1	9.8	585	252
			2	1.54	23.5	12.2	11.3	604	291
			3	1.62	23.6	12.4	11.2	637	303
B.K.	M.R.	II	1	3.44	12.7	6.8	5.3	728	304
			2	3.26	12.1	6.2	5.9	658	320
			3	2.79	13.8	7.0	6.8	642	316
J.P.	M.R.	III	1	1.53	27.3	18.6	8.7	696	222
			2	1.44	26.7	18.3	8.4	642	202
			3	1.50	27.0	18.9	8.1	676	203
H.B.	A.S.	II	1	2.97	11.1	5.4	5.7	550	282
			2	3.21	11.2	5.6	5.6	600	299
			3	2.83	11.9	5.5	6.4	561	302
D.C.	A.S.	III	1	3.32	11.0	5.5	5.5	610	304
			2	3.50	10.9	5.7	5.2	635	304
			3	3.20	10.2	5.0	5.2	545	278
D.R.	A.S.	III	1	2.80	14.8	6.5	8.3	680	390
			2	2.64	14.5	6.3	8.2	662	360
			3	2.71	14.5	6.3	8.2	642	354
L.N.	A.R.	II	1	3.16	12.3	8.2	4.1	648	216
	M.R.		2	3.34	12.3	8.6	3.7	686	206
			3	3.46	12.3	7.9	4.4	710	255
W.M.	A.R.	II	1	2.94	21.6	12.7	8.9	1060	242
			2	3.12	22.7	12.9	9.8	1110	289
			3	2.87	25.5	15.3	10.2	1220	277
B.H.	I.C.	II	1	1.75	21.0	11.7	9.3	570	254
			2	1.50	21.8	11.2	10.6	555	270
			3	1.75	20.3	11.3	9.0	533	234
S.N.	I.C.	II	1	2.50	13.1	7.4	5.7	540	237
			2	2.92	10.9	6.6	3.3	530	208
			3	2.91	10.8	6.9	3.9	521	189
W.H.	C.P.	IV	1	2.38	13.7	8.2	5.5	525	261
			2	2.50	12.9	7.1	5.8	540	242
			3	2.48	13.9	7.1	6.8	572	280
S.S.	T.P.H.	II	1	2.28	15.2	8.9	6.3	576	249
			2	2.44	15.7	8.9	6.8	631	274
			3	2.26	15.0	8.5	6.5	564	246
F.R.	H.T.	II	1	2.32	14.9	7.5	7.4	576	285
			2	2.36	14.8	8.0	6.8	532	268
			3	2.43	14.4	7.2	7.2	584	291

F.C. = Functional classification
M.S. = Mitral stenosis
E.H. = Essential hypertension
M.R. = Mitral regurgitation
T.R. = Tricuspid regurgitation
A.S. = Aortic stenosis

A.R. = Aortic regurgitation
I.C. = Idiopathic cardiomyopathy
C.P. = Constrictive pericarditis
T.P.H. = Thromboembolic pulmonary hypertension
H.T. = Hypothyroidism

Other symbols and abbreviations are the same as those used in Table 8-1.

TABLE 8-3 Hemodynamic Data, "Central," Total Pulmonary and Pulmonary Capillary Blood Volumes in "Normal" Subjects

Name	Age	Sex	BSA	Blood Flow CI	HR	SI	Pressures (mm Hg) RAm	PAm	LAm	Pd	LV (S/D)	BA (S/D,m)	PVR (dynes·sec/cm⁵)	Blood Volume (ml/M²) CBV	PBV	LHV	Vc	C (ml/M²/mm Hg)
J.M.	21	M	2.05	3.10	96	32	1	9	4	6.5	125/5	125/80,90	63	530	257	273	63	39.3
W.H.	45	M	1.90	3.67	60	61	4	10	8	9	120/8	140/80,110	23	772	257	515	61	28.5
R.S.	21	M	1.84	4.40	80	55	1	11	3	7	144/5	140/84,108	79	594	286	308	—	40.9
J.D.	27	F	1.77	3.24	74	44	2	12	4	8	120/5	124/70,88	111	568	282	286	—	35.2
R.C.	23	M	1.92	3.78	83	46	2	12	8	10	144/8	130/80,96	44	618	296	322	58	29.6
L.W.	14	M	1.99	3.22	70	46	5	12	9	10.5	140/12	130/81,104	37	440	204	236	—	19.4
T.D.	20	F	1.59	3.03	79	38	4	13	7	10	132/7	134/74,94	96	585	267	319	44	26.7
J.B.	20	F	1.77	3.53	90	39	4	13	8	10.5	112/11	108/64,75	64	558	264	294	—	25.2
F.H.	45	M	2.20	2.74	60	46	5	14	6	10	100/6	96/55,66	106	679	314	365	—	31.4
G.G.	24	M	1.74	4.04	90	45	4	15	8	12.5	126/6	128/80,96	68	728	249	479	45	19.9
B.B.	21	F	1.53	3.16	80	39	5	15	9	12	120/11	133/75,90	99	596	248	348	62	20.6
J.C.	24	M	17.4	3.30	74	45	4	15	11	13	125/10	125/75,100	56	616	291	325	39	22.4
L.G.	20	M	1.83	2.70	73	37	3	16	7	11.5	105/10	112/90,100	152	645	301	344	54	26.2
R.L.	40	F	1.72	3.16	100	32	1	16	8	12	125/7	125/75,95	118	485	234	251	66	19.5
D.G.	17	M	1.86	3.49	60	58	5	17	12	14.5	125/13	130/80,90	62	599	291	308	—	20.0
Mean	25.5		1.83	3.37	77.7	44.6	3.3	13.3	7.6	10.5	123/8	125/76,93	78.5	601	271	329	54	26.5
±S.E.	±2.5		±0.05	±0.12	±3.2	±2.4	±0.3	±0.6	±0.7	±0.6	±2.7/0.6	±4/27.4	±9.0	±22	±8.1	±19.8		±1.9

CI = Cardiac index (L/min/M²)
HR = Heart rate (beats)
SI = Stroke index (ml/beat/M²)
RA = Right atrial mean pressure
PAm = Pulmonary arterial mean pressure
LAm = Left atrial mean pressure
Pd = Pulmonary distending pressure $\left(\dfrac{PAm + LAm}{2}\right)$
LV = Left ventricular pressure

BA = Systemic arterial pressure
S = systolic, D = diastolic, and m = mean
PVR = Pulmonary vascular resistance
CBV = "Central" blood volume
PBV = Pulmonary blood volume
LHV = Left heart and aortic blood volume
Vc = Pulmonary capillary blood volume
C = Relative compliance (PBV/Pd)

Studies were undertaken as part of an evaluation for a systolic murmur. These subjects were free of cardiorespiratory symptoms, and no cardiovascular abnormalities were demonstrated by clinical, electrocardiographic, hemodynamic and angiocardiographic studies. They were considered normal hemodynamically. Hemodynamic data, CBV, PBV and Vc from 15 such normal patients are presented in Table 8-3.[9]

The CI varied from 2.7 to 4.4 L/min/M[2] and the stroke index (SI) from 32 to 61 ml/beat/M[2]. The intracardiac and intravascular pressures of all patients were within normal limits. The average pulmonary vascular resistance (PVR) for the entire group was 78.5 ±9 (mean ±S.D.) dynes · sec/cm[5].

The CBV ranged from 440 to 772 ml/M[2] with a mean of 601 ml/M[2], and the PBV varied from 204 to 314 ml/M[2] with a mean of 271 ml/M[2]. In general, the PBV of normal subjects was slightly less than half the CBV, and experimental changes in CBV usually reflected altered PBV rather than effects on left heart-aortic volume.

The Vc was estimated in the recumbent position in only nine patients, and the values varied from 39 to 66 ml/M[2] with a mean of 54 ml/M[2]. Chapter 14 reports the Vc of 16 additional normal subjects and the results are within the same range, with an identical mean value.

The values for PBV and Vc in our normal subjects compare favorably with those reported by other investigators.[11-21] Accepting the total blood volume in normal subjects as about 2.7 L/M[2], the CBV constitutes about 22%, PBV about 10% and Vc about 2% of the total blood volume.

The ratio of PBV to Pd may be considered as a static or relative compliance (C) of the pulmonary vascular bed.[1] Since no tissue pressure was measured, the value of Pd could not be taken as true transmural pressure. In this group of normal subjects the value of C was 26.5 ± 1.9 ml/M[2]/mm Hg.

Mitral Valve Disease

Table 8-4 summarizes the hemodynamic data, CBV and PBV in 128 patients with predominant mitral stenosis.

From class II to class IV, patients with mitral stenosis showed a progressive reduction in both CI and SI on the one hand, and a linear increase in PAm and LAm on the other. The mean values for PVR were significantly higher in all three groups of patients with predominant mitral stenosis than in the normal group. The respective values were 138 for class I-II, 361 for class III and 989 dynes · sec/cm[5] for class IV patients.

TABLE 8-4 Hemodynamic Data and Pulmonary Blood Volume in Patients with Predominant Mitral Stenosis

F.C.	No. of Patients	Age	BSA	CI	HR	SI	PAm	LAm	Pd	CBV	PBV	LHV	C	PVR
I and II	33	39.3*	1.66	2.65	84.4	32.4	22.1	14.9	18.5	601	287	314	16.3	138
		±2.1	±0.03	±0.10	±3.6	±1.6	±1.0	±0.7	±0.8	±17.4	±9.1	±14.9	±0.8	±14.8
III	87	41.7	1.64	2.19	81.5	27.7	34.6	20.7	27.6	653	310	342	12.1	361
		±1.2	±0.02	±0.06	±1.8	±1.0	±1.4	±0.6	±0.9	±13.7	±7.6	±9.6	±0.5	±40.9
IV	8	49.9	1.54	1.47	78.5	20.1	44.4	23.1	33.8	554	216	338	7.0	989
		±3.8	±0.06	±0.19	±5.1	±3.1	±6.0	±1.5	±3.7	±31.1	±17.2	±25.0	±1.0	±279.6

F.C. = Functional classification according to the criteria adopted by the New York Heart Association
Other symbols and abbreviations are the same as those used in Table 8-3
* = Mean ± S.E.

The mean CBV and PBV for class II patients were 601 ml/M² and 287 ml/M², respectively, values which closely approximate the normal. The respective mean CBV and PBV for class III patients were 653 ml/M² and 310 ml/M² respectively. The PBV in class III patients was significantly higher than normal (p < 0.01). For class IV patients the mean CBV and PBV were 554 ml/M² and 216 ml/M². Both the CBV and PBV in this class of patients were significantly lower than normal (p < 0.01).

Nine (27%) of 33 class I-II patients and 37 (42%) of 87 class III patients had a PBV greater than 315 ml/M², the upper limit of normal. Only five patients in class I and II and one patient in class III had a PBV less than 204 ml/M², the lower limit of normal. In contrast, the PBV was either normal or decreased in class IV patients.

For the group of patients with mitral stenosis as a whole, the LAm in 42 of 46 patients with elevated PBV was higher than 15 mm Hg. This is understandable because the elevated LAm and PAm pressures in many class II and class III patients undoubtedly tend to increase the PBV by passive distention of pulmonary arteries and veins. In later stages of the disease, however, when marked increase in PAm and PVR has occurred, the blood volume in the pulmonary vascular bed may return to normal, as reported here and by others.[17] This reduction of a previously elevated PBV most likely results from structural thickening and restriction of the pulmonary vessels, functional vasoconstriction or thromboembolism or combinations of such factors.[22-24] The postulation of functional vasoconstriction is supported by the reduction of PAm and the concomitant increase in PBV observed during acetylcholine infusion.[10] The importance of thromboembolism as a factor in reducing the PBV is substantiated by the post-mortem demonstration of multiple pulmonary emboli in three of our class IV patients. Mean C (PBV/Pd) in class I-II, III and IV patients with predominant mitral stenosis was 16.3, 12.1 and 7.0 ml/M²/mm Hg, respectively, progressively lower from class I-II to class IV. In all three groups the value of C was significantly low compared with normal (p < 0.01).

The changes in pulmonary blood flow, pressures and volumes in 62 patients with predominant mitral regurgitation are summarized in Table 8-5. In general, the CI and SI in these patients were comparable to those observed in patients with predominant mitral stenosis, although the PAm and LAm were slightly lower. The PVR was 130, 371 and 462 dynes · sec/cm⁵ in class I-II, III and IV, respectively. Compared with observations in normal subjects, the PVR was increased significantly in class III and IV (p < 0.01).

The average PBV was normal in 21 class II patients, but the average

TABLE 8-5 Hemodynamic Data and Pulmonary Blood Volume in Patients with Predominant Mitral Regurgitation

F.C.	No. of Patients	Age	BSA	CI	HR	SI	PAm	LAm	Pd	CBV	PBV	LHV	C	PVR
I and II	21	40.0	1.81	2.67	86.4	32.0	18.7	11.8	15.2	722	279	444	20.7	130
		±3.1	±0.05	±0.11	±4.5	±1.9	±1.7	±1.4	±1.5	±36.9	±11.1	±31.0	±1.6	±19.2
III	39	42.3	1.69	2.09	89.7	24.2	34.1	20.4	27.1	752	312	439	12.6	371
		±1.7	±0.03	±0.11	±3.3	±1.3	±2.4	±1.2	±1.7	±20.3	±15.6	±17.2	±0.8	±59.6
IV	2	47.0	1.57	1.38	80.5	17.0	39.5	22.0	30.7	522	215	312	7.5	462

Symbols and abbreviations are the same as those used in Tables 8-3 and 8-4

PBV in 39 class III patients was significantly higher than in normal subjects (p < .01). With only two class IV patients, we can note only that both showed a low normal PBV. Altogether, 20 patients had a PBV greater than 314 ml/M², the upper limit of normal, and two patients (one class I-II and one class IV) had a PBV less than 204 ml/M², the lower limit of normal.

The CBV in class I-III patients with predominant mitral regurgitation was generally higher than in the corresponding classes of patients with predominant mitral stenosis. The increase was mainly due to the augmented left heart-aortic volume, most likely a result of the more dilated left atrium and left ventricle. C (PBV/Pd) was progressively smaller from class I-II to class IV patients. The mean values (ml/M²/mm Hg) were 20.7 for class I-II, 12.6 for class III and 7.5 for class IV. All these values were significantly less than normal (p < 0.01).

Aortic Valve Disease

The hemodynamic data and PBV in 55 patients with predominant aortic stenosis and in 38 patients with predominant aortic regurgitation are summarized in Tables 8-6 and 8-7 respectively. Mean CI and SI were lower and mean PAm and LAm were higher in class III patients with predominant aortic stenosis than in class I and II patients. The PVR in patients with aortic stenosis was either normal or slightly increased, except in severe cases.

The mean PBV was 267 ml/M² for class I and II patients with aortic stenosis, and 301 ml/M² for class III patients. The mean PBV in class III patients was significantly higher than normal (p < 0.05). For the entire group, the PBV was greater than 315 ml/M² in 20 patients and less than 204 ml/M² in only two patients.

The mean CBV in class III patients was 712 ml/M², 111 ml more than the normal mean. This increase was mainly a result of enlargement of the left heart-aortic volume.

The C was minimally reduced in these patients, indicating an approximately normal pressure-volume relationship in the pulmonary vascular bed

TABLE 8-6   Hemodynamic Data and Pulmonary Blood Volume in Patients with Predominant Aortic Stenosis

F.C.	No. of Patients	Age	BSA	CI	HR	SI	PAm	LAm	Pd	CBV	PBV	LHV	C	PVR
I and II	20	35.9	1.80	2.92	75.6	38.9	16.6	9.4	13.0	647	267	380	21.9	133
		±4.0	±0.03	±0.16	±2.8	±2.1	±0.8	±0.7	±0.7	±23.3	±11.1	±24.7	±1.7	±18.6
III	35	48.8	1.82	2.76	78.7	32.8	20.4	12.5	16.3	712	301	411	21.0	144
		±1.5	±0.03	±0.10	±1.9	±1.8	±1.2	±1.0	±1.0	±19.2	±10.8	±15.4	±1.5	±17.0

Symbols and abbreviations are the same as those used in Tables 8-3 and 8-4.

TABLE 8-7   Hemodynamic Data and Pulmonary Blood Volume in Patients with Predominant Aortic Regurgitation

F.C.	No. of Patients	Age	BSA	CI	HR	SI	PAm	LAm	Pd	CBV	PBV	LHV	C	PVR
I and II	19	34.3	1.90	2.84	76.3	37.8	15.7	8.6	12.2	736	300	436	26.0	112
		±2.6	±0.04	±0.14	±2.8	±2.6	± 1.2	±0.9	±1.0	±28.6	±11.9	±22.5	±1.6	±10.7
III	19	40.3	1.78	2.38	77.1	31.3	22.2	13.8	18.0	803	290	512	20.6	223
		±3.3	±0.05	±0.15	±3.0	±2.0	±2.5	±1.8	±2.1	±46.4	±19.5	±33.6	±3.1	±62.4

Symbols and abbreviations are the same as those used in Tables 8-3 and 8-4.

at rest. This relationship became markedly abnormal during exercise, however (see Chapter 18).

Only three class IV patients with predominant aortic stenosis were studied. In these the mean CI was 1.9 L/min/M² and the mean SI 20 ml/beat /M². The LAm was greater than 20 mm Hg and the PAm greater than 35 mm Hg in all three. The PBV in these three patients was respectively 335, 320 and 295 ml/M². Thus, the high pulmonary vascular pressures and volumes in class IV patients with aortic stenosis resembled those observed in class III patients with mitral valve disease. Furthermore, because the severe pulmonary venous and arterial hypertension was not as long standing as in patients with mitral disease, the structural changes of the pulmonary vessels and the degree of hypoxemia and functional vasoconstriction which might result from such changes would be expected to be less.[25] This may be one important explanation for the absence of a decreased PBV in class IV patients with aortic valve disease.

Observations in patients with predominant aortic regurgitation were similar to those in predominant aortic stenosis, with the exception of CBV and LHV. The mean CBV in class I-II and in class III patients with predominant aortic regurgitation was 736 and 803 ml/M², respectively, and the respective mean values of LHV were 436 and 512 ml/M². In class I-II patients the mean PBV was 300 ml/M², significantly higher than the normal. In the entire group, PBV was greater than 314 ml/M² in 12 patients and lower than 204 ml/M² in only two patients.

In almost half the patients the ratio of CBV/PBV was greater than 3 to 1 instead of the normal of about 2 to 1, indicating a much larger volume in the left side of the heart and aorta

and its tributaries than in the pulmonary vascular bed. This finding is consistent with the characteristic and considerable dilatation of the left ventricle and ascending aorta in most of these patients. In patients with severe aortic regurgitation, the indicator-dilution curves were usually so distorted that the reliability of measurements of CBV and PBV was questioned.[10,26] C was normal in class I-II patients and slightly low in class III patients.

Primary Myocardial Disease

A series of 24 patients with primary myocardial disease or cardiomyopathy has been studied in our laboratory. In one patient (F.S.) of the restrictive group, the cause was proven amyloidosis, and in one case in the congestive group (J.M.), hemochromatosis was the cause. In most patients, however, the etiology of the myocardial disease was unknown.

These patients were divided into four hemodynamic groups: (1) compensated, (2) obstructive, (3) restrictive and (4) congestive. The characteristics of each group have been described in detail elsewhere.[27,28] Briefly, patients in the compensated group showed no evidence of congestive cardiac failure, restriction to ventricular filling, or obstruction to left ventricular outflow. Their CI and SI were normal or slightly reduced and their PAm and LAm were essentially normal. With one exception, pressures in the right heart were also normal. Patients in the obstructive group had a distinct systolic pressure gradient from the body of the left ventricle to the subvalvular zone or aorta, either at rest or induced by inotropic drugs, exercise, and the Valsalva maneuver. Characteristic angiocardiographic features were demonstrated in each case. Patients in the restrictive group all showed marked elevation of the right atrial and jugular venous pressures, with a high plateau and rapid "y" descent. The right ventricular pressure tracing displayed an early diastolic dip followed by a sharp, early rise to a high diastolic plateau. The left ventricular diastolic and left atrial mean pressures were also elevated, but the early diastolic dip and a subsequent high plateau were not as obvious as in the right ventricular pressure tracing because of the much higher left ventricular systolic pressure. Patients in the congestive group had markedly reduced CI and SI and moderately elevated LAm and PAm. The left ventricular end-diastolic pressure was markedly elevated in 8 patients in whom that chamber was entered. In most of these patients the right ventricular end-diastolic and right atrial mean pressures were both within normal limits.

The CI, SI, PAm, LAm, mean transit times, PBV and CBV of patients in these four groups are presented in Table 8-8. With one exception (R.W.), the PBV was either normal or slightly subnormal. The CBV in the obstructive group was normal or low, partly due to the obliterated left ventricular cavity. In the congestive group, 4 of the 10 patients had an increased CBV because of a dilated left ventricular cavity.

Ischemic Heart Disease

Four patients with ischemic heart disease have been studied in our labo-

TABLE 8-8 Hemodynamic Data and Pulmonary Blood Volume in Patients with Various Types of Cardiomyopathy

Patients	Age	Sex	BSA	Blood Flow			Pressures (mm Hg)				Tm (seconds)			Blood Volume (ml/M²)	
				CI	HR	SI	PAm	LAm	Pd	BAm	PA–BA	LA–BA	PA–LA	CBV	PBV
A. "Compensated" Group															
D.J.	35	M	1.90	4.08	68	60	14	6	10	100	9.7	5.9	3.8	660	258
L.G.	20	M	1.82	3.50	75	47	15	12	13.5	100	11.2	5.9	5.3	662	307
H.C.	29	M	2.05	2.40	84	28	15	8	11.5	92	16.6	11.9	5.7	665	228
C.H.	47	M	2.06	2.26	46	49	17	8	12.5	85	19.5	11.7	7.8	732	294
T.D.	23	M	1.68	4.49	79	57	17	12	14.5	105	10.0	5.8	4.2	748	318
R.S.	48	M	1.89	2.49	63	40	18	12	15	88	12.1	8.2	3.9	500	160
B. Obstructive Group															
P.C.	39	M	2.16	2.38	75	29	10	5	7.5	80	14.3	7.3	7.0	560	275
F.McM.	62	F	1.67	1.86	78	20	17	8	12.5	85	14.5	7.2	7.3	366	190
H.M.	49	F	1.73	2.31	108	21	27	20	23.5	75	17.4	9.5	7.9	673	308
C. Restrictive Group															
D.P.	45	F	1.45	1.53	71	26	22	16	19	100	17.8	9.8	8.0	459	205
B.B.	72	M	18.5	0.96	103	9	24	20	22	88	34.5	25.6	8.9	1020	263
W.O.'B.	57	M	1.92	1.85	100	19	27	24	25.5	50	22.0	12.0	10.0	680	310
R.W.	38	M	1.80	2.32	130	18	35	23	29	85	22.2	12.3	9.9	856	384
G.D.	42	M	1.63	1.35	110	12	40	28	34	85	29.5	16.9	12.6	668	284
D. Congestive Group															
M.B.	42	F	1.50	2.09	81	26	17	15	16	85	14.7	6.5	8.2	499	285
R.M.	59	M	1.84	1.40	72	20	23	14	18.5	93	34.6	21.8	12.8	810	298
S.C.	44	M	2.02	1.42	70	20	28	20	24	115	24.2	12.3	11.9	573	286
R.F.	38	M	1.80	2.32	138	17	26	22	24	104	16.6	8.5	8.1	641	312
J.McE.	28	M	1.75	1.75	120	15	28	25	62.5	94	23.7	14.7	9.0	694	259
J.M.	35	M	1.85	0.89	68	13	30	26	28	78	37.4	25.9	11.5	555	170
G.Z.	56	F	1.58	1.48	82	18	34	28	31	88	40.6	31.4	9.2	882	200
J.H.	50	M	1.68	1.87	90	21	38	23	30.5	80	24.7	15.5	9.2	766	284
S.R.	53	M	1.71	1.47	96	15	40	25	32.5	77	34.0	21.4	12.6	834	309
G.D.	42	M	1.63	1.29	112	12	43	30	36.5	85	30.2	17.2	13.0	650	279
M.L.	40	M	1.98	1.34	66	20	45	26	35.5	115	29.4	19.8	9.6	656	214

Symbols and abbreviations are the same as those used in Tables 8-2 and 8-3.

TABLE 8-9   Hemodynamic Data and Pulmonary Blood Volume in Patients with Ischemic Heart Disease

Patients	Age	Sex	BSA	Blood Flow			Pressures (mm Hg)				Tm (seconds)			Blood Volume (ml M²)		Remarks
				CI	HR	SI	PAm	LAm	Pd	BAm	PA-BA	LA-BA	PA-LA	CBV	PBV	
W.P.	57	M	1.83	2.53	79	32	15	3	9	107	21.2	14.8	6.4	835	254	A
L.B.	35	M	1.92	1.68	70	24	15	7	11	100	14.0	6.8	7.2	392	197	A
S.N.	55	M	2.06	2.50	85	29	15	10	12.5	85	13.1	6.4	5.7	530	228	A
A.O.	61	M	1.83	2.14	60	35	17	6	11.5	85	14.7	8.5	6.2	534	226	A
M.A.	68	M	1.82	1.85	70	26	22	16	19	77	20.0	10.8	9.2	666	308	P
T.S.	50	M	1.85	1.85	85	21	27	14	20.5	87	17.5	10.0	7.5	808	241	A
R.C.	46	M	1.84	1.08	110	10	41	32	36.5	94	27.2	15.6	11.6	478	204	A, P

A = Coronary arterial angiograms   P = Postmortem examination
Other symbols and abbreviations are the same as those used in Table 8-2 and 8-3.

ratory. The diagnosis was established by coronary arterial angiogram or postmortem examination or both. Data on the pulmonary blood flow, pressures and volumes are summarized in Table 8-9. The CI and SI were both diminished in all patients. The LAm and PAm were either normal or elevated, depending upon the functional status of the left ventricle. With the exception of patient W.P., the CBV was within normal limits. The PBV was either normal or decreased, regardless of the LAm and PAm.

McGaff and co-workers measured PBV in three patients with ischemic heart disease and the mean value was only 153 ml/M². [18] The reason for the subnormal PBV in these patients was obscure.

Idiopathic or Thromboembolic Pulmonary Hypertension

This section includes data from patients with marked pulmonary hypertension, either idiopathic (primary) or secondary to thromboembolism. The thromboembolic pulmonary hypertension under consideration here is caused principally by repeated diffuse pulmonary embolization with small thrombi. Clinical and hemodynamic differentiation of idiopathic from this kind of thromboembolic pulmonary hypertension is sometimes extremely difficult,

if not impossible. [29-31] Both conditions may be associated with angiocardiographic changes characterized by enlargement of the main pulmonary arteries and obliteration of their terminal branches. Pulmonary embolization of a main pulmonary artery or a lobar branch can be readily demonstrated by angiocardiography and lung scanning, [32-39] but the bilateral diffusetype usually escapes detection by such methods. In some cases, even lung biopsy or post-mortem examination fails to settle the final diagnosis conclusively. In both conditions, the structural changes are confined mainly to the small pulmonary arterial branches, resulting in a progressive increase in the pulmonary vascular resistance and a corresponding elevation of the pulmonary artery pressure. [30,40-49] The physiologic consequences and hemodynamic derangements are so similar in the two conditions that changes in PBV would not be expected to differ greatly.

We have studied 10 such patients, 5 probably idiopathic and 5 probably secondary to thromboembolism. In half of these patients no information concerning PBV is available because left heart catheterization was not performed. The hemodynamic data, CBV and PBV on these 10 patients are summarized in Table 8-10.

The CI was decreased in all patients, ranging from 1.76 to 2.60 L/M²/

TABLE 8-10   Hemodynamic Data and Pulmonary Blood Volume in Patients with Idiopathic or Thromboembolic Pulmonary Hypertension

Patients	Age	Sex	BSA	Blood Flow			Pressures (mm Hg)				Tm (seconds)			Blood Volume (ml/M²)		Remarks
				CI	HR	SI	PAm	LAm	Pd	BAm	PA-BA	LA-BA	PA-LA	CBV	PBV	
A. Idiopathic Pulmonary Hypertension																
R.S.	39	F	1.55	2.06	84	26	54	9*	31.5	111	15.3	—	—	525	—	Autopsy
V.S.	27	F	1.37	1.90	63	30	60	8	34.0	100	14.5	7.5	7.0	456	222	
L.T.	24	F	1.50	2.31	64	36	62	—	—	65	12.4	—	—	480	—	
M.R.	30	F	1.62	1.76	66	27	67	7*	37	85	14.4	—	—	425	—	
J.H.	35	M	1.88	2.10	108	19	76	10	43	76	15.5	9.7	5.8	545	202	
B. Thromboembolic Pulmonary Hypertension																
S.S.	19	M	1.82	2.28	68	34	43	7	25	57	15.2	8.6	6.6	576	—	1. Angio** 2. Lung Biopsy
M.M.	67	F	1.50	2.08	76	27	45	2	23.5	110	16.8	9.7	7.1	581	246	1. Angio
C.K.	64	M	1.92	2.76	86	32	45	10*	27.5	100	13.8	—	—	635	—	1. Angio 2. Autopsy
J.H.	55	M	1.77	2.13	120	19	65	15	40	90	15.4	9.7	5.7	547	202	1. Angio 2. Autopsy

* = Pulmonary wedge pressure
** = Pulmonary arterial angiogram
Other symbols and abbreviations are the same as those used in Tables 8-1, 8-2 and 8-3

min. The SI was usually subnormal. The PAm was uniformly markedly elevated, and the LAm or the pulmonary wedge pressure was within normal limits. In patient J.H. the LAm was slightly elevated during the study (15 mm Hg), but disease involving the left side of the heart was absent clinically and at post-mortem examination.

In this group of patients, the most characteristic feature other than pre-capillary pulmonary hypertension was the finding of normal or subnormal CBV and PBV. The CBV was less than 600 ml/M² and the PBV less than 250 ml/M² in all patients. This finding is consistent with the invariable histologic demonstration of considerable oblitera-tion of the pulmonary vessels, particu-larly the small arteries and arterioles. We and others[16,50] have observed mark-ed reduction in pulmonary capillary blood volume, further substantiating the reduction of the pulmonary vascular bed in these patients.

The normal LAm and pulmonary wedge pressure would also tend to keep the PBV within normal limits. The question of the existence and signif-icance of a strong element of concomi-tant functional vasoconstriction re-mains unsettled in these patients.[40-43,51] Subsequently (Chapter 12), we shall review our observations that acetyl-choline infusion failed to induce a significant change in either the pulmo-nary vascular pressure or volume, lead-ing us to question the presence and importance of functional vasoconstric-tion in these patients.

Chronic Pulmonary Disease

The PBV has been studied in only a few patients with chronic pulmonary disease in our laboratory. The PBV and hemodynamic data are presented in Table 8-11. These patients had some reduction in vital capacity and a moder-ate increase in residual volume. Mean expiratory flow rate and forced expir-atory volume were significantly reduced. The CI was low normal or slightly reduced. While the PAm was slightly or moderately elevated, the LAm usu-ally remained normal.

As a rule, the CBV and PBV were both either normal or slightly

TABLE 8-11   Hemodynamic Data and Pulmonary Blood Volume in Patients with Chronic Pulmonary Disease

Patients	Age	Sex	BSA	Blood Flow			Pressures (mm Hg)				Tm (seconds)			Blood Volume (ml/M²)	
				CI	HR	SI	PAm	LAm	Pd	BAm	PA-BA	LA-BA	PA-LA	CBV	PBV
A.V.	71	M	1.48	2.06	80	26	13	6*	9.5	100	18.0	—	—	622	—
H.B.	59	F	1.80	2.97	84	35	18	8	12	90	11.1	5.4	5.7	550	282
M.B.	17	F	1.40	3.12	118	26	22	4*	13	86	8.6	—	—	450	—
A.K.	52	F	1.46	2.82	100	28	29	4	15.5	86	13.2	10.5	2.7	600	127
R.N.	48	M	2.05	2.68	75	36	30	8	19	100	10.8	5.0	5.8	485	255

* = Pulmonary wedge pressure
Other symbols and abbreviations are the same as those used in Tables 8-2 and 8-3

subnormal. It is assumed that the parenchymal tissue of these patients is variably distorted, associated with loss of alveolar-capillary interface and reduction of the pulmonary vascular bed. Utilizing the technique of quantitative radiocardiography, Giuntini and associates reported a mean PBV of 270 ml/M² in 7 patients with chronic bronchitis and emphysema.[52] The low or normal PBV is consistent with our finding of low Vc in many patients with chronic pulmonary disease.[53]

Pericardial Disease

We have studied the PBV in 2 patients with pericardial disease, one with constrictive pericarditis and the other with pericardial effusion. Table 8-12 summarizs the pertinent data.

The CI was normal or slightly subnormal. Both the PAm and LAm were normal or minimally elevated at rest.

The PAm was significantly elevated during exercise in both patients. Exercise induced a marked increase in LAm in only one patient (I.K.). The CBV and PBV of patient L.V. were normal at rest and increased to a small extent during exercise. The PBV of patient I.K. was high normal at rest, although the CBV was moderately increased. The mechanism for the increased CBV is unknown. The increase in CBV and PBV during exercise was modest in view of the disproportionate change in the pulmonary vascular pressure. Thus, the distensibility of the pulmonary vascular bed was somewhat compromised.

TABLE 8-12   Hemodynamic Data and Pulmonary Blood Volume in Patients with Pericardial Disease

Patients	Age	Sex	BSA	Diagnosis	Condition	Blood Flow			Pressures (mm Hg)				Tm (seconds)			Blood Volume (ml/M²)	
						CI	HR	SI	PAm	LAm	Pd	BAm	PA-BA	LA-BA	PA-LA	CBV	PBV
I.K.	41	F	1.56	C.P.	R	3.38	72	47	21	16	18.5	99	14.1	9.4	4.7	890	298
					E	5.12	100	51	30	26	28	148	12.0	8.2	3.8	1020	325
L.V.	51	F	1.57	P.E.	R	2.35	84	28	18	8	13	96	8.8	4.7	4.1	543	254
					E	3.74	128	29	28	9	18.5	120	6.8	3.6	3.2	610	273

C.P. = Constrictive pericarditis
P.E. = Pericardial effusion
R   = At rest
E   = During exercise
Other symbols and abbreviations are the same as those used in Tables 8-2 and 8-3

REFERENCES

1. Milnor, W.R., Jose, A.D., and McGaff, C.J.: Pulmonary vascular volume, resistance and compliance in man. Circulation, *22*, 130, 1960.

2. Ross, J., Braunwald, E., and Morrow, A.G.: Left heart catheterization by the transseptal route. A description of the technic and its applications. Circulation, *22*, 927, 1960.

3. Brockenbrough, E. C., Braunwald, E., and Ross, J.: Transseptal left heart catheterization. A review of 450 studies and description of an improved technic. Circulation, *25*, 15, 1962.

4. Yu, P.N., Glick, G., Schreiner, B.F., and Murphy, G.W.: Effects of acute hypoxia on the pulmonary vascular bed of patients with acquired heart disease, with special reference to the demonstration of active vasomotion. Circulation, *27*, 541, 1963.

5. Schreiner, B.F., Murphy, G.W., and Yu, P.N.: Pulmonary blood volume in congestive heart failure. Circulation, *34*, 249, 1966.

6. Stewart, G.N.: The pulmonary circulation time, the quantity of blood in the lungs and the output of the heart. Am. J. Physiol., *58*, 20, 1921.

7. Hamilton, W.F., Moore, J.W., Kinsman, J.M., and Spurling, R.G.: Studies on the circulation. IV. Further analysis of the injection method, and of changes in hemodynamics under physiologic and pathologic conditions. Am. J. Physiol., *66*, 534, 1932.

8. Ogilvie, C.M., Forster, R.E., Blakemore, W.S., and Morton, J.W.: A standardized breath holding technique for clinical measurement of the diffusing capacity of the lung for carbon monoxide. J. Clin. Invest. 36, 1, 1957.

9. Gazioglu, K., and Yu, P.N.: Pulmonary blood volume and pulmonary capillary blood volume in valvular heart disease. Circulation, *35*, 701, 1967.

10. Oakley, C., Glick, G., Luria, M.N., Schreiner, B.F., and Yu, P.N.: Some regulatory mechanisms of the human pulmonary vascular bed. Circulation, *25*, 917, 1962.

11. Dock, D.S., Kraus, W.L., McQuire, L.B., Hyland, J.W., Haynes, F.W., and Dexter, L.: The pulmonary blood volume in man. J. Clin. Invest., *40*, 317, 1961.

12. McGaff, C.J., Roveti, G.C., Glassman, E., and Milnor, W.R.: The pulmonary blood volume in rheumatic heart disease and its alteration by isoproterenol. Circulation, *27*, 77, 1963,

13. Samet, P., Bernstein, W.H., Medow, A., and Levine, S.: Transseptal left heart dynamics in thirty-two normal subjects. Dis. Chest, *47*, 632, 1965.

14. Roy, S.B., Bhardwaj, P., and Bhatia, M.L.: Pulmonary blood volume in mitral stenosis. Brit. Med. J., *2*, 1466, 1965.

15. Freitas, F.M. de, Faraco, E. Z., Azevedo, D.F. de, Zaduchliver, J., and Lewin. I.: Behavior of normal pulmonary circulation during changes of total blood volume in man. J. Clin. Invest., *44*, 366, 1965.

16. McNeill, R.S., Rankin, J., and Forster, R.E.: The diffusing capacity of the pulmonary membrane and the pulmonary capillary blood volume in cardiopulmonary disease. Clin. Sci., *17*, 465, 1958.

17. Lewis, B.M., Lin, T.H., Noe, F.E., and Kamisaruk, R.: The measurement of pulmonary capillary blood volume and pulmonary membrane diffusing capacity in normal subjects; the effects of exercise and position. J. Clin. Invest., *37*, 1061, 1958.

18. Ross, J.C., Maddock, G.E., and Ley, G.D.: Effect of pressure suit inflation on pulmonary capillary blood volume. J. Appl. Physiol., *16*, 674, 1961.

19. Daly, W.J., Ross, J.C., and Behnke, R.H.: The effect of changes in the pulmonary vascular bed produced by atropine, pulmonary engorgement, and positive pressure breathing on diffusing and mechanical properties of the lung. J. Clin. Invest., *42*, 1083, 1963.

20. Daly, W.J., Giammona, S.T., and Ross, J.C.: The pressure-volume relationship of the normal pulmonary bed. J. Clin. Invest., *44*, 1261, 1965.

21. Johnson, R.L., Taylor, H.F., and Lawson, W.H.: Maximal diffusion capacity of the lung for carbon monoxide. J. Clin. Invest., *44*, 349, 1965.

22. Parker, F., and Weiss, S.: The nature and significance of the structural changes in the lungs in mitral stenosis. Am. J. Pathol., *12*, 573, 1936.

23. Short, D.S.: The arterial bed of the lung in pulmonary hypertension. Lancet, *2*, 12, 1957.

24. Heath, D., and Edwards, J.E.: Histological changes in the lung in diseases associated with pulmonary venous hypertension. Brit. J. Dis. Chest, *53*, 8, 1959.

25. Smith, R.C., Burchell, H.B., and Edwards, J.E.: Pathology of the pulmonary vascular tree. IV. Structural changes in the pulmonary vessels in chronic left ventricular failure. Circulation, *10*, 801, 1954.

26. Yu, P.N., Finlayson, J.K., Luria, M.N., Stanfield, C.A., Schreiner, B.F., and Lovejoy, F.W.: Indicator dilution curves in valvular heart

disease; after injection of indicator into the pulmonary artery and the left ventricle. Am. Heart J., *60*, 503, 1960.

27. Yu, P.N., Cohen, J., Schreiner, B.F., and Murphy, G.W,: Hemodynamic alterations in primary myocardial disease. Prog. Cardiovasc. Dis., *7*, 125, 1964.

28. Yu, P.N., Schreiner, B.F., Cohen, J., and Murphy, G.W.: Idiopathic cardiomyopathy. A study of left ventricular function and pulmonary circulation in 15 patients. Am. Heart J., *71*, 330, 1966.

29. Owen, W.R., Thomas, W.A., Castleman, B., and, Bland, E.F.: Unrecognized emboli to the lungs with subsequent cor pulmonale. New Eng. J. Med., 249, 919, 1953.

30. Kuida, H., Dammin, G.J., Haynes, F.W., Rapaport, E., and Dexter, L.: Primary pulmonary hypertension. Am. J. Med., *23*, 166, 1957.

31. Dexter, L., Dock, D.S., McQuire, L.B., Hyland, J.W., and Haynes, F.W.: Pulmonary embolism. Med. Clin. North Amer., *44*, 1251, 1960.

32. Sasahara, A.A., Stein, M., Simon, M., and Littman, D.: Pulmonary angiography in diagnosis of thromboembolic disease. New Eng. J. Med., 270, 1075, 1964.

33. Björk, L., and Ansusinka, T.: Angiographic diagnosis of acute pulmonary embolism. Acta Radiol., *3*, 129, 1965.

34. Wiener, S.N., Edelstein, J., and Charms, B.L.: Observations in pulmonary embolism and the pulmonary angiogram. Am. J. Roent. Rad. Ther. & Nucl. Med., 98, 859, 1966.

35. Alexander, J.K., Gonzalez, D.A., and Fred, H.L.: Angiographic studies in cardiorespiratory diseases; special reference to thromboembolism. J.A.M.A., *198*, 575, 1966.

36. Lowman, R.M., Reardon, J., Hipona, F.A., Stern, H., and Toole, A.L.: The role of pulmonary angiography in pulmonary embolism. Angiol., *18*, 29, 1967.

37. Wagner, H.N., Sabiston, D.C., McAfee, J.G., Tow, D., and Stern, H.S.: Diagnosis of massive pulmonary embolism in man by radioisotope scanning. New Eng. J. Med., *271*, 377, 1964.

38. Haynie, T.P., Hendrick, C.K., and Schreiber, M.H.: Diagnosis of pulmonary embolism and infarction by photoscanning. J. Nucl. Med., *6*, 613, 1965.

39. Taplin, G.V., Dore, E.K., Poe, N.D., and Swanson, L.A.: Pulmonary embolism—early detection by lung scanning. Clin. Res., *14*, 151, 1966.

40. Dresdale, D.T., Schultz, M., and Michtom, R.J.: Primary pulmonary hypertension. I. Clinical and hemodynamic study. Am. J. Med., *11*, 686, 1951.

41. Shephard, J.T., Edwards, J.E., Burchell, H.B., Swan, H.J.C., and Wood, E.H.: Clinical, physiological, and pathological considerations in patients with idiopathic pulmonary hypertension. Brit. Heart J., *19*, 70, 1957.

42. Wood, P.: Pulmonary hypertension, with special reference to the vasoconstrictive factor. Brit. Heart J., *20*, 557, 1958.

43. Yu, P.N.: Primary hypertension: Report of six cases and review of literature. Ann. Int. Med., *46*, 1138, 1958.

44. Whitaker, W., and Heath, D.: Idiopathic pulmonary hypertension: Etiology, pathogenesis, and treatment. Prog. Cardiovasc. Dis., *1*, 380, 1959.

45. Sleeper, J.C., Orgain, E.S., and McIntosh, H.D.: Primary pulmonary hypertension. Review of clinical features and pathologic physiology with a report of pulmonary hemodynamics derived from repeated catheterization. Circulation, *26*, 1358, 1962.

46. Farrar, J.F.: Idiopathic pulmonary hypertension. Am. Heart J., *66*, 128, 1963.

47. Wilhelmsen, L., Selander, S., Söderholm, B., Paulin, S., Varnauskas. E., and Werkö, L.: Recurrent pulmonary embolism. Medicine, *42*, 335, 1963.

48. Goodwin, J.F., Harrison, C.V., and Wilcken, E.L.: Obliterative pulmonary hypertension and thromboembolism. Brit. Med. J., *1*, 777, 1963.

49. Rosenberg, S.A.: Study of etiologic basis of primary pulmonary hypertension. Am. Heart J., *68*, 484, 1964.

50. Gazioglu, K., and Yu, P.N.: Pulmonary capillary volume in patients with thromboembolic or idiopathic pulmonary hypertension. Unpublished data.

51. Samet, P., Bernstein, W.H., and Widrich, J.: Intracardiac infusion of acetylcholine in primary pulmonary hypertension. Am. Heart J., *60*, 433, 1960.

52. Giuntini, C., Lewis, A.S., and Harvey, R.M.: A study of the pulmonary blood volume in man by quantitative radiocardiography. J. Clin. Invest., *42*, 1589, 1963.

53. Gazioglu, K., and Yu, P.N.: Pulmonary diffusing capacity and pulmonary capillary blood volume in chronic pulmonary disease. To be published.

CHAPTER 9

Pulmonary Blood Volume in Congestive Heart Failure and Pulmonary Edema[*]

In this chapter discussion of changes in pulmonary blood volume(PBV) will be centered on patients with congestive heart failure and pulmonary edema associated with mitral stenosis or secondary to myocardial disease. For a number of years the early manifestations of heart failure in these patients have been recognized as usually respiratory rather then cardiac.[1-6] The presenting symptoms and signs commonly include cough, exertional or nocturnal dyspnea, pulmonary rales and radiologic abnormalities in the lungs. More recently, the early recognition of such cardiac findings as gallop rhythm and pulsus alternans has been emphasized.[7-10] One of the most dramatic features of heart failure in these patients is the development of episodes of acute pulmonary edema.[11-14] These episodes occur most often in recumbency at night; or they may be provoked by strenuous exertion, unusual excitement or the rapid intravenous infusion of blood or fluids. After appropriate and effective therapy, clinical and radiologic improvement may be striking within a few hours, particularly with reference to pulmonary congestion.

Pulmonary function studies in these patients have consistently demonstrated (*a*) a decrease in vital capacity; (*b*) an increase in the ratio of residual volume to total lung capacity, with or without an increase in absolute residual volume; and (*c*) a decrease in static pulmonary compliance $(\triangle V/\triangle P)$.[15-21] The pulmonary capillary blood volume (Vc) may be elevated, normal or slightly reduced, depending upon the nature of the cardiac disease and the stage of decompensation.[22-25]

Hemodynamically, both cardiac output and ventricular work are less than in the compensated state. The left ventricular end-diastolic (LVd) pressure is invariably elevated in patients with failure secondary to myocardial disease, and left atrial (LAm) pressure is always elevated in patients with failure associated with mitral stenosis or secondary to myocardial disease. Some degree of pulmonary venous and arterial hypertension is almost always encountered. An elevated LVd may not, however, be an indication of left ventricular decompensation *per se*. For instance, an elevated LVd is frequent in patients with aortic stenosis with no manifestations of congestive failure, presumably as an effect of reduced ventricular compliance.[26]

In considering the pathogenesis of the pulmonary congestion associated with congestive heart failure associated

---

[*]Much of the work summarized in this chapter was done by my colleagues, Drs. Bernard F. Schreiner and Gerald W. Murphy.

with mitral stenosis or myocardial disease, many workers have suggested that a significant increase in the PBV may be important.[27-31] Others have postulated that vital capacity and total lung capacity decline in congestive heart failure largely because of increased pulmonary blood volume, the distended blood vessels encroaching on the alveoli and displacing air.[17,32-35] The presumed dominant role of PBV has depended upon such indirect evidence as clinical examination, interpretation of the chest roentgenograms, and measurements of pulmonary vascular pressures and intrathoracic or central blood volumes (CBV). On the other hand, some investigators reported only slightly elevated CBV in patients with severe mitral stenosis or with heart failure,[36-40] and others found no correlation between the diminished vital capacity or pulmonary compliance and the elevation of pulmonary wedge or pulmonary arterial pressure.[41-43] Whether the increased CBV in some patients with left ventricular failure

was related to an increase in PBV or to augmented left heart and aortic volume was uncertain.

In this context, Ebert offered the explanation that absence of a consistent large elevation in PBV with congestive heart failure may be a result of altered pressure-volume characteristics of the pulmonary vascular bed.[44] More precise measurements of the PBV by Varnauskas and associates[45] confirmed the earlier findings of Lagerlöf and co-workers[38,46] that the pulmonary circulation in heart failure is characterized not by an increase in PBV but by elevation of pressure in the pulmonary vessels. Varnauskas and associates further stated that the high pulmonary capillary pressure causes transudation of fluid into the alveoli and interstitium, especially in the dependent portions of the lungs.[45] Elevated pulmonary vascular pressures and the presence of interstitial edema impair the elastic properties of the lungs, thus restricting the potential volume of the pulmonary vessels.

TABLE 9-1   Hemodydamic Data and Pulmonary Blood Volume in Patients with Severe Mitral Stenosis and Congestive Heart Failure

Patients	CI	SI	PAm	LAm	Pd	PVR	CBV	PBV	C
M.P.	2.23	30	25	18	21.5	177	624	212	9.9
M.G.	2.15	27	28	18	23	275	698	258	11.2
P.M.	1.30	23	35	24	29.5	485	482	252	8.5
J.P.	1.83	25	38	24	31	390	630	248	8.0
F.M.	1.28	19	40	20	30	1200	494	183	6.1
M.K.	1.19	16	42	27	34.5	378	500	197	5.3
H.G.	1.00	13	52	26	39	1350	518	171	4.4
G.R.	0.80	8	67	25	46	2245	442	135	2.9
E.G.	1.55	21	68	24	46	2270	478	220	4.7
E.K.	1.20	12	70	30	50	1700	547	269	5.4
F.S.	2.19	12	71	40	55.5	707	656	306	5.5
E.W.	1.63	22	72	27	49.5	1520	491	233	4.7

CI   = Cardiac index (L/min/M^2)
SI   = Stroke index (ml/beat/M^2)
PAm = Pulmonary arterial mean pressure (mm Hg)
LAm = Left atrial mean pressure (mm Hg)
Pd   = Pulmonary distending pressure $\left(\dfrac{PAm + LAm}{2}\right)$
PVR = Pulmonary vascular resistance (dynes · sec/cm^5)
CBV = "Central" blood volume (ml/M^2)
PBV = Pulmonary blood volume (ml/M^2)
C   = Relative compliance, PBV/Pd (ml/M^2/mm Hg)

TABLE 9-2   Hemodynamic Data and Pulmonary Blood Volume in Patients with Myocardial
Disease and Congestive Heart Failure

Patients	CI	SI	PAm	LAm	Pd	PVR	CBV	PBV	B
R.M.	1.40	20	23	14	18.5	216	810	298	16.2
R.F.	2.32	17	26	22	24	77	641	312	12.0
W.O'B.	1.85	19	27	24	25.5	31	680	310	11.3
S.C.	1.42	20	28	20	24	223	656	214	11.9
J. McE.	1.75	15	28	25	26.5	78	694	259	9.8
G.Z.	1.48	18	34	28	31	204	882	200	6.5
R.W.	2.32	18	35	23	28.5	230	856	384	13.2
J.H.	1.87	21	38	23	30.5	384	766	284	9.3
S.R.	1.47	15	40	25	32.5	475	834	309	9.5
E.G.	1.61	15	40	26	33	350	792	280	8.5
G.D.	1.29	12	43	30	31.5	496	650	279	7.6
M.L.	1.34	20	45	26	35.5	272	640	259	6.0

Symbols and abbreviations are the same as those in Table 9-1

Data from our laboratory are in essential agreement with the postulation of Ebert and the findings of Varnauskas.[47] This series included 12 patients with congestive heart failure asscoiated with severe mitral stenosis and 12 patients with congestive heart failure secondary to primary myocardial disease. The data summarized in Tables 9-1 and 9-2 have been published previously or included in Chapter 8. Patients with mitral stenosis in heart failure had marked dyspnea on slight exertion and showed radiologic evidence of pulmonary venous congestion with engorged vascular roots and interstitial edema. Patient F.S. was studied during an episode of acute pulmonary edema. Those patients with myocardial disease in heart failure showed clinical and radiologic evidence of pulmonary congestion during the study or had had recent cardiac decompensation.

The cardiac and stroke indices of all patients were low, and their LAm and PAm were moderately or markedly elevated. Pulmonary hypertension was usually more severe in patients with mitral stenosis than in those with primary myocardial disease. The LVd was less than 10 mm Hg in all 8 patients with mitral stenosis in whom it was measured. The left ventricle was entered in 10 patients with myocardial disease and cardiac failure and the LVd was markedly elevated in all, averaging 30 mm Hg.

The PVR was increased in all patients with mitral stenosis and cardiac failure, severely so in 6 patients with values ranging from 1200 to 2270 dynes · sec/cm⁵. In contrast, the PVR in patients with myocardial disease and cardiac failure was either normal or only moderately elevated. The PVR of these patients did not exceed 500 dynes · sec/cm⁵.

The most surprising findings were the values of PBV and CBV. In patients with mitral stenosis the mean PBV was 228 ml/M², and the mean CBV was 537 ml/M². Neither mean value differed significantly from normal. The relative pulmonary vascular compliance (C or PBV/Pd) was less then one third of normal, and the mean for the group as a whole was 6.4 ml/M²/mm Hg.

Patient F.S. was especially interesting because she was studied during an episode of acute pulmonary edema. PAm and LAm were both markedly elevated, but the PBV and CBV were within normal limits, measuring 306 ml/M² and 656 ml/M² respectively. A previous report by Finlayson and co-workers from our laboratory further documented the extreme pressure changes observed in patients with valvular heart disease studied during acute pulmonary edema.[48] The mean control PAm was 57 mm Hg in 6 patients; during pulmonary edema, 76 mm Hg (3 patients); and following recovery, 37 mm Hg (5 patients). The pulmonary wedge pressure in 2 patients during pulmonary edema averaged 39 mm Hg.

The PBV was also normal in all but one patient with myocardial disease and cardiac failure. The mean for the group was 282 ml/M^2, a value which was not significantly different from normal. The CBV, however, was increased in 5 patients to values exceeding 780 ml/M^2, the upper limit of normal. In the remaining 7 patients the CBV was normal. The mean CBV for the group was 742 ml/M^2, significantly higher than the normal mean. The augmented CBV clearly was attributable to an increase in left heart and aortic volume, most probably as a consequence of a dilated left ventricle. For the group, C averaged 10.1 ml/M^2/mm Hg, less than half the normal value.

Before the values of CBV and PBV determined in patients with congestive heart failure can be considered valid and reliable, the potential sources of error in this method should be reexamined with attention to the possible effects of pulmonary venous hypertension and cardiac failure. A major concern is uneven blood flow through the lungs which may alter both rate of blood flow and the mean transit time from the pulmonary artery to the systemic artery (Tm_{PA-BA}), as measured by the present method. Indicator which traverses a vascular segment where the flow velocity is slow may arrive late at the sampling site. This will prolong the downslope of the indicator-dilution curve and increase the

Tm_{PA-BA}. Thus, assuming that the cardiac index remained unchanged, the estimated CBV would be larger than if the indicator had traveled more rapidly through a normal pulmonary vascular bed.

Another source of error may arise whenever indicator is lost from the pulmonary circulation after it is injected into the pulmonary artery. It may escape through the pulmonary capillary wall, a phenomenon which very likely occurs during acute pulmonary edema, or it may return to the systemic venous system through bronchopulmonary venous anastomoses, an effect which is common in mitral stenosis. The area under the indicator-dilution curve would be reduced and the cardiac output calculated would be larger than that derived from a paired curve after left atrial injection of indicator. If Tm_{PA-BA} remained constant, the calculated CBV would again be increased.

Either possibility would result in an overestimation of PBV, because the calculation of blood volume between the left atrium and the systemic artery would not be affected. Such effects would tend to minimize or cancel out our results, not exaggerate them. Furthermore, if indicator were lost from the lungs during its primary circulation, a systematic difference in the calculated cardiac output between the PA and LA curves would be expected. We have not found such a discrepancy.

A third possible source of error may arise from incomplete mixing of the dye because of sluggish flow or stagnation of blood in a segment of the pulmonary vascular bed. Blood in such a segment would not be included in the calculated CBV and PBV, causing a falsely low calculated PBV. The existence of such a hypothetical pathophysiologic state of stagnation is doubtful in the presence of chronic pulmonary venous hypertension. According to Harris and Heath, although medial hypertrophy and intimal fibrosis of pulmonary arteries and veins are characteristically associated with pulmonary venous hypertension, extensive and complex arterial "dilation" lesions were not observed.[49] From the pathologic observations of these authors and the hemodynamic observations of moderate and marked elevation of pulmonary arterial pressure, severe stagnation of blood in the pulmonary vascular bed is unlikely as an important source of error.

An added safeguard in our study is the use of computerized programming. Our criteria for accepting or rejecting an indicator-dilution curve were described in Chapter 8. Furthermore, our technique is sensitive enough to detect larger than normal PBV in many class II and III patients with mitral stenosis and significantly altered PBV during certain physiologic interventions and during the administration of several pharmacologic agents, even in the presence of pulmonary venous hypertension.[50-55]

If our results and those of others in patients with cardiac failure are valid, several points require explanation: (a) the mechanism by which PBV remains relatively normal, (b) the role of PBV in congestive heart failure and its relationship to pulmonary vascular pressure, (c) the nature of the clinical and pathologic manifestations of pulmonary congestion, and (d) the mechanism of some of the pulmonary functional abnormalities.

Progressive pulmonary vascular obstructive disease is well known in association with chronic pulmonary venous hypertension, especially that associated with severe mitral stenosis.[49,56-58] The pathophysiologic alterations may be summarized as follows:

(a) medial hypertrophy and intimal proliferation and fibrosis in pulmonary arteries and veins; (b) dilatation of the proximal pulmonary arteries and narrowing of the distal pulmonary arteries and arterioles, frequently accompanied by atheromatous changes; (c) dilatation and distention of pulmonary lymphatics and increased lymphatic drainage from the lungs; (d) interstitial and alveolar edema and interstitial fibrosis; (e) thrombosis and thromboembolism; and (f) functional vasoconstriction because of hypoxemia. PBV may be reduced on the basis of any or all of these changes which eventually lead to progressive obliterative vascular disease and a contracted pulmonary vascular bed. PBV may be augmented or unchanged by the redistribution of blood flow toward the superior or upper portions of the lungs, partly as a result of increased pulmonary vascular resistance in the inferior or lower portions.[59,60]

Many of the same pathologic changes occur in patients with left ventricular failure and pulmonary venous hypertension. Less prominent changes in the pulmonary vessels and in the interstitium would be expected in these patients than in patients with severe mitral stenosis, since the duration of cardiac failure is a matter of months rather than years as in the case of mitral stenosis. Nevertheless, pulmonary vascular volume may be reduced by a number of the pathophysiologic mechanisms mentioned.

Recent findings suggest that reappraisal of the pulmonary vascular pressure-volume relationship in patients with congestive heart failure is appropriate. Increased PBV would be predicted from the traditional interpretations of the clinical and pathologic manifestations of pulmonary congestion. The data reported by Varnauskas and from our laboratory, however, indicate that an elevated PBV is not *sine qua non* in either pulmonary congestion or edema in patients with chronic pulmonary venous hypertension. We measured PBV in only one patient with acute pulmonary edema, and a generalization is accordingly improper about the possibility that PBV would be increased in pulmonary edema if more such patients were studied. Elevated PBV and high pulmonary vascular pressures are possible in patients with compensated cardiovascular disease or with nearly normal cardiovascular function who develop acute left ventricular failure following the injudicious administration of intravenous salt solutions or blood transfusion. This possibility has received support from experimental studies in the dog recently reported by Levine and associates.[61]

The observations of Guyton and Lindsay in experimentally produced acute pulmonary edema are of special interest.[62] Initially, they maintained LAm at various levels from O to 45 mm Hg for 30 minutes. When LAm was less than 24 mm Hg, no significant transudation from the pulmonary capillaries to alveoli was observed. When LAm was maintained higher than 24 mm Hg, fluid transudates from the capillary bed were directly proportional to the additional pressure. The second part of the experiment was conducted with LAm maintained at elevated levels for as long as three hours. No animal died of pulmonary edema if the LAm was 24 mm Hg or less, whereas all animals with LAm of 26 mm Hg or higher failed to survive the three hours of elevated pressure. In the third part of the experiment, serum protein was decreased to about half the control value before the effects of elevation of LAm were studied. Pulmo-

nary edema was absent when LAm was maintained at less than 12 mm Hg. Pulmonary edema developed, however, when LAm was elevated to 12 mm Hg or above.

Pressure elevation rather than augmented PBV appears to be the dominant hemodynamic feature of congestive cardiac failure. Long-standing pulmonary venous hypertension results in the structural and functional changes which progressively restrict the pulmonary vascular bed. A disproportionate increase in the pulmonary vascular pressure evolves, accompanied by a marked reduction in pulmonary vascular compliance.[63,64] In other words, the pressure-volume characteristics of the pulmonary vascular bed in these patients are significantly altered and are represented by the upper steep portion of the canine pulmonary vascular pressure-volume curve as described by Sarnoff and Berglund[65] (Figure 9-1). Thus, a large increase in pulmonary vascular pressure is associated with a relatively slight increase in PBV. When pulmonary venous and capillary pressures are elevated above the colloid osmotic pressure, either acutely or chronically, significant transudation of fluid from the capillaries to the alveoli would be expected, followed by accumulation of fluid in the small air passages, bronchioles and interstitial spaces.

The concept that increased PBV *per se* is important in producing pulmonary edema is further compromised by the hemodynamic observations in patients with left to right intracardiac shunts. For instance, most patients with sizable atrial septal defects and large elevations in the pulmonary capillary blood volume and presumably the total pulmonary blood volume almost always have normal pulmonary venous and capillary pressures.[23,66-68]

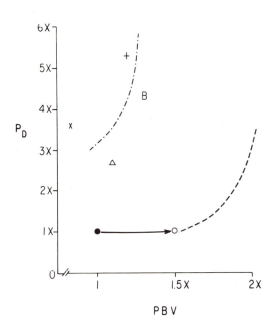

Figure 9-1. The relationship between pulmonary distending pressure (Pd) and pulmonary blood volume (PBV). Line A shows response of "normal" persons to two successive levels of exercise. PBV increases moderately with little or no change in Pd. Line B is a hypothetical pressure-volume curve derived from data presented in this chapter. △ represents the mean resting value for patients with primary myocardial disease and cardiac failure; × is the mean resting value for patients with heart failure associated with mitral stenosis; and + is the value obtained from patient F.S. during an episode of acute pulmonary edema.

Acute pulmonary edema is rarely encountered in these patients.

If the pulmonary vascular volume is not appreciably increased in patients with congestive heart failure, how can pulmonary "congestion," impaired pulmonary function and reduced pulmonary compliance be explained? We believe that "congestion" is primarily extravascular rather than intravascular, resulting from the accumulation of fluid in air passages and interstitial tissues. Fluid in these areas may prevent the expansion of alveoli with inspiration and obstruct bronchioles, often leading to atelectasis. This complication may explain the absence of pulmonary rales in some patients when clinical and radiologic manifestations of pulmonary congestion are evident.

In this regard, the recent experimental observations reported by Staub and associates on sequence of fluid accumulation in dog lungs during pulmonary edema are of special interest.[69] They produced pulmonary edema in dogs (a) by augmenting capillary hydrostatic pressure with rapid transfusion of blood and dextran, or (b) by increasing capillary permeability after intravenous injection of Alloxan. Based upon studies of the rapidly frozen lungs, both types of pulmonary edema showed the same sequence of fluid accumulation in various compartments of the lung. Fluid appeared first in the interstitial connective tissue around the large blood vessels and airways. This was followed by alveolar wall thickening and fluid accumulation in the alveolar sacs. Atelectasis was uncommon but the total volume of each fluid-filled alveolus was reduced.

In the isolated dog lung, West and associates have demonstrated a great increase in pulmonary vascular resistance in dependent zones, where pulmonary venous pressure was elevated.[70] This increased vascular resistance was attributed to perivascular edema, one factor which might interfere with the normal opening of pulmonary vessels.

The impairment of pulmonary function and the reduction of pulmonary compliance in patients with congestive heart failure clearly reflect alterations in the elastic properties of the lungs. In these patients a change in intrathoracic pressure produces less change in lung volume than in normals.[19-21,43,71]

Although pulmonary compliance is reduced in most patients with high pulmonary venous and capillary pressures, it has been observed to correlate poorly with pulmonary arterial or pulmonary wedge pressure.[41-43] In animal experiments, on the other hand, compliance declined progressively, associated with a gradual increase in pulmonary venous pressure.[72,73] Compliance returned toward normal when the pressure was lowered. The changes in compliance were rather small in relation to the large increase in pressure, however. Thus, the magnitude of pulmonary vascular pressures did not appear to act as a dominant determinant in the reduction of pulmonary compliance.

Recently, the surface tension of the fluid lining the alveoli has been studied as it might contribute to the maintenance of the elastic properties of the lungs. The reader is referred to Comroe's excellent description of the historical background and other important aspects of this fascinating subject.[74] In 1929, Von Neergaard found that less than half as much pressure was required to distend fluid-filled lungs to a given volume than when the lungs were filled with air.[75] He introduced the concept that a special film may line the alveoli, tending to retract or recoil just as a bubble does. The fluid-air interface is eliminated by filling the lungs with fluid and the fluid-filled interface has no surface tension. Therefore, the recoil pressure of the air-filled lung measures the elastic properties of the elastic tissue and the surface film, while the recoil pressure of fluid-filled lungs represents only that of the elastic tissue. These studies have been confirmed and extended by Radford and associates,[76,77] who considered that two important factors govern the elastic or static mechanical properties of the lungs. These two factors are the fibrous proteins (such as elastin, collagen and reticulin) and surface tension.

The work of Pierce and Hocutt further substantiated the contribution of alveolar surface tension to the elastic properties of the lungs.[78] After the elastin of the canine lung is destroyed chemically, elastic properties of the lung are well preserved in air-filled lungs but entirely lost in fluid-filled lungs.

Clements and co-workers expanded this concept and measured the surface tension of extracts of the lung.[79,80] In order to explain why alveoli do not collapse during expiration, he postulated that the surface tension of the alveolar film increases during inflation and decreases during deflation of the lungs.

The law of LaPlace states that $T = Pr$, where T = tension, P = pressure and r = radius. It is assumed that the alveolar pressure is equal throughout the lungs. Thus, tension in the alveolar wall must vary with the radius of the alveolus. Unless tension in the walls of the smaller alveoli is lower, they would tend to collapse toward larger alveoli with higher tension. This would shortly result in all alveoli being completely collapsed or markedly distended. In a healthy subject, however, the lung contains hundreds of millions of stable alveoli of varying sizes. This fact makes necessary the postulation of a special surface-active material lining the alveoli which regulates the surface tension at rest and with the respiratory cycle. This surface-active material, known as surfactant, maintains the patency of the alveoli under all physiologic conditions. Surfactant is not plasma, saline or ordinary tissue fluid. Its origin, exact chemical nature and structure are still unknown. It is believed to be a complex material, containing protein, lecithin, and highly saturated phospholipids. Conditions which tend to depress the activity of surfactant include (a) immature lungs; (b) atelectasis; (c) decrease in local blood supply; (d) the presence of fibrin and fibrinogen; and (e) tobacco smoke.

The lungs of patients with congestive heart failure would no longer be free of fluid, and new fluid-air interfaces in the alveolar ducts or respiratory bronchioles would be expected. The accumulation of excessive fluid in the lungs and extensive pulmonary vascular changes would be expected to depress the activity of the surfactant appreciably. The elastic properties of the lung would be altered by interference with surfactant activity together with possible changes in the elastic tissues. Impaired elastic properties in turn would interfere with the normal expansion of the lung, reduce the vital capacity, and impair the static pressure-volume relationship or lung compliance.

An excellent review on mechanical properties of the lungs was recently published by Mead.[81]

To summarize, from a clinical point of view, the pulmonary "congestion" and respiratory symptoms associated with congestive cardiac failure cannot be specifically related to increase in pulmonary vascular volume. We suggest that the factors crucial to the pathogenesis of the syndrome of pulmonary "congestion" are those which elevate pulmonary vascular pressures and those which increase the rate of transfer of fluid from the vascular compartment to extravascular sites within the lungs. Reduced vascular compliance at increased pressures makes possible the induction of congestive manifestations by provocative pressure changes without appreciable change in intravascular volume. Accumulation of fluid in the terminal respiratory tract and in the interstitial tissue is largely responsible for the manifestations of "congestion." This accumulated fluid not only accentuates the pulmonary vascular resistance but also alters the elastic properties and compliance of the lung by interfering with the surfactant activity and possibly by causing parenchymal changes.

This hypothesis implies that the treatment of the pulmonary congestion and edema of cardiac failure will be most effective if it causes a fall in pulmonary venous and capillary pressures. With lower pressure the extravascular fluid will tend to return to the vascular compartment. In view of the altered pulmonary vascular pressure-volume relationships in these patients, therapy which reduces the PBV even slightly may cause a much larger decrease in the pulmonary vascular pressure. This explains the effectiveness of such measures as upright position, phlebotomy, and tourniquet application to the extremities in the treatment of acute pulmonary edema.[82-85] The use of ganglionic blocking agents has been equally effective in the treatment of acute pulmonary edema in patients with mitral stenosis or with hypertensive cardiovascular disease.[86-89] These drugs lower the pulmonary vascular pressures in these patients, presumably by shifting blood from the pulmonary to the systemic circulation. Morphine also has been shown to lower the PBV and pulmonary vascular pressures.[90]

Pharmacologic agents which augment left ventricular function or reduce heart rate in the presence of tachycardia are also useful.[91-99] They tend to lower the LVd and, in turn, the pulmonary capillary pressure, thus promoting return of extravascular fluid to the capillaries. One well-known example is the use of rapidly acting digitalis preparations.[91,94,95,97]

In patients with cardiac failure and chronic pulmonary "congestion," salt restriction and use of newer diuretics may drastically lower the total extracellular and intravascular volumes.[100-104]

To the relatively small extent that such measures decrease the PBV, the pulmonary capillary pressure may decline significantly.

REFERENCES

1. Peabody, F.W.: Clinical studies on respiration. III. A mechanical factor in the production of dyspnea in patients with cardiac disease. Arch. Int. Med., 20, 433, 1917.

2. Peabody, F.W., Wentworth, J.A., and Barker, B.I.: Clinical studies on the respiration. V. The basal metabolism and the minute-volume of the respirations of patients with cardiac disease. Arch. Int. Med., 20, 468, 1917.

3. Christie, R.V.: Dyspnea: A review. Quart. J. Med., 7, 421, 1938.

4. Altschule, M.D., Zamcheck, N., and Iglaner, A.: The lung volume and its subdivisions in the upright and recumbent positions in patients with congestive failure: Pulmonary factors in the genesis of orthopnea. J. Clin. Invest., 22, 805, 1943.

5. Harrison, T.R. Harrison, WG., Calhoun, J.A., and March, J.P.: Congestive heart failure. XVII. The mechanism of dyspnea on exertion. Arch. Int. Med., 50, 690, 1932.

6. Donald, K.W.: Disturbances in pulmonary function in mitral stenosis and left heart failure. Prog. Cardiovasc. Dis., 1, 298, 1958.

7. Warren, J.V., Leonard, J.J., and Weissler, A.M.: Gallop rhythm. Ann. Int. Med., 48, 580, 1958.

8. Crevasse, L., Wheat, M.W., Wilson, J.R., Leeds, R.F., and Taylor, W.J.: The mechanism of the generation of the third and fourth heart sounds. Circulation, 25, 635, 1962.

9. Gleason, W.L., and Braunwald, E.: Studies on Starling's law of the heart. VI. Relationships between left ventricular end-diastolic volume and stroke volume in man, with observations on the mechanics of pulsus alternans. Circulation, 25, 841, 1962.

10. Mitchell, J.H., Sarnoff, S.J., and Sonnenblick, E.H.: The dynamics of pulsus alternans: Alternating end-diastolic fiber length as a causative factor. J. Clin. Invest., 42, 55, 1963.

11. Stead, E.A.: Edema and dyspnea of heart failure. Bull. N.Y. Acad. Sci., 28, 159, 1952.

12. Richards, D.W.: The nature of cardiac and of pulmonary dyspnea. Circulation, 7, 15, 1953.

13. Altschule, M.D.: *Acute Pulmonary Edema.* New York, Grune & Stratton, 1954.

14. Comroe, J.H.: Dyspnea. Mod. Conc. Cardiovasc. Dis., 25, 347, 1956.

15. Peters, J.P., and Barr, D.P.: Studies of respiratory mechanism in cardiac dyspnea. II. A note of the effective lung volume in cardiac dyspnea. Am. J. Physiol., 54, 335, 1920.

16. Binger, C.A.L.: The lung volume in heart disease. J. Exp. Med., 38, 445, 1923.

17. Lundsgaard, C.: Determination and interpretation of changes in lung volume in certain heart lesions. J.A.M.A., 80, 163, 1923.

18. Christie, R.V., and Meakins, J.C.: The intrapleural pressure in congestive heart failure and its clinical significance. J. Clin. Invest., 13, 323, 1934.

19. Brown, C.C., Fry, D.L., and Ebert, R.V.: The mechanics of pulmonary ventilation in patients with heart disease. Am. J. Med., 17, 438, 1954.

20. Frank, N.R., Lyons, H.A., Siebens, A.A., and Nealon, T.F.: Pulmonary compliance in patients with cardiac disease. Am. J. Med., 22, 516, 1957.

21. Sharp, J.T., Griffith, G.T., Bunnell, I.L., and Greene, D.G.: Ventilatory mechanics in pulmonary edema in man. J. Clin. Invest., 37, 111, 1958.

22. McNeill, R.S., Rankin, J., and Forster, R.E.: The diffusing capacity of the pulmonary membrane and the pulmonary capillary blood volume in cardiopulmonary disease. Clin. Sci., 17, 465, 1958.

23. Flatley, F.J., Constantine, H., McCredie, R.M., and Yu, P.N.: Pulmonary diffusing capacity and pulmonary capillary blood volume in normal subjects and in cardiac patients. Am. Heart J., 64, 159, 1962.

24. Palmer, W.H., Gee, J.B.L., Mills, F.C., and Bates, D.V.: Disturbances of pulmonary function in mitral valve disease. Canad. Med. Ass. J., 89, 744, 1963.

25. McCredie, R.M.: The pulmonary capillary bed in various forms of pulmonary hypertension. Circulation, 33, 854, 1966.

26. Braunwald, E., and Ross, J.: The ventricular end-diastolic pressure: Appraisal of its value in the recognition of ventricular failure in man. Am. J. Med., 34, 147, 1963.

27. Wood, P.: *Diseases of the Heart and Circulation*, 2nd ed., Philadelphia, J.B. Lippincott Co., 1956, p. 270.

28. Rushmer, R.F.: *Cardiovascular Dynamics*, 2nd ed., Philadelphia, W.B. Saunders Co., 1961, p. 463.

29. Harrison, T.R., Adams, R.D., Bennett, I.L., Resnik, W.H., Thorn, G.W., and Wintrobe, M.M.: *Principles of Internal Medicine*, 4th ed., New York, McGraw-Hill Book Co., 1962, p. 98.

30. Beeson, P.B., and McDermott, W.: *Cecil-Loeb Textbook of Medicine*, 11th ed., Philadelphia, W.B. Saunders Co., 1963, p. 620.

31. Muller, C.: *Cardiopulmonary Hemodynamics in Health and Disease.* Springfield, Charles C Thomas, 1965.

32. Drinker, C.K., Peabody, F.W., and Blumgart, H.L.: The effect of pulmonary congestion on the ventilation of the lungs. J. Exp. Med., *35*, 77, 1922.

33. Dow, P.: The venous return as a factor affecting vital capacity. Am. J. Physiol., *127*, 793, 1939.

34. Glaser, E.M., and McMichael, J.: Effect of venesection on the capacity of the lungs. Lancet, *2*, 230, 1940.

35. Sjöstrand, T.: Über die Bedeutung der Lungen als Blutdepot bein Menschen. Acta Physiol. Scand., *2*, 231, 1941.

36. Hamilton, W.F., Moore, J.W., Kinsman, J.M., and Spurling, R.G.: Study on the circulation. IV. Further analysis of the injection method and of changes in hemodynamics under physiological and pathological conditions. Am. J. Physiol., *99*, 534, 1932.

37. Borden, C.W., Ebert, R.W., Wilson, R.H., and Wells, H.S.: Studies of the pulmonary circulation. II. The circulation time from the pulmonary artery to the femoral artery and the quantity of blood in the lungs in patients with mitral stenosis and in patients with left ventricular failure. J. Clin. Invest., *28*, 1138, 1949.

38. Lagerlöf, H., Werkö, L., Bucht, H., and Holmgren, A.: Separate determination of the blood volume of the right and left heart and the lungs in man with the aid of the dye injection method. Scand. J. Clin. & Lab. Invest., *1*, 114, 1949.

39. Kopelman, H., and Lee, G. de J.: The intrathoracic blood volume in mitral stenosis and left ventricular failure. Clin. Sci., *10*, 383, 1951.

40. Rapaport, E., Kuida, H., Haynes, F.W., and Dexter, L.: The pulmonary blood volume in mitral stenosis. J. Clin. Invest., *35*, 1393, 1956.

41. Borden, C.W., Ebert, R.V., Wilson, R.H., and Wells, H.S.: Pulmonary hypertension in heart disease. New Eng. J. Med., *242*, 529, 1950.

42. Saxton, G.A., Rabinowitz, M., Dexter, L., and Haynes, F.: The relationship of pulmonary compliance to pulmonary vascular pressures in patient switch heart disease. J. Clin. Invest., *35*, 611, 1956.

43. White, H.C., Butler, J., and Donald, K.W.: Lung compliance in patients with mitral stenosis. Clin. Sci., *17*, 667, 1958.

44. Ebert, R.V.: The lung in congestive heart failure. Arch. Int. Med., *107*, 450, 1961.

45. Varnauskas, E., Forsberg, S.A., Widimsky, J., and Paulin, S.: Pulmonary blood volume and its relation to pulmonary hemodynamics in cardiac patients. Acta Med. Scand., *173*, 529, 1963.

46. Werkö, L.: Current status, unsolved problems and future directions in congestive heart failure research. Am. Heart J., *70*, 402, 1965.

47. Schreiner, B.F., Murphy, G.W., and Yu, P.N.: Pulmonary blood volume in congestive heart failure. Circulation, *34*, 249, 1966.

48. Finlayson, J.K., Luria, M.N., Stanfield, C.A., and Yu, P.N.: Hemodynamic studies in acute pulmonary edema. Ann. Int. Med., *54*, 244, 1961.

49. Harris, P., and Heath, D.: *Human Pulmonary Circulation*, Chapter 19, Baltimore, The Williams & Wilkins Co., 1962.

50. Oakley, C., Glick, G., Luria, M.N., Schreiner, B.F., and Yu, P.N.: Some regulatory mechanisms of human pulmonary vascular bed. Circulation, *26*, 217, 1962.

51. Yu, P.N., Glick, G., Schreiner, B.F., and Murphy, G.W.: Effects of acute hypoxia on the pulmonary vascular bed in patients with acquired heart disease: With special reference to the demonstration of active vasomotion. Circulation, *27*, 541, 1963.

52. Schreiner, B.F., Murphy, G.W., Glick, G., and Yu, P.N.: Effects of exercise on the pulmonary blood volume in patients with acquired heart disease. Circulation, *27*, 559, 1963.

53. Gazioglu, K., and Yu, P.N.: Pulmonary blood volume and pulmonary capillary blood volume in valvular heart disease. Circulation, *35*, 701, 1967.

54. Yu, P.N., Murphy, G.W., Schreiner, B.F., and James, D.H.: Distensibility characteristics of the human pulmonary vascular bed: Study of the pressure-volume response to exercise in patients with and without heart disease. Circulation, *35*, 710, 1967.

55. Schreiner, B.F., Murphy, G.W., James, D.H., and Yu, P.N.: The effects of isoproterenol

upon the pulmonary blood volume in patients with valvular heart disease and primary myocardial disease. Circulation, *37*, 220, 1968.

56. Parker, F., and Weiss, S.: The nature and significance of the structural changes in the lungs in mitral stenosis. Am. J. Path., *12*, 573, 1936.

57. Heath, D., and Edwards, J.E.: Histological changes in the lung in diseases associated with pulmonary venous hypertension. Brit. J. Dis. Chest, *53*, 8, 1959.

58. Daley, R., Goodwin, J.P., and Steiner, R.E.: *Clinical Disorders of the Pulmonary Circulation*, Boston, Little, Brown and Co, 1960, p. 136.

59. West, J.B.; Perivascular edema, a factor in pulmonary vascular resistance. Am. Heart J., *70*, 570, 1965.

60. Hughes, J.M.B., Glazier, J.B., Maloney, J.E., and West, J.B.: Effect of interstitial pressure on pulmonary blood flow. Lancet, *1*, 192, 1967.

61. Levine, O.R., Mellins, R.B., and Fishman, A.P.: Quantitative assessment of pulmonary edema. Circ. Res., *17*, 414, 1965.

62. Guyton, A.C., and Lindsey, A.W.: Effect of elevated left atrial pressure and decreased plasma protein concentration on the development of pulmonary edema. Circ. Res., *7*, 649, 1959.

63. Little, R.C.: Volume elastic properties of the right and left atrium. Am. J. Physiol., *158*, 237, 1949.

64. Gorlin, R., Lewis, B.M., Haynes, F.W., Spiegl, R.J., and Dexter, L.: Factors regulating pulmonary "capillary" pressure in mitral stenosis. Am. Heart J., *41*, 834, 1951.

65. Sarnoff, S.J., Berglund, E., and Sarnoff, L.C.: Neurohemodynamics of pulmonary edema. III. Estimated changes in pulmonary blood volume accompanying systemic vasoconstriction and vasodilation. J. Appl. Physiol., *5*, 367, 1953.

66. Bucci, G., Cork, C.D., and Hamann, J.F.: Studies of respiratory physiology in children. VI. Lung diffusing capacity of the pulmonary membrane and pulmonary capillary blood volume in congenital heart disease. J. Clin. Invest., *40*, 1431, 1961.

67. Bedell, G.N: Comparison of pulmonary diffusing capacity in normal subjects and in patients with intracardiac septal defect. J. Lab. & Clin. Med., *57*, 269, 1961.

68. McCredie, R.M., Lovejoy, F.W., and Yu, P.N.: Pulmonary diffusing capacity and pulmonary capillary blood volume in patients with intracardiac shunts. J. Lab. & Clin. Med., *63*, 914, 1964.

69. Staub, N.C., Nagano, H., and Pearce, M.L.: Pulmonary edema in dogs, especially sequence of fluid accumulation in lungs. J. Appl. Physiol., *22*, 227, 1967.

70. West, J.B., Dollery, C.T., and Heard, B.E.: Increased pulmonary vascular resistance in the dependent zone of the isolated dog lung caused by perivascular edema. Circ. Res., *17*, 191, 1965.

71. Christie, R.V., and Meakins, J.C.: The intrapleural pressure in congestive heart failure and its clinical significance. J. Clin. Invest., *13*, 323, 1934.

72. Borst, H.G., Berglund, E., Whittenberger, J.L., Mead, J., McGregor, M., and Collier, C.: The effect of pulmonary vascular pressures on the mechanical properties of the lungs of anesthetized dogs. J. Clin. Invest., *36*, 1708, 1957.

73. Hughes, R., May, A.J., and Widdicombe, J.G.: The effect of pulmonary congestion and oedema in lung compliance. J. Physiol., *142*, 306, 1958.

74. Comroe, J.H.: *Physiology of Respiration*, Chapter 10, Chicago, Year Book Medical Publishers, Inc., 1965.

75. von Neergaard, K.: Neue Auffassungen über einen Grundbegriff der Atemmechanik: Die Retraktionskraft der Lunge, Abhängig von der oberflachenspannung in den Alveolen. Ztschr. Ges Exper. Med., *66*, 373, 1929.

76. Radford, E.P.: Method for estimating respiratory surface area of mammalian lungs from their physical characteristics. Proc. Soc. Exp. Biol. Med., *87*, 58, 1954.

77. Mead, J., Whittenberger, J.L., and Radford, E.P.: Surface tension as a factor in pulmonary volume-pressure hysteresis. J. Appl. Physiol., *10*, 191, 1957.

78. Pierce, J.A., and Hocutt, J.M.: Studies on the collagen and elastin content of the human lung. J. Clin. Invest., *36*, 8, 1960.

79. Clements, J.A.: Surface tension of lung extracts. Proc. Soc. Exp. Biol. Med., *95*, 170, 1957.

80. _____ Surface phenomena in relation to pulmonary function. Physiologist, *5*, 11, 1962.

81. Mead, J.: Mechanical properties of lungs. Physiol. Rev., *41*, 281, 1961,

82. Weiss, S., and Robb, G.P., The treatment of cardiac asthma (paroxysmal cardiac dyspnea). Med. Clin. N. Amer., *16*, 961, 1933.

83. Ebert, R.V., and Stead, E.A.: The effect of the application of tourniquets on the hemodynamics of the circulation. J. Clin. Invest., *19*, 561, 1940.

84. Kountz, W.B., Smith, J.R., and Wright, S.T.: Observations on the effect of tourniquets on acute cardiac crises, normal subjects and chronic heart failure. Am. Heart J., *23*, 624, 1942.

85. Stead, E.A., and Hickam, J.B.: Heart failure. *Disease-A-Month*, January, 1955.

86. Sarnoff, S.J., Goodale, W.T., and Sarnoff, L.C.: Graded reduction of arterial pressure in man by means of a thiophanium derivative (RO 2-2222): Preliminary observations on its effect in acute pulmonary edema. Circulation, *6*, 63, 1952.

87. Kelley, R.T., Fries, E.D., and Higgins, T.F.: The effects of hexamethonium on certain manifestations of congestive heart failure. Circulation, *7*, 196, 1952.

88. Ellestad, M.H.: Use of intravenously given ganglionic blocking agents for acute pulmonary edema. J.A.M.A., *161*, 49, 1956.

89. Yu, P.N., Nye, R.E., Lovejoy, F.W., Schreiner, B.F., and Yim, B.J.B.: Studies of pulmonary hypertension. IX. The effects of intravenous hexamethonium on pulmonary circulation in patients with mitral stenosis. J. Clin. Invest., *37*, 194, 1958.

90. Roy, S.B., Singh, I., Bhatia, M.L., and Khanna, P.K.: Effect of morphine on pulmonary blood volume in convalescents from high altitude pulmonary edema. Brit. Med. J., *27*, 876, 1965.

91. Bloomfield, R.A., Rapoport, B., Milnor, J.P., Long, W.K., Mebane, J.G., and Ellis, L.B.: Effects of cardiac glycosides upon dynamics of circulation in congestive heart failure; Ouabain. J. Clin. Invest., *27*, 588, 1948.

92. Lagerlöf, H., and Werkö, L.: Studies on circulation in man; the effect of Cedilanid (lanatoside C) on cardiac output and blood pressure on the pulmonary circulation in patients with compensated and decompensated heart disease. Acta Cardiol., *4*, 1, 1949.

93. Harvey, R.M., Ferrer, M.I., Cathcart, R.T., Richards, D.W., and Cournand, A.: Some effects of digoxin upon the heart and circulation in man; digoxin in left ventricular failure. Am. J. Med., *7*, 439, 1949,

94. Ahmed, S., Bayliss, R.I.S., Briscoe, W.A., and McMichael, J.: Action of Ouabain (g-strophanthin) on the circulation in man, and a comparison with digoxin. Clin. Sci., *9*, 1, 1950.

95. Yu, P.N., Nye, R.E., Lovejoy, F.W., Macias, de J., Schreiner, B.F., and Lux, J.J.: Studies of pulmonary hypertension. VIII. Effects of acetyl strophanthidin on pulmonary circulation in patients with cardiac failure and mitral stenosis. Am. Heart J., *54*, 235, 1957.

96. Ferrer, M.I., Conroy, R.J., and Harvey, R.M.: Some effects of digoxin upon the heart and circulation in man: Digoxin in combined (right and left) ventricular failure. Circulation, *21*, 372, 1960.

97. Mason, D.T., and Braunwald, E.: Studies on digitalis. IX. Effects of Ouabain on the non-failing human heart. J. Clin. Invest., *42*, 1105, 1963.

98. Weissler, A.M., Gamel, W.G., Grode, H.E., Cohen, S., and Schoenfield, C.D.: The effect of digitalis on ventricular ejection in normal human subjects. Circulation, 29, 721, 1964.

99. Murphy, G.W., Schreiner, B.F., Bleakley, P.L., and Yu, P.N.: Left ventricular performance following digitalization in patients with and without heart failure. Circulation, 30, 358, 1964.

100. Cannon, P.J., Heinemann, H.O., Stason W.B., and Laragh, J.H.: Ethacrynic acid. Effectiveness and mode of diuretic action in man. Circulation, *31*, 5, 1965.

101. Stason, W.B., Cannon, P.J., Heinemann, H.O., and Laragh, J.H.: Furosemide, a clinical evaluation of its diuretic action. Circulation, *34*, 910, 1966.

102. Reubi, F.C.: Clinical use of Furosemide. Ann. N.Y. Acad. Sci., *139*, 433, 1966.

103. Goldberg, M.: Ethacrynic acid: Site and mode of action. Ann. N.Y. Acad. Sci., *139*, 443, 1966.

104. Laragh, J.H.: The proper use of newer diuretics. Ann. Int. Med., *67*, 606, 1967.

CHAPTER 10

Relationship of Pulmonary Blood Volume to Other Variables

Table 10-1 presents the coefficients of correlation between pulmonary blood volume (PBV) and a number of variables in 15 normal subjects and in 281 patients with valvular heart disease studied in our laboratory. These relationships are discussed in the following sections.

Cardiac Output

Many investigators have reported a positive correlation between cardiac output (CO) and intrathoracic or central blood volume (CBV) at rest, during exercise, and during induction of anesthesia.[1-7] With the newer technique of measuring PBV, some but not all workers found a positive correlation between CO and PBV.[8-11]

In our series of patients with various types of valvular heart disease, PBV correlated positively with cardiac index (CI) in class III predominant mitral stenosis, class III predominant mitral regurgitation, class II predominant aortic stenosis and class III predominant aortic regurgitation (Table 10-1). Milnor and others have pointed out that such a positive correlation may not be artificial, even though cardiac output enters into the calculation of PBV.[12] No correlation between PBV and CI was observed in normal patients, in class II patients with either

mitral valvular disease or aortic regurgitation, or in class III aortic stenosis. As shown in Figure 10-1, the PBV of many patients with CI varying between 2.0 and 3.5 L/M²/min was greater than

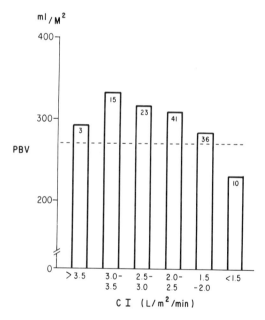

Figure 10-1. Mean pulmonary blood volume (PBV) in 128 patients with predominant mitral stenosis arranged according to their resting cardiac indices (CI). The figures at the top of each column denote the number of patients. In many patients with CI varying between 2.0 and 3.5 L/M²/min, the PBV was greater than the mean normal of 271 ml/M² (dotted line), while in all 10 patients with a CI less than 1.5 L/M²/min, the mean PBV was only 230 ml/M².

109

TABLE 10-1   Coefficients of Correlation between Pulmonary Blood Volume and Various Variables

Patients	No.	CI	SI	PAm	LAm	Pd	PVR	C	LHV
"Normal"	15	−0.071	0.266	0.256	−0.044	0.110	0.242	0.383	0.067
M.S.									
II	33	0.166	0.106	0.285	0.394*	0.352*	−0.162	0.273	−0.035
III	87	0.364*	0.193	0.124	0.193	0.165	−0.027	0.454*	0.217
IV	8	0.553	0.563	−0.316	0.036	−0.252	0.596	0.672⁺	0.053
M.R.									
II	21	0.314	0.225	0.100	−0.026	0.044	0.145	0.438⁺	0.424⁺
III	39	0.336*	0.214	0.035	0.243	0.121	0.185	0.522*	−0.228
A.S.									
II	20	0.501**	0.575*	−0.452*	−0.049	−0.296	−0.346	0.752*	0.016
III	35	0.290	0.484*	0.167	0.235	0.186	−0.157	0.424*	0.037
A.R.									
II	19	0.321	0.272	0.272	0.339	0.308	−0.146	0.168	0.398
III	19	0.573*	0.612*	0.062	0.164	0.108	−0.251	0.435*	0.535**

M.S. = Mitral stenosis
M.R. = Mitral regurgitation
A.S. = Aortic stenosis
A.R. = Aortic regurgitation
CI   = Cardiac index (L/min/M²)
SI   = Stroke index (ml/bcat/M²)
PAm = Pulmonary arterial mean pressure (mm Hg)
LAm = Left atrial mean pressure (mm Hg)
Pd   = Pulmonary distending pressure (mm Hg)
PVR = Pulmonary vascular resistance (dynes · sec/cm⁵)
C   = Relative pulmonary vascular compliance (ml/M²/mm Hg)

LHV = Left heart and aortic volume (ml/M²)
*   = p < 0.01
**   = p < 0.02
⁺   = p < 0.05

271 ml/M², while the mean PBV was only 230 ml/M² in all 10 patients with CI less than 1.5 L/M²/min.

Stroke Volume

Almost all workers who have studied the relationship between PBV and stroke volume (SV) have found a positive correlation.[8-13] Forsberg reported a positive correlation between PBV and SV only when SV was 70 ml or greater.[10] On the other hand, Freitas observed an inverse relationship between PBV and SV in patients with pulmonary hypertension, but not in those with normal pulmonary arterial pressure.[14]

In our series, PBV and stroke index (SI) showed no correlation in patients with mitral valvular disease but a significant correlation was demonstrated in patients with predominant aortic stenosis and in class III predominant aortic regurgitation (Table 10-1).

The PBV has been described as a blood reservoir, available for regulation of the left ventricular output in the normal circulation.[15] Accordingly, the volume and elasticity of the pulmonary vascular bed would contribute to the regulation of cardiac output. However, inasmuch as we found no significant correlation between PBV and CI or between PBV and SI in normal subjects and in many patients with mild valvular heart disease, we consider the applicability of such a postulation to normal subjects or to many patients with cardiac disease unsettled.

Mean Transit Time

Dock and associates observed a direct correlation between PBV and mean transit time through the pulmonary vascular bed, Tm$_{(PA-LA)}$.[16]

Similar results were reported by Freitas and co-workers[14] and by Oakley from our laboratory.[17] On the other hand, Forsberg and Fermoso and their respective associates failed to find a significant correlation between the two variables.[10,13] The reason for this discrepancy is not clear. $Tm_{(PA-LA)}$ is one of the two components in the calculation of PBV, a circumstance which might be expected to favor such a correlation.

Pulmonary Arterial Pressure

Studies of correlation between PBV and pulmonary arterial pressure (PAm) have not yielded uniform results. Dock and associates found a positive correlation between PBV and PAm in patients with marked pulmonary hypertension, but the correlation was insignificant if all cases were included.[16] Roy also reported a correlation between the two variables in patients with PAm up to 25 mm Hg.[18] Forsberg observed no correlation between PBV and PAm except when the PAm was greater than 20 mm Hg.[10] No correlation between PBV and PAm was reported by Freitas and associates.[14]

With the exception of class II aortic stenosis, our patients showed no correlation between PBV and PAm (Table 10-1). The absence of correlation in most of these patients is understandable because the tendency of an increased PAm to augment PBV may be countered by restrictive structural changes in the pulmonary vascular bed and reduction in PBV resulting from long-standing pulmonary hypertension.

Left Atrial Pressure

Dock and associates reported no correlation between PBV and left atrial pressure (LAm) if all their patients were included.[16] PBV and LAm were directly and significantly correlated, however, if those patients were excluded whose pulmonary vascular resistance (PVR) exceeded 500 dynes · sec/cm[5]. The mean PBV was 277 ml/M^2 in their patients whose LAm was 15 mm Hg or less, and the mean PBV was 357 ml/M^2 in those whose LAm exceeded 15 mm Hg.

McGaff and co-workers observed a positive correlation between PBV and LAm in patients with both high and low PVR.[8] In general, patients with high PVR had a smaller PBV than those with low PVR.

Forsberg and Varnauskas found a mean PBV of 693 ml in patients whose

TABLE 10-2   Pulmonary Blood Volume in Patients with Valvular Heart Disease

Diagnosis	Functional Classification	LAm ≤ 13 mm Hg		LAm > 13 mm Hg		p value
		No. of Patients	PBV	No. of Patients	PBV	
M.S.	I – II	13	256 ± 13.5	20	306 ± 10.2	< 0.01
	III	7	259 ± 24.4	80	315 ± 7.9	< 0.05
M.R.	I – II	16	279 ± 14.3	5	288 ± 11.3	N.S.
	III	9	310 ± 21.7	30	313 ± 19.4	N.S.
A.S.	I – II	17	264 ± 12.0	3	284 ± 34.5	N.S.
	III	21	293 ± 13.3	14	311 ± 18.4	N.S.
A.R.	I – II	17	297 ± 13.0	2	322 ± 24.5	N.S.
	III·	11	276 ± 23.6	8	310 ± 33.4	N.S.
Total Group		111	280 ± 5.6	162	307 ± 5.8	< 0.01

LAm = Left atrial mean pressure
PBV = Pulmonary blood volume (ml/M^2) mean ± S.E.
N.S. = Not significant
Other symbols and abbreviations are identical to those used in Table 10-1.

LAm was greater than 13 mm Hg and 585 ml in those whose LAm was less than 13 mm Hg.[10,19] No correlation between PBV and LAm was observed in their patients except for those whose LAm exceeded 13 mm Hg.

Roy reported good correlation between PBV and LAm in patients with LAm up to 27 mm Hg.[18] Fermoso, Freitas and respective associates, on the other hand, found no correlation between these two variables.[13,14]

Table 10-2 shows the PBV in our series of 273 patients with valvular heart disease, listed according to whether the LAm was 13 mm Hg or less on the one hand, or greater than 13 mm Hg on the other. When the predominant valvular disease and the functional classification were the same, the mean PBV was always greater in the group of patients with the higher LAm. The difference between the two groups of patients as a whole was statistically significant ($p < 0.01$), as it was for the subgroup of patients with predominant mitral stenosis (for class I-II patients, $p < 0.01$; for class III patients, $p < 0.05$). The difference was not statistically significant for the subgroups of patients with predominant mitral regurgitation and aortic valve disease. Table 10-1 shows that no significant correlation was demonstrated between PBV and LAm in the various groups of patients except for class II patients with mitral stenosis ($p < 0.05$).

McGaff and associates pointed out that the wide scatter of values for PBV at all levels of LAm suggests that differences in the elastic properties of pulmonary vessels are superimposed on the simple pressure-volume relationship.[8] Thus, although the mean PBV is generally greater in patients with high LAm, because of augmented distending pressure, the patients in this group tend to have a relatively low volume-pressure ratio. When the LAm has been elevated for a prolonged period, associated with marked pulmonary hypertension, the PBV may return to normal or become subnormal. This apparently paradoxical reduction in PBV in advanced cases most likely results from structural and functional changes in the pulmonary vascular bed, causing a considerable increase in PVR. The large difference in PBV observed between patients in class III and class IV reported in Chapter 8 could not be explained by arteriolar narrowing alone, inasmuch as maximal constriction of the pulmonary arterioles would reduce the total PBV only very little. Therefore, the restriction of the pulmonary vascular bed manifested by marked reduction in the PBV in the presence of structural as well as functional changes must include both pulmonary arteries and veins.

Pulmonary Vascular Resistance

Forsberg, Freitas, Dock and Varnauskas and their respective coworkers found no correlation between PBV and PVR.[10,14,16,19] On the other hand, McGaff, Roy and their respective associates reported an inverse relationship between PBV and PVR.[8,18] Varnauskas pointed out that the major portion of the PBV may be located in the most compliant regions of the pulmonary vascular bed, i.e., capillaries and veins, while a much smaller volume may be found in the less compliant portions of the vascular bed, i.e., the arteries and arterioles, in patients with elevated PVR and pulmonary vascular pressures.[19] These divergent results are not surprising, since the studies included little specific information regarding the magnitude of distending pressure and the extent of the vascular changes.

TABLE 10-3   Pulmonary Blood Volume in Patients with Valvular Heart Disease

Diagnosis	Functional Classification	PVR < 500* No. of Patients	PVR < 500* PBV	PVR ≥ 500* No. of Patients	PVR ≥ 500* PBV	p value
M.S.	III	72	306 ± 8.2	15	330 ± 20.8	N.S.
	IV	4	242 ± 10.3	4	190 ± 28.4	N.S.
M.R.	III	33	317 ± 18.2	6	286 ± 17.7	N.S.
A.R.	III	17	299 ± 20.6	2	216 ± 29.0	N.S.
Total Group		126	297 ± 4.4	27	289 ± 14.7	N.S.

$*$ = dynes · sec/cm^5
The symbols and abbreviations are identical to those used in Tables 10-1 and 10-2

In 126 patients with valvular heart disease studied by us, no significant difference in PBV was observed between the patients with PVR less than 500 dynes · sec/cm^5 and those with PVR greater than 500 dynes · sec/cm^5 (Table 10-3).

Volume of the Left Atrium

By angiographic studies, Arvidsson estimated the left atrial volume (LA volume) in patients with various types of valvular heart disease.[20] The results are reproduced in Table 10-4. In general, the LA volume was smaller with predominant mitral stenosis than with predominant mitral regurgitation. Further, the LA volume was smaller with normal sinus rhythm than with atrial fibrillation in the same type of valvular disease. The presence of aortic stenosis did not materially affect the LA volume.

Utilizing indicator-dilution curves,

LA volume = V(PA − LA) + V(LA − BA) − V(PA − BA)

Where V(PA−LA) = volume determined by injecting indicator into the pulmonary artery and sampling blood from the left atrium

V(LA−BA) = volume determined by injecting indicator into the left atrium and sampling blood from a systemic artery

V(PA−BA) = volume determined by injecting indicator into the pulmonary artery and sampling blood from a systemic artery

Fujimoto and associates estimated the LA volume in patients with mitral valvular disease by the following formula.[21]

In their patients with predominant mitral stenosis the estimated LA volume averaged 111 ml/M^2, ranging from 45 to 173 ml/M^2. In those with predominant mitral regurgitation the average LA volume was 171 ml/M^2, ranging from 96 to 256 ml/M^2.

TABLE 10-4   Left Atrial Volume Determined by Angiocardiographic Method (after Arvidsson)

Diagnosis	Rhythm	No. of Cases	Maximum LA Volume Range	Maximum LA Volume Average	Average Volume Variation
MS	NSR	18	75 − 265	145	35
MS	AF	7	150 − 400	230	16
MR	NSR	7	120 − 200	155	80
MR	AF	3	610 − 980	770	125
MS & MR	NSR	9	150 − 270	210	60
MS & MR & AS	NSR	4	130 − 220	165	80
MS & MR	AF	8	160 − 1230	380	60

NSR = Normal sinus rhythm
AF = Atrial fibrillation
LA Volume = Left atrial volume in ml/M^2
Other symbols and abbreviations are identical to those used in Table 10-1.

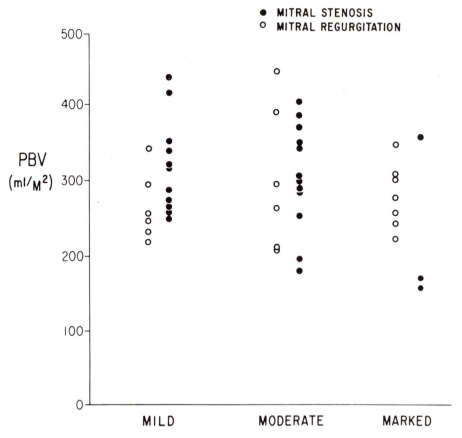

Figure 10-2.   The pulmonary blood volume in patients with mitral valve disease grouped according to the size of the left atrium estimated by selective angiocardiographic study. No correlation between the pulmonary blood volume and the left atrial size was observed.

In all published reports, including our own studies, no correlation was found between PBV and estimated LA volume, or its size by roentgenogram.[10,13,16,17] Forsberg further stated that patients with the largest left atria did not have the largest PBV.[10]

We have studied at random the left atrial size estimated by selective angiocardiograms in patients with mitral valvular disease in order to correlate PBV and left atrial size.* Enlargement of the left atrium was

arbitrarily estimated as mild, moderate or marked. The PBV values are plotted according to the estimated left atrial size in Figure 10-2. The results confirm the previous report of Oakley from our laboratory in a separate series of patients that PBV fails to correlate with the size of the left atrium.[17] Present methods for estimating PBV by indicator-dilution technique include an indeterminate portion of left atrial blood volume, but the lack of correlation between PBV and left atrial size suggests that this fraction of LA volume probably is not a major source of technical error in the determination of PBV by such methods.

*I am indebted to Dr. Elliot O. Lipchik, Associate Professor of Radiology, for information concerning the estimated size of the left atrium in these patients.

Relative Pulmonary Vascular Compliance (C)

No significant correlation between PBV and C was observed in normal subjects and in class II patients with either mitral stenosis or aortic regurgitation (Table 10-1). On the other hand, a positive correlation was found between PBV and C in all class III patients with valvular heart disease, in class II patients with mitral regurgitation or with aortic stenosis, and in class IV patients with mitral stenosis. The lack of correlation in normal subjects and in class II patients with mitral stenosis or aortic regurgitation was unexpected. In patients with more severe valvular disease, structural and functional changes usually cause a corresponding decrease in both C and PBV. Thus, a positive correlation between C and PBV would be expected in these patients.

Total Blood Volume

The techniques for estimating total blood volume (TBV) and the range of normal values have been described in Chapter 4. In normal subjects the TBV is about 2600 ml/M² or 70 ml/Kg, usually somewhat greater in men than in women of the same age group.

Utilizing different techniques, various workers have reported that the PBV in patients without cardiovascular abnormalities and in those with mild cardiopulmonary disease is about 10% of TBV.[9-12,22] In our laboratory nearly simultaneous determinations of TBV and PBV have been made in a series 200 patients.* In a small number of normal subjects and in patients with

*The technical assistance of Mr. Dennis Edwards in the determination of total blood volume in these patients is gratefully acknowledged.

mild cardiovascular abnormalities the value of PBV was appoximately 10% of that of TBV, thus confirming the findings of others. The results also agree with the classical direct estimates and analog computer analysis of PBV in dogs.[23-25]

As shown in Figures 10-3 to 10-7, no correlation was observed between PBV and TBV in patients with mitral regurgitation and in those with aortic valve disease. These two variables were directly and significantly correlated, however, in patients with predominant mitral stenosis ($p < 0.02$), and in those with cardiomyopathy ($p < 0.005$). In several patients with cardiomyopathy and congestive heart failure, however, a marked increase in TBV was not accompanied by a corresponding augmentation of PBV. Thus, a PBV/TBV ratio of 0.7 to 0.8 was not uncommon in these patients. Similar observations have been made in patients with mitral valve disease complicated by congestive

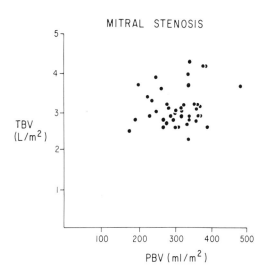

Figure 10-3. Pulmonary blood volume (PBV) plotted against total blood volume (TBV) in patients with predominant mitral stenosis. A positive correlation was observed between the two variables (n = 43, r = 0.36, and p < 0.02).

heart failure. The mechanisms of such changes have been described in detail in the preceding chapter. After appro-

priate therapy, the PBV/TBV ratio usually returns toward the normal value of 0.1.

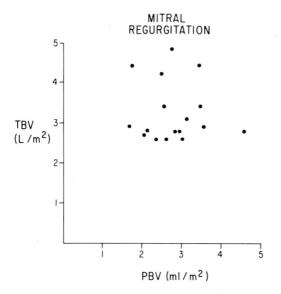

Figure 10-4.   PBV plotted against TBV in patients with predominant mitral regurgitation. No correlation was observed between these two variables (n = 17, r = −0.07).

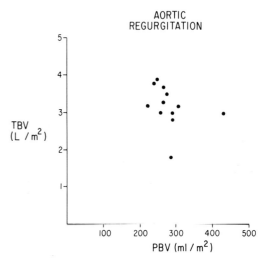

Figure 10-6.   PBV plotted against TBV in patients with predominant aortic regurgitation. No correlation exists between the two variables (n = 12, r = 0.06).

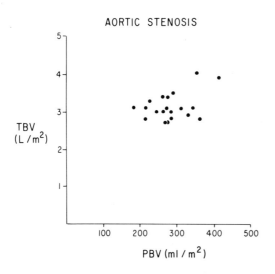

Figure 10-5.   PBV plotted against TBV in patients with predominant aortic stenosis. No significant correlation was observed between these two variables (n = 20, r = 0.38, and 0.05 < p < 0.1).

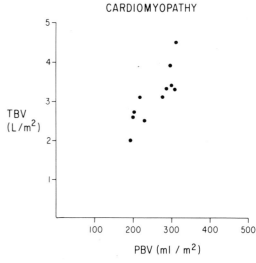

Figure 10-7.   PBV plotted against TBV in patients with cardiomyopathy. There was a significantly positive correlation between the two variables (n = 11, r = 0.83. and p < 0.005).

Central Blood Volume (CBV)

In normal subjects or in patients with minimal or no cardiovascular abnormality, the PBV/CBV ratio is about 0.45, and the two measurements correlate closely.

In patients with predominant mitral stenosis the PBV/CBV ratio usually remains about normal because any increase in LA volume is balanced by an augmented PBV (Figure 10-8). Thus, a highly significant correlation was observed between these two variables (p < 0.005).

some of these patients (Figures 10-9 to 10-12).

Unless CBV and PBV are both measured, the possibility must be considered that changes in CBV may

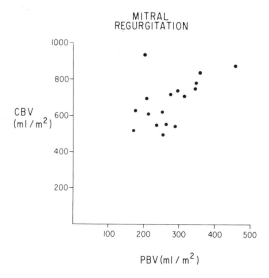

Figure 10-9. PBV plotted against CBV in patients with predominant mitral regurgitation. There was a positive correlation between these two variables (n = 43, r = 0.61, and p < 0.005).

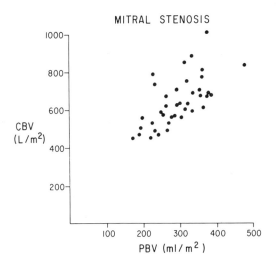

Figure 10-8. PBV plotted against "central" blood volume (CBV) in patients with predominant mitral stenosis. A highly positive correlation was observed between these two variables (n = 43, r = 0.61 and p < 0.005).

In patients with predominant mitral regurgitation, in those with aortic valve disease, and in those with cardiomyopathy, CBV increased disproportionately as a result of augmented left ventricular and aortic volume, although a positive correlation between PBV and CBV was still observed. The PBV/CBV ratio may be reduced to 0.33 in

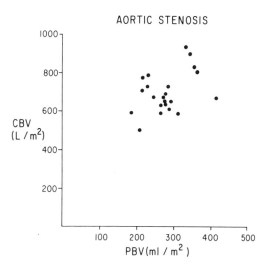

Figure 10-10. PBV plotted against CBV in patients with predominant aortic stenosis. A positive correlation was observed between the two variables (n = 22, r = 0.64, and p < 0.05).

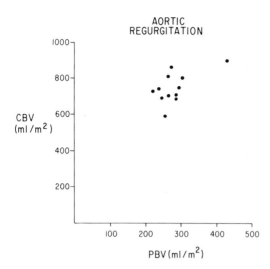

Figure 10-11. PBV plotted against CBV in patients with predominant aortic regurgitation. The two variables correlate positively (n = 12, r = 0.58, and p < 0.05).

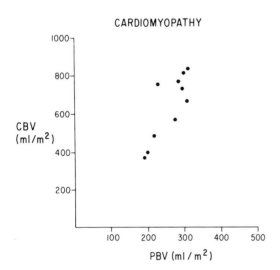

Figure 10-12. PBV plotted against CBV in patients with cardiomyopathy. There was a positive correlation between the two variables (n = 10, r = 0.82 and p < 0.01).

represent changes in PBV such as are observed during exercise or other interventions, or merely a redistribution of blood flow in the peripheral arteries

as demonstrated during a study of the effects of local hyperemia from heat application to a limb.

Left Heart-Aortic Blood Volume

Left heart-aortic blood volume (LHV) is estimated by subtracting PBV from CBV. In normal subjects and in patients with minimal or no cardiopulmonary disease the PBV is usually slightly lower than LHV and the PBV/LHV ratio is about 0.90. A close correlation between the two variables is usual. In most patients with predominant mitral stenosis the proportion between PBV and LHV is unaltered. In patients with predominant mitral regurgitation, and in those with an enlarged left ventricle or dilated aorta due to aortic valvular disease or to other etiological factors, the LHV may be disproportionately increased. In these patients the value of LHV may often reach twice that of PBV. Varnauskas found no correlation between PBV and radiographic heart volume.[19]

Pulmonary Capillary Blood Volume*

The relationship between PBV and pulmonary capillary blood volume (Vc) has been studied in a series of 100 patients in our laboratory.[26] The Vc was estimated by the carbon monoxide diffusing technique, using two oxygen concentrations.

In normal subjects the mean PBV was 270 ml/M², and the mean Vc was 54 ml/M². Thus, the Vc/PBV ratio was approximately 0.20. The resting PBV and Vc in normal subjects are maintained in a narrow range, constituting, respectively, approximately 10% and

*I am grateful to Dr. Kuddusi Gazioglu for his time and assistance in estimating the pulmonary capillary blood volume.

2% of the TBV. During exercise, an appreciable increase in both Vc and PBV has been reported by many workers, and in some instances the percentage increase in Vc was much greater than that for PBV.

In patients with predominant mitral valvular disease, PBV and Vc correlated positively for the group as a whole ($p < 0.01$), although no significant correlation was found between these two variables in any individual class of patients. In class II and III patients, the PBV was either normal (62%) or increased (33%), while the value of Vc varied considerably (increased, normal or decreased). In general, increased PBV was associated with increased or normal Vc, and normal PBV was associated with normal or decreased Vc. Markedly increased PBV associated with reduced Vc is unusual, however, in a given patient. Most patients with moderate mitral valvular disease appear to store their increased pulmonary blood volume in either the pulmonary arteries or the pulmonary veins or both.

PBV and Vc were both markedly reduced in patients with class IV mitral valvular disease, the respective mean values being 228 ml/M^2 and 27 ml/M^2. Similar observations were also reported by Palmer and associates.[27] The decrease in PBV and Vc in these patients implies marked narrowing of the pulmonary vascular bed as a consequence of structural changes and probably functional vasoconstriction.

The PBV was usually normal with class I and class II aortic valvular disease, but was increased in 40% of class III patients. Vc was essentially unchanged in all three classes of these patients, although an increased Vc was observed in a small number of class III patients. PBV and Vc correlated positively in patients with aortic valvular disease as a group ($p < 0.02$). A more significant correlation ($p < 0.01$) between these two variables was observed for the class III patients with aortic valvular disease.

Body Surface Area and Body Weight

Forsberg found a significant positive correlation between PBV and body weight or body surface area (BSA).[10] The following regression formula was proposed, relating PBV to BSA.

$$PBV = 687 \times BSA - 683$$

Using the data obtained by quantitative radiocardiography, Giuntini and associates also found a positive correlation between PBV and body surface area.[9]

Varnauskas found a positive correlation between PBV and height in subjects with normal left atrial pressure, but no correlation was demonstrable in those with left atrial pressure above 13 mm Hg.[19]

Dock and co-workers failed to find

TABLE 10-5 Correlation between Body Surface Area (BSA) and Pulmonary Blood Volume (PBV) in Normal Subjects and in Patients with Valvular Heart Disease

Group	No. of Cases	BSA (M^2) mean $\pm$ S.E.	PBV (ml) mean $\pm$ S.E.	C.C.	p value
Normal	15	1.83 $\pm$ 0.04	497 $\pm$ 21.5	0.714	< 0.005
M.S.	128	1.64 $\pm$ 0.02	480 $\pm$ 15.5	0.472	< 0.005
M.R.	60	1.72 $\pm$ 0.03	517 $\pm$ 22.1	0.490	< 0.005
A.S.	55	1.82 $\pm$ 0.02	531 $\pm$ 17.3	0.544	< 0.005
A.R.	38	1.84 $\pm$ 0.03	552 $\pm$ 26.2	0.680	< 0.005

C.C. = Correlation coefficient
Other symbols and abbreviations are identical to those used in Table 10-2.

significant correlation between PBV and BSA.[16] Forsberg explained the discrepancy between his observations and those of Dock and co-workers on the basis of severity of disease.[10] He felt that patients in Dock's series in general had more advanced disease than those in his own study.

As shown in Table 10-5, our own analysis of a series of 15 normal subjects and 281 patients with valvular heart disease showed a highly positive correlation between the PBV and BSA. Thus, we suggest that the expression of PBV per square meter of BSA would lend uniformity to the reporting of future data from various laboratories.

REFERENCES

1. Ball, J.D., Kopelman, H., and Witham, A.C.: Circulatory changes in mitral stenosis at rest and on exercise. Brit. Heart J., *14*, 363, 1952.

2. Doyle, J.T., wilson, J.S., Lépine, C., and Warren, J.V.: An evaluation of the measurement of the cardiac output and of the so-called pulmonry blood volume by the dye-dilution method. J. Lab. & Clin. Med., *41*, 29 1953.

3. Rapaport, E., Kuida, H., Haynes, F.W., and Dexter, L.: The pulmonary blood volume in mitral stenosis. J. Clin. Invest., *35*, 1393, 1956.

4. Warren, J.V., and Weissler, A.M.: Cenl blood volume as a factor in the regulation t. of the circulation. Circulation,*18*, 793, 1958 ra

5. Braunwald, E., and Kelly, E.R.: The effects of exercise on central blood volume in man. J. Clin. Invest., *39*, 413, 1960.

6. Johnson, S.R.: The effect of some anesthetic agents on the circulation in man. Acta Chir. Scand., Suppl. 158, 1951.

7. Etsten, B., and Li, T.H.: Hemodynamic changes during thiopental anesthesia in humans: Cardiac output, stroke volume, total peripheral resistance and intrathoracic blood volume. J. Clin. Invest., *34*, 500, 1955.

8. McGaff, C.J., Roveti, G.C., Glassman, E., and Milner, W.R.: The pulmonary blood volume in rheumatic heart disease and its alteration by isoproterenol. Circulation, *27*, 77, 1963.

9. Giuntini, C., Lewis, M.L., Sales Luis, A., and Harvey, R.M.: A study of the pulmonary blood volume in man by quantitative radiocardiography. J. Clin. Invest., *42*, 1589, 1963.

10. Forsberg, S.A.: Pulmonary blood volume in man. Acta Med. Scand., *175*, Suppl. 410, 1964.

11. Levinson, G.E., Frank, M.J., and Hellems, H.K.: The pulmonary vascular volume in man. Measurement from atrial dilution curves. Am. Heart J., *67*, 734, 1964.

12. Milnor, W.R., Jose, A.D., and McGaff, C.J.: Pulmonary vascular volume, resistance and compliance in man. Circulation, *12*, 130, 1960.

13. Fermoso, J.D., Aramendia, P., and Taquini, A.C.: Volumen sanquineo pulmonar em la estenosis mitral. Medicina (B. Air), *21*, 161, 1961.

14. Freitas, F.M. de, Faraco, E.Z., Nedel, N., Azévedo, D.F. de, and Zaduchliver, J.: Determination of pulmonary blood volume by single intravenous injection of one indicator in patients with normal and high pulmonary vascular pressures. Circulation, *30*, 370, 1964.

15. Sjöstrand, T.: Volume and distribution of blood and their significance in regulating the circulation. Physiol. Rev., *33*, 202, 1953.

16. Dock, D.S., Kraus, W.L., McQuire, L.B., Hyland, J.W., Haynes, F.W., and Dexter, L.: The pulmonary blood volume in man. J. Clin. Invest., *40*, 317, 1961.

17. Oakley, C., Glick, G., Luria, M.N., Schreiner, B.F., and Yu, P.N.: Some regulatory mechanisms of the human pulmonary vascular bed. Circulation, *26*, 917, 1962.

18. Roy, S.B., Bhardwaj, P., and Bhatia, M.L.: Pulmonary blood volume in mitral stenosis. Brit. Med. J., *2*, 1466, 1965.

19. Varnauskas, E., Forsberg, S.A., Widimsky, J., and Paulin, S.: Pulmonary blood volume and its relation to pulmonary hemodynamics in cardiac patients. Acta Med. Scand., *173*, 529, 1963.

20. Arvidsson, H.: Angiocardiographic observations in mitral stenosis. Acta Radiol. Scand., Suppl. 158, 1958.

21. Fujimoto, K., Kunieda, R., and Shiba, T.: Lung blood volume in acquired valvular disease. Jap. Heart J., *1*, 442, 1960.

22. Lewis, M.L., Giuntini, C., Donato, L., Harvey, R.M., and Cournand, A.: Quantitative radiocardiography. III. Results and validation of theory and method. Circulation, *26*, 189, 1962.

23. Heger, P., and Spehl, E.: Recherches sur la fistule peri-cardique chez le lepin. Arch. Biol. (Liege), *2*, 154, 1881.

24. Plumier, L.: La circulation pulmonaire chez le chien. Arch. Int. Physiol., *1*, 176, 1904.

25. Parrish, D., Hayden, D.T., Garrett, W., and Huff, R.L.: Analog computer analysis of flow characteristics and volume of the pulmonary vascular bed. Circ. Res., *7*, 746, 1959.

26. Gazioglu, K., and Yu, P.N.: Pulmonary blood volume and pulmonary capillary blood volume in valvular heart disease. Circulation, *35*, 701, 1967.

27. Palmer, W.H., Gee, J.B.L., Mills, F.C., and Bates, D.V.: Disturbances of pulmonary function in mitral valve disease. Canad. Med. Ass. J., *89*, 744, 1963.

Chapter 11

Effects of Physiologic, Mechanical or Chemical Interventions or Stresses on Pulmonary Blood Volume

The effects of various mechanical interventions and physiological stresses on pulmonary blood volume are discussed in this chapter. Most of the data presented were obtained in our laboratory, but considerable information is included which was derived from the work of many other investigators.

Our methodology is described in detail in Chapter 8. The initial control studies were conducted after a steady state had been established. Cardiac output (CO) was determined by the Fick procedure and by indicator-dilution curves, and pressures were recorded from various sites. Central blood volume (CBV) and pulmonary blood volume (PBV) were calculated respectively as the product of CO and specific mean transit times $Tm_{(PA-BA)}$ and $Tm_{(PA-LA)}$. Similar measurements were made during such experimental interventions as change of posture, exercise, inhalation of low oxygen, etc. A third set of data was obtained during a recovery period in some instances.

Postural Effects

When the standing upright position is assumed following a period of re-cumbency, a sequence of hemodynamic changes occurs.[1] Venous return and end-diastolic ventricular volume decline, resulting in a decrease in stroke volume (SV). Although heart rate (HR) usually increases 10 to 20 beats per minute, CO may actually decrease by as much as one third.[2-8] Lesser degrees of head-up tilting from the recumbent position cause a smaller reduction in CO. The reduction in CO is manifested by widening of the arteriovenous oxygen difference without alteration of the oxygen uptake.

Systemic arterial systolic pressure remains unchanged, but diastolic and mean pressures both rise. Thus, the systemic arterial pulse pressure narrows. Reduced CO and elevated mean systemic arterial pressures (BAm) result in increased calculated total systemic resistance.

Pulmonary arterial pressure (PAm) has been reported to fall in normal subjects and more so in patients with cardiopulmonary disease.[6-9] Information about left atrial pressure (LAm) is scanty, but a slight decline in the pulmonary wedge pressure (Pw) has been observed in normal subjects.[6,9]

Various workers have reported a marked diminution in pulmonary vascular perfusion at the apex of the lungs in the erect position.[10-16] Most of the intrathoracic blood moves to the lower limbs, even though blood volume in the basal regions of the lungs may not change or may even increase slightly. Overall, the volume of blood in the cardiac chambers and pulmonary vascular bed may fall as much as 25%, compared with values determined in recumbency.[17-20] Thus, the intrathoracic vessels may function as a reservoir.[17,18] Blood stored in the thorax is especially important for rapid mobilization into the systemic circuit after a sudden change from recumbent to upright posture when CO temporarily exceeds venous return.

The positional reduction in CO and related changes may be largely eliminated if the blood volume displacement is prevented by an antigravity pressure suit or by immersion of the body in water up to the diaphragm.[1,8,18,21]

During such maneuvers as head-down tilting, raising the legs in the recumbent position, application of an antigravity suit or immersion of the body in water up to the neck, blood moves from the lower limbs and abdomen into the thorax, increasing CBV and pulmonary capillary blood volume (Vc).[17-19,22-24] In patients with myocardial or valvular heart disease, LAm and PAm rise significantly, usually in association with a decrease in vital capacity and total lung volume.

We have studied pulmonary blood flow, pressures and volume in relation to postural changes in 8 patients. In 3, studies were conducted before and after 45° heap-up tilting; and in 5, before and after raising the legs on a bicycle ergometer in the recumbent position. The results are summarized in Tables 11-1 and 11-2.

Cardiac index (CI) declined, despite an increase in HR during head-up tilting in all three subjects (Table 11-1). PAm, LAm and BAm uniformly decreased. A definite reduction in CBV was observed consistently. PBV also decreased in the 2 patients in whom it was measured. A proportionate decrease in the Vc determined by the carbon monoxide diffusing method was observed in the single subject studied.

When both legs of recumbent subjects were raised on a bicycle ergometer, CI and stroke index (SI) rose in all 5 (Table 11-2). LAm, PAm and BAm all increased slightly but definitely. CBV and PBV increased in 2 but no appreciable change in these volumes was detected in the other 3 subjects.

Some uncertainty must be recognized in comparing PAm and LAm in the recumbent and head-up tilting positions, because the location of the zero reference is necessarily somewhat conjectural. We attached the strain gauge to the fluoroscopic table and adjusted it to the mid-thoracic position as the zero reference point. Thus, when the patients were tilted to the 45° head-up position, the reference point of the strain gauge was almost unchanged. Nevertheless, minor reservations remain in the interpretation of pressure changes in the pulmonary circulation during such maneuvers.

Respiratory Cycle

During inspiration in animals the venous return to the right heart and the pulmonary blood flow increase, accompanied by dilatation of the pulmonary vessels.[25-31] Blood is probably stored in the pulmonary vascular bed and left atrium because the left ventricular output actually decreases. During expiration these changes are reversed.

In man, the PAm and Pw both decrease during inspiration and increase during expiration.[32,33] The difference

Table 11-1   Effect of 45° Head-Up Tilt on Pulmonary Blood Volume

Patient	Age	BSA	Diagnosis	FC	Condition	Blood Flow			Pressures (mm Hg)				Tm (seconds)			Blood Volume (mL/M²)		
						CI	HR	SI	PAm	LAm	P_t	BAm	PA-BA	LA-BA	PA-LA	CBV	PBV	Vc
P.V.H.	30 M	1.58	MS	II	R	2.35	75	30	38	26	32.0	84	18.1	6.3	11.8	710	463	96
					T	1.43	90	16	—	—	—	—	19.5	8.2	11.3	464	270	52
E.R.	52 F	1.79	IC	III	R	1.41	88	16	14	6	10.0	105	19.5	12.0	7.5	460	172	—
					T	1.01	101	10	12	5	8.5	95	24.6	15.0	9.1	415	150	—
					R	1.21	90	13	14	7	10.5	—	21.7	12.7	9.0	440	184	—
J.R.	23 M	1.85	PH	I	R	2.70	45	60	16	—	—	82	16.1	—	—	726	—	—
					T	2.26	96	24	14	—	—	78	12.1	—	—	457	—	—
					R	2.35	41	57	17	—	—	80	18.6	—	—	728	—	—

BSA = Basal surface area (M²)
FC   = Functional capacity
Tm   = Mean transit time
CI   = Cardiac index (L/min/M²)
HR   = Heart rate (beats/min)
SI   = Stroke index (ml/beat/M²)
PAm = Pulmonary arterial mean
LAm = Left atrial mean
P_d = Pulmonary distending
BAm = Systemic arterial mean

PA-BA = Pulmonary artery to systemic artery
LA-BA = Left atrium to systemic artery
PA-LA = Pulmonary artery to left atrium
CBV   = Central blood volume
PBV   = Pulmonary blood volume
Vc   = Pulmonary capillary blood volume
MS   = Mitral stenosis
IC   = Idiopathic cardiomyopathy
PH   = Postural hypotension of unknown etiology
R   = Recumbent position
T   = Tilting position (45° head up)

Table 11-2   Effect of Leg Raising on Pulmonary Blood Volume

Patient	Age	BSA	Diagnosis	FC	Condition	Blood Flow			Pressures (mm Hg)				Tm (seconds)			Blood Volume (mL/M²)	
						CI	HR	SI	PAm	LAm	P_d	BAm	PA-BA	LA-BA	PA-LA	CBV	PBV
B.B.	25 F	1.53	N	I	A	3.15	79	40	13	7	10.0	88	11.0	6.2	4.8	578	252
					B	3.28	75	44	15	8	11.5	97	10.4	5.9	4.5	568	246
F.H.	61 F	1.93	AS	III	A	2.76	87	32	13	7	10.0	95	11.8	6.7	5.1	542	235
					A	2.15	54	40	34	20	27.0	97	22.6	11.7	10.9	812	330
					B	2.43	45	54	34	22	28.0	—	22.2	9.4	12.8	900	517
R.C.	49 F	1.44	MS	III	A	1.93	56	34	32	20	26.0	—	25.2	14.2	11.0	810	356
					A	1.90	112	17	33	26	29.5	91	22.2	14.4	7.8	720	247
					B	1.93	95	20	35	28	31.5	91	24.3	13.6	10.7	780	320
J.S.	52 F	1.46	MS	III	A	1.72	100	17	33	27	30.0	86	25.0	14.7	10.3	675	294
					A	2.00	60	34	22	15	18.5	82	16.2	9.4	6.8	540	228
					B	2.18	60	34	26	16	21.0	90	15.3	8.5	6.8	565	247
N.G.	36 F	1.79	MS	III	A	2.42	82	29	30	18	24.0	85	14.4	7.8	6.6	590	252
					B	2.64	84	31	35	25	30.0	—	14.4	8.4	6.0	630	258

A = Legs down   AS = Aortic stenosis
B = Both legs up on a bicycle ergometer

N = Normal subject
Other symbols and abbreviations are identical to those used in Table 11-1

between PAm and intraesophageal (or intrapleural) pressure, however, increases during inspiration and decreases during expiration.[33]

Utilizing body plethysmographic technique, DuBois and Marshall estimated pulmonary capillary blood flow and gas exchange throughout the respiratory cycle in man.[34] They suggested that during inspiration there was an increased flow through the right ventricle and pulmonary arteries associated with a decreased flow through the pulmonary veins and the left heart. During expiration the flow through the pulmonary veins and the left heart was augmented, while the right ventricular and pulmonary arterial flow was reduced. The pulmonary capillary blood flow was not materially influenced by either inspiration or expiration.

Recent studies of the pulmonary venous flow in dogs by chronically implanted probes, however, have indicated that the peak and mean pulmonary venous flows may be slightly augmented during inspiration.[35-37] Such a flow record obtained by Dr. Edwin Kinnen in our laboratory is shown in Figure 11-1. Apparently, flow increases throughout the pulmonary vascular bed

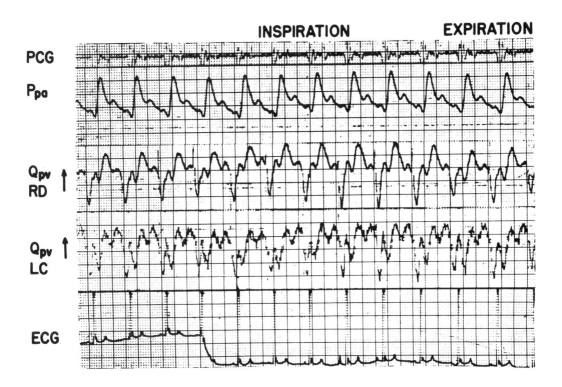

INSPIRATION   **EXPIRATION**

PCG

P$_{pa}$

Q$_{pv}$ RD

Q$_{pv}$ LC

ECG

Figure 11-1. Pulmonary venous flow waveforms recorded in an anesthetized dog with spontaneous respirations. From top to bottom: PCG = phonocardiogram, P$_{PA}$ = pulmonary arterial pressure, Q$_{PV}$ RD = pulmonary venous flow recorded in right diaphragmatic lobe, Q$_{PV}$ LC = pulmonary venous flow recorded in left cardiac lobe, ECG = electrocardiogram. Note increased peak pulmonary venous flow during inspiration.

during inspiration and blood is probably stored in both left atrium and left ventricle.

We have studied the effects of inspiration and expiration on the pulmonary circulation in two patients with valvular heart disease (Table 11-3). During inspiration CI increased slightly and pulmonary vascular pressure decreased minimally. The CBV and PBV were both greater during inspiration than expiration, again suggesting expansion of the pulmonary vascular bed during inspiration.

Forced Expiration (Valsalva)

Forced expiration, the Valsalva maneuver, is characterized by an act of closing the glottis and forcibly expiring to increase intrathoracic pressure, by blowing against a manometer to about 40 mm Hg.

In normal subjects the response of the BAm to the Valsalva maneuver may be divided into four stages: (*a*) an initial rise of BAm, (*b*) a precipitous fall in BAm and tachycardia, (*c*) a further brief fall in BAm in the immediate poststrain period, and (*d*) a rapid rise or "overshoot" of BAm and bradycardia after release of the forced intrathoracic pressure.[38,39] PAm and LAm (or Pw) both rise during the period of increased intrathoracic pressure.[33,34,40]

Considerable reduction in CO during the Valsalva maneuver was reported by two groups of workers. Elisberg and associates, employing a ballistocardiographic technique, found a 50% reduction in the control CO during the period of increased intrathoracic pressure.[41] Using the indicator-dilution technique, McIntosh and co-workers found a 47% reduction in CO during the period when the fall in BAm was maximal.[42] The reliability of either method is doubtful in the determination of CO during the Valsalva maneuver. The ballistocardiogram may be greatly distorted by the marked straining and muscular movement of the subject.[43] Determinations of CO from indicator-dilution curves recorded during the maneuver may be unreliable because of the constantly changing blood flow.[44,45]

Recently, Fox and associates estimated thoracic aortic flow before, during and after 15-second periods of Valsalva maneuver by the constant-rate injection indicator-dilution technique.[43] This is a convenient method for measuring changes in blood flow during non-steady state conditions because the results are not affected by changing blood flow. According to these authors, thoracic aortic flow comprises 45% of total CO. The mean thoracic blood flow of eight healthy subjects during the control period and during the four stages of the Valsalva maneuver were 4.2, 4.1, 1.6, 1.5 and 5.0 L/min, respectively. Thus, the thoracic aortic flow decreased to about 35% of the control flow during forced expiration and then increased to a value 19% above control during the period of "overshoot."

CBV and Vc have both been reported to diminish during the Valsalva maneuver.[19,46,47] The several contributing factors include blood volume squeezed from the thorax, a net reduction in the pulmonary vascular transmural pressure and impaired venous return to the right heart and pulmonary vessels.

We studied the effects of the Valsalva maneuver in a 19-year-old patient with idiopathic cardiomyopathy. After control measurements of pulmonary blood flow, pressures and volume, the Valsalva maneuver was performed twice, with the forced expiration kept constant at 40 mm Hg. During the first

Table 11-3 Changes in Pulmonary Blood Volume During Inspiration and Expiration

Patient	Age	Sex	BSA	Diagnosis	Condition	Blood Flow			Pressures (mm Hg)				Tm (seconds)			Blood Volume (mL/M²)	
						CI	HR	SI	PAm	LAm	P_d	BAm	PA-BA	LA-BA	PA-LA	CBV	PBV
R.Z.	22	F	1.47	MS	I	2.92	85	36	27	22	24.5	72	15.4	7.0	8.4	750	409
					E	2.82	85	35	27	24	25.5	68	15.4	7.7	7.7	724	363
M.A.	36	M	1.85	AS	I	2.65	75	35	14	10	12.0	110	15.4	8.1	7.3	680	323
					E	2.35	74	32	15	11	13.0	110	15.3	8.7	6.6	600	258

I = inspiration; E = expiration
Other symbols and abbreviations are identical to those used in Tables 11-1 and 11-2

Table 11-5 Effects of Positive Pressure Breathing on Pulmonary Blood Volume

Patient	Age	BSA	Diagnosis	FC	Condition	Blood Flow			Pressures (mm Hg)				Tm (seconds)			Blood Volume (mL/M²)	
						CI	HR	SI	PAm	LAm	P_d	BAm	PA-BA	LA-BA	PA-LA	CBV	PBV
M.T.	51	1.75	MS	III	C	1.93	108	18	40	26	33.0	130	22.2	11.3	10.9	720	352
					P	2.22	110	20	41	25	33.0	125	19.1	11.7	7.4	710	274
					C	1.77	100	18	40	28	34.0	130	19.3	—	—	550	—
M.Th.	48	1.80	MS	II	C	2.25	96	23	18	11	14.5	110	15.4	8.4	7.0	575	262
					P	2.18	100	22	18	13	15.5	100	15.2	8.1	7.1	550	258
					C	2.18	70	30	14	8	11.0	108	15.4	7.1	7.4	560	277

C = Control period
P = Period of positive pressure breathing
Other symbols and abbreviations are identical to those used in Table 11-1

Table 11-4 Effects of Forced Expiration (Valsalva Maneuver) on Pulmonary Blood Volume

Condition	CI	Tm (seconds)			Blood Volume (ml/M²)	
		PA-BA	LA-BA	PA-LA	CBV	PBV
Control						
1	3.20	11.9	5.7	6.2	634	330
2	2.95	13.0	5.9	7.1	638	347
Valsalva maneuver	1.15	18.3	10.6	7.7	345	148

The symbols and abbreviations are identical to those used in Table 11-1

trial a dilution curve was inscribed with the indicator injected into the main pulmonary artery and blood sampled from the brachial artery through a cuvette densitometer. A few minutes later, during the second trial, a dilution curve was inscribed with the indicator injected into the left atrium. The technical limitations are admittedly formidable, especially with reference to the reliability of the CO and of the Tm determinations. Nevertheless, striking reductions in CI, CBV and PBV were demonstrated (Table 11-4). The decrease in CI during the period of forced expiration was almost identical to the mean reduction reported by Fox and associates.[43]

Positive and Negative Pressure Breathing

In both closed and open chest animals positive pressure breathing causes a fall in CO and BAm.[48-50] In both animals and man, CO declines about 20% as measured by the Fick procedure or by the indicator-dilution method.[47-58] The mechanisms most commonly cited as responsible include diminished venous return to the thorax resulting from elevated intrathoracic pressures, augmented intravascular resistance, and possibly decreased force of ventricular contraction as a result of limited ventricular diastolic volume.

A substantial reduction (average 35%) in CBV accompanied the fall in CO and BAm.[55-59] This has been ex-

plained by impairment of the return of blood to the thorax resulting from a smaller pressure gradient in the absence of simultaneous interference with the outflow of blood from the thorax.

Many workers have reported an increase in pulmonary vascular resistance (PVR) during positive pressure breathing.[49,53,60] In the anesthetized dog, however, Linde found no significant change in the PVR, even though CO was reduced.[50]

Roncoroni and co-workers studied the hemodynamic effects of positive pressure breathing in normal subjects and in patients with chronic pulmonary disease.[58] PAm and PVR rose in normal subjects, with no appreciable reduction in CO. In patients with chronic pulmonary disease, however, changes in the arterial blood carbon dioxide tension apparently complicated the effects of positive pressure breathing.

Braunwald and co-workers reported that metaraminol (Aramine) elevated the reduced CBV during positive pressure breathing.[56] The beneficial effects were interpreted as the results of drug-induced enhancement of peripheral venous and arteriolar tone and myocardial contractility. Blood volume in the lung is a reciprocal function of the tone of peripheral blood vessels. Increase in peripheral vascular tone is associated with a diminished peripheral vascular volume and augmented PBV. Thus, any measure which increases peripheral vascular tone is likely to diminish depletion of the CBV during positive pressure breathing.

The effects of negative pressure breathing are opposite to those reported during positive pressure breathing. Huggett first demonstrated increased CO by an average of 37% during negative pressure breathing with inspiratory obstruction in cats.[61] Other investigators have reported similar changes in animals and man.[57,62,63]

In man, negative pressure breathing decreases intrathoracic pressure, reduces central venous pressure and augments the flow gradient from the periphery. The CBV increases only slightly, probably because pulmonary compliance decreases by as much as 50% secondary to pulmonary congestion.[64]

Kilburn and Sieker reported that continuous negative pressure breathing in normal subjects increased CO, SV and, to a lesser extent, CBV.[57] In contrast, continuous positive pressure breathing decreased both CO and CBV. If hyperventilation, either voluntary or induced by breathing 5% CO_2, accompanied positive pressure breathing, however, no significant reduction in CO, SV or CBV was observed. Thus, the diminished intrathoracic pressures resulting from hyperventilation probably facilitate the entry of blood into the central venous reservoir, counteracting the effect of positive pressure breathing. The authors concluded that decreased intrathoracic pressure is important in maintaining or increasing the volume of blood available to the heart in man, particularly during circulatory stress.

We studied 2 patients with cardiac disease during positive pressure breathing. The results are presented in Table 11-5. The CI, PAm, LAm and BAm were not notably affected. A significant decrease in the PBV was observed in 1 patient but not in the other. It is likely that the reduction of PBV during positive pressure breathing is entirely mechanical, resulting from compression of the pulmonary vascular bed.

Exercise

Many workers have studied the hemodynamic effects of exercise in normal subjects. Earlier reports by Hickam, Riley, Dexter, Donald and their respective associates have been repeatedly quoted.[25-69] Light exercise (oxygen uptake less than 400 ml/M^2/min) usually caused a small rise in the PAm, and larger increases occurred in subjects performing heavier exercise (oxygen uptake greater than 400 ml/M^2/min).

Sancetta and co-workers studied the PAm during prolonged mild steady state exercise in the recumbent position.[70] They found that the PAm rose slightly but rapidly at the start, and generally began to decline after the sixth and seventh minute of exercise. They recognized that a part of the initial pressure rise might be attributed to redistribution of blood resulting from elevation of the legs when a bicycle ergometer was employed.

Slonim and associates observed (a) a prompt rise in PAm following the abrupt start of exercise, (b) the achievement of a steady state pressure which was higher than the resting control value, and (c) a prompt fall in pressure to a level lower than the resting control value following the abrupt cessation of exercise.[71] These findings were confirmed by Barrett-Boyes and Wood.[72]

Harris and Heath noted that the difference between the PAm and pulmonary wedge pressures (PAm-Pw) tended to increase during exercise.[73]

They found that the increase in PAm-Pw was proportionately greater than the increase in pulmonary blood flow and that the calculated PVR was accordingly higher during exercise. In general, pulmonary blood flow increases appreciably during exercise depending on the severity of exertion. Donald and associates found that the PAm in normal subjects did not rise more than 30 mm Hg when the exercise CI was less than 7.9 L/M²/min.[69] Wang and associates reported that for a given person the stroke volume increases only slightly once exercise has begun, regardless of whether the person is supine or standing.[74]

Many investigators have demonstrated an increase in intrathoracic or CBV in normal subjects during exercise, using indicator-dilution technique. [75-78] The validity of using peripheral arterial sampling for the calculation of CBV during exercise has been challenged by some workers on the basis that local hyperemia and redistribution of arterial blood during exercise may cause spuriously high estimates of the Tm and CBV.[79,80] Exercise studies using aortic root sampling, however, have shown that threefold increases in CO over resting values may be associated with no significant augmentation of the calculated CBV.[79]

Utilizing precordial radioisotope dilution curves, some workers have found that exercise increases CO without increasing the CBV in the majority of normal subjects.[81,82] The precordial dilution technique is considered to approximate the conditions of aortic root sampling which may provide a more accurate estimation of central circulating blood volume than the peripheral arterial sampling technique. The blood volume so determined, however, includes the four heart chambers as well as the pulmonary vascular bed.

The responses of patients with cardiac disease to exercise were characterized by a more marked rise in the LAm, PAm and sometimes left ventricular diastolic pressure and less augmentation of the CO or pulmonary blood flow.[83-91]

Our own previous reports clearly indicate that both CBV and PBV increased during exercise in normal subjects, in patients with valvular heart disease and in those with cardiomyopathy.[92,93] We have shown that the reliability of the PBV measurement was not affected by local hyperemia and arterial blood distribution. Recent studies by Korsgren and associates also demonstrated that local hyperemia did not affect the validity of the PBV determination.[94]

In this section we present data obtained during exercise in 57 patients. Five had a functional systolic murmur and are considered normal. Forty-four had valvular heart disease and 8 myocardial or pericardial disease. Some patients reported previously are also included. The group included 37 men and 20 women, varying in age from 15 to 61 years. The patients with valvular heart disease included 8 with predominant aortic regurgitation, 8 with predominant aortic stenosis, 9 with predominant mitral regurgitation and 19 with predominant mitral stenosis. After control observations, the patients performed leg exercise in the supine position, using a bicycle ergometer. The work load was sufficient to increase oxygen consumption to two to three times the resting value. Measurements of oxygen uptake and pulmonary blood flow, pressures and volumes were repeated between the sixth and twelfth minutes of exercise. In 10 patients (3 normal subjects, 2 with aortic regurgitation, 4 with aortic stenosis and 1 with mitral stenosis), exercise was repeated with a heavier work load in order to ascertain whether the PBV could be further augmented. The results are summarized in Tables 11-6 to 11-11.

A statistically significant increase in oxygen uptake and CI occurred in all groups. The increase in the average oxygen uptake during exercise varied from 3.6 times the resting control values in normal subjects to 1.9 times control in patients with myocardial or pericardial disease. The average increase in CI during exercise varied from 40% of the control value in patients with predominant mitral stenosis to 62% of the resting value in those with predominant aortic regurgitation (Figure 11-2). The average SI did not change appreciably in any group. Thus, the augmented CI was achieved almost entirely by increases in the HR.

In normal subjects and in patients with predominant aortic regurgitation, a slight to moderate rise in PAm was associated with a slightly decreased LAm. The increase in the pulmonary distending pressure (P_d) was slight and statistically insignificant. The only exception in the aortic regurgitation group was patient T.M., who had resting LAm and PAm of 21 and 32 mm Hg respectively. During exercise the LAm rose to 29 mm Hg and the PAm to 47 mm Hg. In patients with predominant aortic stenosis, in those with mitral valve disease, and in those with either myocardial or pericardial disease, PAm, LAm and P_d all rose significantly. The increase was particularly pronounced in patients with predominant mitral stenosis or predominant aortic stenosis.

The BAm rose during exercise in all groups, and the increase was statistically significant in all but the normal group.

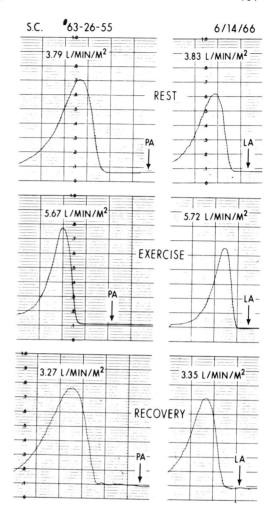

Figure 11-2. Indicator-dilution curves inscribed respectively from injections into the pulmonary artery and left atrium at rest, during exercise and during recovery in a patient with mild aortic regurgitation. Note the substantial increase in the cardiac index during exercise.

The increased rate of blood flow resulted in a uniform decrease in the mean transit times from the pulmonary artery to the systemic artery $Tm_{(PA-BA)}$, from the left atrium to the systemic artery $Tm_{(LA-BA)}$, and from the pulmonary artery to the left atrium $Tm_{(PA-LA)}$. These reductions were

(*Text Continued p. 138*)

10

Table 11-6   Changes in Hemodynamics and Pulmonary Blood Volume During Exercise in Normal Subjects

Patient	Age	Sex	BSA	Condition	$\dot{V}_{O_2}$	Blood Flow		Pressures (mm Hg)				Tm (seconds)			Blood Volume (ml M²)	
						CI	SI	PAm	LAm	P_d	BAm	PA-BA	LA-BA	PA-LA	CBV	PBV
R.C.	23	M	1.91	R	125	3.76	45	12	8	10.0	96	9.8	5.1	4.7	614	296
				E	534	5.53	46	13	6	9.5	100	8.0	4.5	3.5	737	323
				R'	170	3.49	45	10	6	8.0	92	10.9	4.7	6.2	634	361
				E'	624	6.60	49	16	5	10.5	108	9.2	4.5	4.7	1010	516
L.W.	15	M	1.98	R	135	3.22	46	12	9	10.5	96	8.2	4.4	3.8	440	204
				E	717	6.02	35	14	4	9.0	92	6.3	3.1	3.2	630	320
J.B.	20	F	1.77	R	113	3.36	37	13	8	10.5	70	8.6	4.3	4.3	481	241
				E	365	4.18	40	17	5	11.0	80	6.8	3.6	3.2	474	223
				R'	141	3.27	36	14	9	11.5	74	9.8	4.8	5.0	534	272
				E'	488	5.35	42	17	9	13.0	90	7.6	3.9	3.7	674	334
G.G.	23	M	1.74	R	136	4.04	47	15	10	12.5	80	10.8	6.1	4.7	728	269
				E	404	5.71	46	21	8	12.5	107	9.7	5.2	4.5	922	428
D.G.	17	M	1.86	R	139	3.56	58	17	12	14.5	90	10.9	4.8	5.5	601	321
				E	346	5.00	50	20	10	15.0	110	7.9	4.0	3.9	658	320
				R'	135	3.38	48	18	13	15.5	105	10.0	4.6	5.4	563	306
				E'	411	6.11	47	20	12	16.0	125	6.5	3.0	3.5	662	357
Control mean					137	3.51	45.3	13.9	9.4	11.6	87.9	9.9	4.9	5.0	574	284
±S.E.					±5.7	±0.10	±2.42	±0.95	±0.80	±0.87	±4.27	±0.36	±0.20	±0.27	±32.2	±17.2
Exercise mean					486	5.56	44.4	17.3	7.4	12.3	101.5	7.8	4.0	3.8	721	353
±S.E.					±46.5	±0.26	±1.78	±1.03	±1.00	±0.94	±4.97	±0.43	±0.26	±0.20	±60.2	±30.6
p value					<0.01	<0.01	N.S.	<0.02	<0.05	N.S.	<0.10	<0.01	<0.01	<0.02	<0.05	<0.20

R = first control period;
R' = second control period;
E = first exercise period;

E' = second exercise period;
$\dot{V}_{O_2}$ = oxynen uptake (ml/M₂/min);
N.S. = not sinnificant

Unless otherwise indicated, in this and the subsequent five tables the symbols and abbreviations are identical to those used in Table 11-1

Table 11-7 Changes in Hemodynamics and Pulmonary Blood Volume During Exercise in Patients with Predominant Aortic Regurgitation

Patient	Age	Sex	BSA	FC	Condition	$\dot{V}O_2$	Blood Flow CI	SI	Pressures (mm Hg) PAm	LAm	P_d	BAm	Tm (seconds) PA-BA	LA-BA	PA-LA	Blood Volume (mL/M²) CBV	PBV
S.S.	44	M	2.02	II	R	122	2.68	42	8	5	7.5	84	17.4	10.0	7.4	780	330
					E	267	4.26	55	15	6	10.5	100	12.6	6.6	6.0	895	426
E.K.	17	M	1.87	I	R	171	3.38	55	13	8	10.5	110	11.2	5.5	5.7	635	326
					E	450	4.83	49	14	7	10.5	135	8.6	4.4	4.2	690	338
R.Ha.	29	M	1.88	II	R	157	3.41	42	15	7	11.0	105	14.1	7.7	6.4	800	364
					E	264	4.60	43	18	7	12.5	115	10.6	4.7	5.9	815	450
					R'	147	2.75	30	10	4	7.0	115	16.1	10.1	6.0	740	270
					E'	439	5.01	38	18	5	11.5	110	10.2	6.1	4.1	850	342
J.G.	43	M	2.03	II	R	146	2.73	32	16	6	11.0	103	13.0	8.4	4.6	590	208
					E	415	3.84	35	18	7	12.5	120	11.0	6.5	4.5	700	288
R.V.	32	M	1.91	II	R	162	3.10	38	16	10	13.0	104	18.5	11.3	7.2	955	375
					E	365	5.78	58	26	12	19.0	156	13.1	7.3	5.8	1270	555
D.K.	30	M	2.16	II	R	160	2.68	36	17	13	15.0	90	16.2	9.2	7.2	724	321
					E	341	5.00	46	20	13	16.5	115	10.7	6.1	4.6	890	385
					R'	155	2.93	37	14	10	12.0	80	15.8	9.5	6.3	772	308
					E'	461	5.55	48	19	10	14.5	105	9.9	5.5	4.4	926	407
J.T.	16	M	1.85	II	R	156	3.94	72	19	10	14.5	110	13.2	7.2	6.0	868	394
					E	454	6.74	64	23	9	16.0	120	8.7	5.4	3.3	978	371
T.M.	36	M	2.30	III	R	177	2.76	27	32	21	26.5	100	23.0	15.9	7.1	1050	330
					E	330	3.83	29	47	29	38.0	120	19.7	12.9	6.8	1240	430
Control mean						155	3.04	41.1	16.0	9.4	12.8	100.1	15.9	9.5	6.4	792	323
±S.E.						±4.8	±0.13	±4.23	±2.05	±1.55	±1.73	±3.70	±1.06	±0.89	±0.28	±43.8	±16.9
Exercise mean						379	4.94	46.5	21.8	10.5	16.2	119.6	11.5	6.6	5.0	925	399
±S.E.						±24.1	±0.29	±3.40	±3.01	±2.21	±2.58	±5.05	±1.02	±0.76	±0.35	±62.1	±23.3
p value						<0.01	<0.01	N.S.	<0.02	N.S.	<0.05	<0.01	<0.01	<0.01	<0.01	<0.01	<0.01

TABLE 11-8 Changes in Hemodynamics and Pulmonary Blood Volume During Exercise in Patients with Predominant Aortic Stenosis

Patient	Age	Sex	BSA	FC	Condition	V̇o₂	Blood Flow		Pressures (mm Hg)				Tm (seconds)			Blood Volume (ml/M²)	
							CI	SI	PAm	LAm	P_d	BAm	PA-BA	LA-BA	PA-LA	CBV	PBV
W.S.	43	M	2.17	II	R	110	1.73	26	7	3	5.0	90	18.9	11.9	7.0	545	202
					E	260	3.04	33	16	6	11.0	98	13.8	8.1	5.7	698	286
F.W.	44	M	2.12	I	R	138	2.33	31	10	6	8.0	100	16.3	10.1	6.2	630	230
					E	312	3.36	32	18	11	14.5	136	12.1	7.7	4.4	680	247
J.S.	56	M	1.70	II	R	160	3.54	54	13	6	9.5	84	14.7	7.9	6.8	866	401
					E	375	5.51	64	22	14	18.5	100	12.1	7.5	4.6	1110	423
					R'	130	3.52	53	12	8	10.0	88	14.9	8.6	6.3	876	370
					E'	634	5.58	60	28	20	24.0	102	11.2	6.1	5.1	1055	468
A.Bu.	18	F	1.81	II	R	132	3.95	49	16	12	14.0	96	11.5	6.2	5.3	758	349
					E	585	7.25	52	30	20	25.0	108	7.6	3.0	4.6	918	559
					R'	160	3.96	49	16	12	14.0	100	11.3	5.6	5.7	750	378
					E'	737	6.62	47	30	16	23.0	112	7.5	3.5	4.0	827	441
C.W.	53	M	1.92	II	R	127	2.43	40	18	12	15.0	100	12.4	7.5	4.9	502	198
					E	396	3.20	34	33	24	28.5	124	10.8	6.0	4.8	576	256
					R'	105	2.02	36	18	14	16.0	104	12.3	7.3	5.0	412	168
					E'	548	4.14	37	44	40	42.0	124	10.5	5.7	4.8	725	331
V.M.	58	M	2.09	II	R	167	2.26	27	21	11	16.0	98	22.4	11.4	11.0	866	414
					E	299	2.90	28	48	38	43.0	102	20.7	11.8	8.9	900	430
R.Hu.	44	M	1.84	II	R	93	2.89	36	21	13	17.0	98	11.0	6.1	4.9	530	224
					E	214	4.34	41	26	13	19.5	118	8.9	5.5	3.4	642	245
					R'	—	2.80	34	16	8	12.0	110	11.7	6.8	4.9	550	228
					E'	401	4.08	34	22	8	15.0	120	8.9	5.5	3.4	604	235
W.L.	57	M	1.74	II	R	137	2.09	33	23	14	18.5	85	24.4	17.8	6.6	850	230
					E	290	3.00	35	40	23	31.5	100	19.2	13.0	6.2	970	310
Control mean						133	2.79	39.0	15.9	9.9	12.9	96.1	15.2	8.9	6.2	678	284
±S.E.						±7.1	±0.22	±2.86	±1.37	±1.04	±1.17	±2.09	±1.21	±0.92	±0.45	±44.7	±24.0
Exercise mean						423	4.22	41.4	29.8	19.8	24.6	112.0	11.9	6.9	5.0	809	353
±S.E.						±52.5	±0.43	±3.38	±2.91	±3.17	±2.95	±3.27	±1.11	±0.79	±0.39	±47.9	±28.6
p value						<0.01	<0.02	N.S.	<0.01	<0.01	<0.01	<0.01	<0.01	<0.02	<0.01	<0.01	<0.05

Table 11-9 Changes in Hemodynamics and Pulmonary Blood Volume During Exercise in Patients with Predominant Mitral Regurgitation.

Patient	Age	Sex	BSA	FC	Condition	$\dot{V}o_2$	Blood Flow		Pressures (mm Hg)				Tm (seconds)			Blood Volume (mL/M²)	
							CI	SI	PAm	LAm	P_d	BAm	PA-BA	LA-BA	PA-LA	CBV	PBV
S.C.	26	M	1.82	II	R	112	3.81	46	12	8	10.0	93	13.6	7.8	5.8	864	369
					E	426	5.70	36	21	13	17.0	112	9.7	5.1	4.6	915	438
D.B.	47	F	1.72	II	R	188	2.77	42	13	7	10.0	90	13.1	8.5	4.6	606	211
					E	342	3.48	32	20	12	16.0	110	11.6	6.7	4.9	675	286
E.McK.	45	M	1.74	II	R	152	1.81	21	17	7	12.0	105	28.0	20.4	7.6	846	230
					E	426	3.16	29	30	12	21.0	120	20.1	13.7	6.4	1060	336
E.P.	56	M	1.87	II	R	118	2.60	30	18	10	14.0	110	27.6	22.4	5.2	1190	226
					E	275	4.83	44	42	30	36.0	115	24.0	18.4	5.6	1940	453
J.R.	46	M	1.88	II	R	152	2.70	33	22	14	18.0	88	12.4	6.9	5.5	558	248
					E	440	4.50	49	40	30	35.0	108	10.3	5.7	4.6	775	345
F.W.	51	M	1.78	II	R	120	2.70	23	23	14	18.5	100	17.5	11.9	5.6	789	254
					E	180	3.60	28	33	23	28.0	114	13.9	7.3	6.6	833	386
K.G.	40	F	1.59	II	R	166	2.10	24	23	15	19.0	88	21.4	10.8	10.6	750	372
					E	324	2.72	30	38	30	34.0	104	19.9	8.7	11.2	900	500
H.F.	54	F	1.70	III	R	126	2.70	31	35	18	26.5	103	13.2	8.2	5.0	596	226
					E	344	3.40	26	60	26	43.0	133	11.1	6.7	4.4	634	308
B.A.	54	F	1.91	III	R	178	2.94	37	42	28	35.0	95	19.1	13.0	5.9	940	290
					E	490	4.56	34	68	34	51.0	110	12.0	6.8	5.2	920	396
Control mean ±S.E.						140 ±7.7	2.68 ±0.18	31.9 ±2.87	22.8 ±3.31	13.4 ±2.24	18.1 ±2.74	96.9 ±2.66	18.4 ±2.05	12.2 ±1.87	6.2 ±0.62	793 ±66.5	269 ±20.5
Exercise mean ±S.E.						361 ±31.9	3.99 ±0.32	34.2 ±2.56	39.1 ±5.39	23.3 ±2.93	31.2 ±3.95	114.0 ±2.81	14.7 ±1.74	8.8 ±1.47	5.9 ±0.71	961 ±130.0	383 ±23.7
p value						<0.01	<0.01	N.S.	<0.01	<0.01	<0.01	<0.01	<0.05	<0.01	N.S.	<0.10	<0.01

Table 11-10　Changes in Hemodynamics and Pulmonary Blood Volume During Exercise in Patients with Predominant Mitral Stenosis

Patient	Age	Sex	BSA	FC	Condition	$\dot{V}o_2$	Blood Flow		Pressures (mm Hg)				Tm (seconds)			Blood Volume (ml/M²)	
							CI	SI	PAm	LAm	P_d	BAm	PA-BA	LA-BA	PA-LA	CBV	PBV
J.I.	39	F	1.65	II	R	150	1.65	29	14	7	10.5	85	14.8	7.0	7.8	407	192
					E	220	2.24	26	18	12	15.0	95	11.7	5.4	6.3	437	202
M.I.	48	F	1.97	II	R	134	2.13	30	14	8	11.0	110	15.4	7.7	7.7	550	275
					E	248	3.15	26	30	22	26.0	120	14.0	7.3	6.7	740	352
G.B.	33	F	1.64	II	R	124	2.90	29	16	10	13.0	104	10.8	6.2	4.6	524	222
					E	305	4.00	33	32	18	25.0	130	10.2	5.3	4.9	684	328
M.B.	45	F	1.62	II	R	113	2.13	21	17	12	14.5	85	14.3	8.0	6.3	510	224
					E	313	2.65	29	21	16	18.5	85	12.6	6.4	6.2	558	274
C.C.	37	F	1.79	II	R	130	2.94	36	20	13	16.5	90	12.1	7.1	5.0	610	246
					E	350	4.48	39	30	20	25.0	92	10.6	5.6	5.0	800	372
S.F.	47	M	1.78	II	R	121	2.28	38	30	15	17.5	90	14.6	7.6	7.0	700	336
					E	216	3.88	35	33	27	30.0	110	12.8	7.1	5.7	810	370
G.C.	43	F	1.66	II	R	105	2.14	29	22	16	19.0	100	15.8	6.0	9.8	564	349
					E	361	3.96	36	55	40	47.5	115	12.1	5.4	6.7	798	441
E.C.	45	F	1.50	III	R	125	2.22	28	24	15	19.5	85	19.8	10.9	8.9	732	330
					E	214	2.37	21	40	23	31.5	90	19.1	9.3	9.8	755	386
M.P.	40	M	1.58	III	R	105	1.99	22	25	22	23.5	90	15.1	8.0	7.1	505	236
					E	309	3.18	18	42	30	36.0	125	11.6	5.9	5.7	616	302
H.C.	39	M	1.82	III	R	145	2.09	26	26	20	23.0	108	20.0	12.1	7.9	695	275
					E	288	2.91	29	59	34	46.5	108	16.7	8.7	8.0	810	388
J.Sm.	51	F	1.46	III	R	100	2.20	35	27	18	22.5	100	17.0	9.6	7.4	625	272
					E	225	2.70	30	42	37	39.5	105	14.5	7.9	6.6	658	297
G.H.	53	M	1.74	III	R	104	1.50	27	27	24	25.5	95	28.3	16.7	11.6	710	292
					E	195	1.83	33	32	26	29.0	100	23.5	12.9	10.6	720	325
E.G.	40	M	1.67	III	R	128	2.11	21	28	18	23.0	77	19.7	9.9	9.8	693	345
					E	366	2.63	20	42	27	34.5	85	17.1	8.3	8.8	750	386
J.Ra.	29	F	1.50	III	R	164	2.75	30	30	12	21.0	88	12.6	5.6	7.0	580	324
					E	255	4.20	35	41	30	35.5	100	12.5	6.1	6.4	870	445
G.F.	50	F	1.70	III	R	126	2.85	38	32	14	23.0	90	14.8	8.5	6.3	695	300
					E	310	4.30	38	60	34	47.0	120	10.6	5.4	4.6	760	331
A.B.	51	M	1.72	III	R	171	1.81	20	32	17	24.5	105	23.2	11.5	11.7	703	354
					E	394	1.98	11	65	38	51.5	105	26.2	9.4	16.8	844	534
R.H.	33	M	1.90	III	R	190	2.15	24	34	20	27.0	118	20.4	9.2	11.2	726	398
					E	440	3.42	21	64	46	55.0	124	17.0	7.2	9.8	969	558
					R'	181	3.05	36	36	24	30.0	118	17.7	11.5	6.2	894	315
					E'	509	4.09	22	88	60	74.0	126	14.1	5.6	8.5	954	580
N.G.	37	F	1.79	III	R	111	2.42	30	35	25	30.0	80	14.4	7.8	6.6	590	252
					E	262	2.98	30	46	30	38.0	100	13.7	7.7	6.0	680	298
M.Ti.	51	F	1.75	III	R	144	1.80	19	40	28	34.0	130	18.3	10.2	8.1	552	243
					E	267	2.50	24	55	32	43.5	130	17.6	9.7	7.9	695	329
Control mean						133	2.26	28.4	26.0	16.9	21.4	97.4	17.0	9.1	7.9	628	289
±S.E.						±5.9	±0.10	±1.35	±1.70	±1.30	±1.43	±3.16	±0.92	±0.59	±0.46	±24.6	±12.1
Exercise mean						302	3.17	27.8	44.8	30.1	37.4	108.3	14.9	7.3	7.6	745	375
±S.E.						±18.3	±0.18	±1.66	±3.82	±2.47	±3.09	±3.32	±0.95	±0.44	±0.62	±28.1	±21.6
p value						<0.01	<0.01	N.S.	<0.01	<0.01	<0.01	<0.01	<0.01	<0.01	N.S.	<0.01	<0.01

TABLE 11-11   Changes in Hemodynamics and Pulmonary Blood Volume During Exercise in Patients with Myocardial or Pericardial Disease

Patient	Age	Sex	BSA	Diagnosis	FC	Condition	$\dot{V}o_2$	Blood Flow		Pressures (mm Hg)				Tm (seconds)			Blood Volume (mL/M²)	
								CI	SI	PAm	LAm	P_d	BAm	PA-BA	LA-BA	PA-LA	CBV	PBV
H.C.	29	M	2.05	IC	II	R	130	2.42	28	15	7	11.0	90	16.6	10.9	5.7	672	232
						E	225	3.35	35	20	8	14.0	100	13.3	8.9	4.4	755	246
A.O.	61	M	1.83	IC	II	R	151	2.18	36	17	6	11.5	85	14.7	8.5	6.2	534	225
						E	321	3.22	40	27	9	18.0	—	12.3	7.0	5.3	662	285
M.De.	57	M	1.48	IC	II	R	172	1.96	23	17	9	13.0	86	22.1	9.7	12.4	730	400
						E	270	3.15	23	31	19	25.0	91	17.4	9.7	7.7	920	406
H.Be.	54	M	1.94	CD	II	R	122	3.69	35	19	13	16.0	120	12.1	6.7	5.4	746	332
						E	393	5.58	39	25	19	22.0	140	9.9	5.2	4.7	920	438
M.A.	68	M	1.82	CD	II	R	—	2.00	30	20	14	17.0	86	20.0	10.8	9.2	666	308
						E	—	2.55	32	26	20	23.0	103	16.0	8.5	7.5	690	318
R.F.	36	M	1.89	IC	III	R	196	2.10	15	28	24	26.0	96	18.2	9.3	8.9	637	312
						E	294	3.15	21	45	42	43.5	120	14.7	7.8	6.9	775	361
L.V.	51	F	1.57	PE	II	R	122	2.35	28	18	8	13.0	93	8.8	4.7	4.1	543	254
						E	246	3.74	29	28	9	18.5	110	6.8	3.6	3.2	610	273
I.K.	41	F	1.56	CP	II	R	125	3.38	47	21	16	18.5	99	14.1	9.4	4.7	890	298
						E	226	5.12	51	30	26	28.0	148	12.0	8.2	3.8	1020	325
Control	mean						145	2.51	30.3	19.4	12.1	15.8	95.7	15.8	8.8	7.1	677	295
	±S.E.						±11.0	±0.23	±3.36	±1.40	±2.12	±1.74	±4.44	±1.53	±0.75	±1.00	±40.8	±20.5
Exercise	mean						282	3.71	33.8	29.0	19.0	24.0	116.0	12.8	7.4	5.4	794	332
	±S.E.						±22.8	±0.37	±3.46	±2.58	±4.01	±3.19	±8.02	±1.20	±0.72	±0.61	±51.2	±23.5
	p value						<0.01	<0.01	<0.05	<0.01	<0.01	<0.01	<0.05	<0.01	<0.02	<0.02	<0.01	<0.02

IC = idiopathic cardiomyopathy;   CD = coronary artery disease;   PE = pericardial effusion;
CP = constrictive pericarditis

statistically significant in all groups with the single exception of Tm_{PA-LA} in patients with mitral valve disease.

During exercise CBV increased significantly in all groups with the exception of patients with predominant mitral regurgitation. Similarly, the increase in PBV was statistically significant in all groups except for the normal subjects. The increase in CBV varied between 117 and 148 ml/M², and the increase in PBV ranged from 37 to 114 ml/M².

During exercise a definite hemodynamic disadvantage was evident in patients with valvular obstruction or left ventricular impairment, compared to normal subjects and to those with a compliant left ventricle. First, work performance and ability to increase CO were reduced. Second, with less increase in pulmonary blood flow and an almost equal augmentation of PBV, the P_d elevation was greater, suggesting decreased distensibility of the pulmonary vascular bed. This topic is discussed in detail in Chapter 17.

Recent studies of changes in extravascular volume during exercise by Varnauskas and associates deserve special comment.[95] They studied pulmonary intravascular and extravascular volumes during exercise in a group of patients with mitral valve disease. PBV was determined by the double injection indicator-dilution technique and the extravascular volume was estimated by a method employing diffusible tritiated water (THO). These patients had elevated LAm and larger than normal extravascular water volumes at rest. With exercise, extravascular water accumulated further. Although any possible relationship between the pulmonary intravascular and extravascular fluid volumes is unclear, the accumulation of a large amount of water in the extravascular space would reduce the compliance of pulmonary vessel walls themselves or compress the vessels by large extravascular sheaths of fluid. Thus, excessive water in the perivascular space may increase pulmonary vascular resistance and may also alter the pressure-volume relationships of the pulmonary vessels.

Vasodepressor Reactions

The monograph entitled "*Fainting*" by Engel is an excellent source of information and references concerning the vasodepressor reaction.[96] Clinically, the vasodepressor reaction is characterized by pallor, profound weakness, diaphoresis, nausea, retching and sometimes syncope. In 1932 Lewis first described bradycardia and hypotension as important features of the vasodepressor reaction.[97] Subsequent reports by other workers also documented consistent bradycardia and arterial hypotension in association with frequent syncope.[98-101] Some investigators have found an increase in blood flow to the skeletal muscles during such syncope, despite the fall in BAm.

We reported pulmonary blood flow, pressures and volume in 2 patients with predominant mitral stenosis who developed vasodepressor reactions during combined right and transseptal left heart catheterization.[92] The data are presented in Table 11-12. A significant decline occurred in CI, HR, pressures in both pulmonary and systemic circuits, and CBV and PBV. In patient E.S., the PBV decreased from 402 to 242 ml/M² while the P_d declined from 18.5 to 10.0 mm Hg. In patient K.V., the PBV and P_d declined from 285 to 247 ml/M² and from 34.0 to 14.0 mm Hg respectively.

Subsequently, we have reported hemodynamic changes during the vaso-

Table 11-12 Effects of Vasodepressor Reactions on Pulmonary Blood Volume

Patient	Age Sex	BSA	Diagnosis	FC	Condition	Blood Flow			Pressures (mm Hg)				Tm (seconds)			Blood Volume (ml/M²)	
						CI	HR	SI	PAm	LAm	P_d	BAm	PA-BA	LA-BA	PB-LA	CBV	PBV
E.S.	46 F	1.50	MS	I	C	4.30	128	34	26	11	18.5	84	9.8	4.2	5.6	704	402
					V	2.30	60	38	16	4	10.0	42	14.2	7.9	6.3	546	242
K.V.	23 F	1.50	MS	II	C	4.50	62	72	36	32	34.0	100	9.2	5.4	3.8	692	285
					V	3.40	48	70	15	13	14.0	54	10.0	4.8	5.2	571	247

C = Control period
V = Period of vasodepressor reactions
Other symbols and abbreviations are identical to those used in Table 11-1

Table 11-14 Hemodynamic Responses to Prolonged Period of Hypoxia and Phlebotomy

Patient	Diagnosis	Age Sex	BSA	Condition	Amount of Blood Removed (ml)	Sa_{O_2}	CI	SI	Pressures (mm Hg)				Tm (sec.)			Blood Volume (ml/M²)	
									PAm	LAm	P_d	BAm	PA-BA	LA-BA	PA-LA	CBV	PBV
J.H.	MR AS	41 M	2.20	C	400	92.4	2.40	28	10	5	7.5	94	20.9	12.3	8.6	840	343
				H(16)		74.0	2.27	28	8	4	6.0	92	18.7	10.4	8.3	710	315
J.B.	MR AR	30 F	1.44	C	350	89.5	2.77	29	20	12	16.0	108	14.3	8.5	5.8	665	267
				H(16)		76.5	2.87	48	13	7	10.0	60	11.4	7.6	3.8	546	182
S.F.	MS	44 M	1.74	C	450	94.8	2.93	34	20	12	16.0	92	10.4	6.0	4.4	510	215
				H(19)		76.0	2.23	32	12	10	11.0	59	11.6	5.5	6.1	432	227
L.M.	MR MS	52 M	1.65	C	480	92.0	2.20	37	30	20	25.0	96	21.1	12.7	8.4	778	310
				H(22)		79.9	1.83	33	28	15	21.5	60	20.0	11.9	8.1	610	247

C = control period; H = period of acute hypoxia and phlebotomy
Figures in parentheses denote duration of hypoxia in minutes
Sa_{O_2} = arterial blood oxygen saturation (%)
Other symbols and abbreviations are identical to those used in Table 11-1

depressor reaction occurring at the time of cardiac catheterization in 13 patients with various types of cardiac disease.[103] The average per cent decrease in the various parameters during vaso-depressor reaction compared with those during the control period were as follows: CI 24%, HR 38%, BAm 40%, PAm 31%, Pw or LAm 31%, total systemic resistance 24%, and PVR 52%. Changes in SI were variable and did not appear to be the primary mechanism producing hypotension.

The derangements observed in vasodepressor reactions are complex and interdependent. The heart, arteries, and veins can all be implicated. During a vasodepressor reaction CI decreased and HR slowed uniformly with or without accompanying cardiac arrhythmias. Ventricular function itself may also be compromised.[104] A *sine qua non* for the vasodepressor reaction is a fall in BAm resulting from the combined effects of a decline in CI and a decrease in total systemic resistance. Venous vasomotion is also probably important.[105-111] Venoconstriction ordinarily enhances venous return and CI. During the vasodepressor reaction, however, impairment of venoconstriction and venous return may precipitate or contribute to hypotension and syncope.

The concomitant reduction in the PAm, LAm and PBV were interpreted as a passive result of decreased resistance, vasodilatation and pooling of blood in the systemic circulation. In other words, pulmonary blood shifted towards the periphery as a result of decreased peripheral vascular tone.

We have postulated that the factor initiating the vasodepressor reaction may be an acute rise in blood pressure and in pulse pressure in the barore-ceptors.[103] This stimulation of the baroreceptors provokes generalized sympathetic inhibition resulting in un-masking and intensification of vagal action.[112] In some cases stimulation of the sympatho-inhibitory areas of the limbic cortex, as a consequence of emotional distress, may contribute to precipitation of the vasodepressor reaction in susceptible persons.[113] All these changes result in bradycardia, arteriolar dilatation and venodilatation, which in turn cause a decrease in CO, a fall in total systemic resistance, hypotension and the classical clinical expression of the vasodepressor reaction.

Respiratory Gases

Low Oxygen. The reader is referred to excellent reviews by Fishman,[114,115] and by Aviado,[116] who have extensively and admirably discussed the hemodynamic effects of acute hypoxia. Up-to-date material is also available in the recently published *Proceedings of the International Symposium on the Cardiovascular and Respiratory Effects of Hypoxia.*[117]

In 1946 Von Euler and Liljestrand reported a rise in PAm during inhalation of low oxygen concentrations in intact anesthetized cats.[118] According to these authors the elevated PAm was a manifestation of pulmonary vaso-constriction resulting from a direct effect of hypoxia on the walls of the vessels. In 1948 Liljestrand stated that the rise in PAm did not depend upon an increase in pulmonary blood flow, back pressure from the left atrium, or nervous control of the lung vessels.[119] Subsequently, other workers also have reported pulmonary pressor effects from acute anoxia in animals.[120-131]

The pulmonary hemodynamic effects of acute hypoxia in man were first reported by Motley and co-workers,[132] and many similar studies have followed.[92,133-139] The pertinent effects of acute hypoxia include a rise in PAm in the absence of corresponding change in Pw or LAm, a modest increase or no change in CO, unaltered CBV, and some increase in calculated PVR. Acute hypoxic pulmonary hypertension has been considered a manifestation of pulmonary vasoconstriction because of (a) a disproportionate increase in the PAm-LAm gradient in relation to the pulmonary blood flow, [133,134,139] (b) diversion of the pulmonary blood flow from hypoxic lung to well-oxygenated lung,[140,141] and (c) pulmonary vasodilatation produced by acetylcholine administration during acute hypoxia.[139,142]

Although the pulmonary arterial pressor response to acute hypoxia was not predominantly related to the action of catecholamines,[143] the effect of hydrogen ion concentration on the response of PAm to acute hypoxia has been recently emphasized.[144-149] At low hydrogen ion concentrations (high pH), the PAm is relatively insensitive to hypoxia, whereas at high hydrogen ion concentrations (low pH), the PAm is extremely sensitive to hypoxia.

The intensity of the response of PAm to acute hypoxia is also related to the oxygen tension.[148] In newborn calves the rise in PAm was small when the alveolar pO_2 was 40 mm Hg or greater. When the pO_2 was lower (20 to 30 mm Hg), elevation of the PAm was marked and precipitous.

In our laboratory the effects of acute hypoxia were studied in 18 patients with cardiac disease (7 with mitral valve disease, 9 with aortic valve disease, and 2 with idiopathic cardiomyopathy). The group included 10 men and 8 women, and their ages ranged from 17 to 54 years. After control studies the inspired gas was changed from room air to 12% oxygen

in nitrogen delivered through an anesthesia bag and a three-way respiratory stopcock. The duration of hypoxia varied from 10 to 15 minutes, during which all the measurements of pulmonary blood flow, pressures and volume were repeated.

The effects of hypoxia are listed in Table 11-13. The average arterial oxygen saturation was 94.2% during the control period and 72.5% during hypoxia. The change was statistically significant. Neither the percentage nor the absolute change in arterial blood oxygen saturation correlated significantly with changes in CI, HR, SI and PAm.

The CI increased more than 11% in 9 cases, decreased in 1 and was unchanged in 8. The average increase in the CI from 2.67 $L/M^2/min$ to 3.03 $L/M^2/min$ was statistically significant. The average HR rose by eight beats per minute, and again the change was significant. The stroke index was not affected, however.

The PAm increased in all but 1 patient, but only by 5 mm Hg or less in 10 of 17 cases. The average PAm rose from 18.6 to 24.4 mm Hg, and the increase was statistically significant. No appreciable change in either the LAm or BAm was observed. In 5 patients in whom the Pw and LAm were recorded simultaneously, the difference between the two did not exceed 2 mm Hg (Figure 11-3). The Pw was slightly higher than the LAm in 2 patients, and the opposite relationship was observed in the other 3.

In most patients the $Tm_{(PA-BA)}$ and $Tm_{(LA-BA)}$ were shortened, and the changes were statistically significant. The $Tm_{(PA-LA)}$ was also reduced significantly from 7.1 second to 5.1 second. The average CBV decreased from 632 to 593 ml/M^2 and the average PBV declined from 288 to 238 ml/M^2.

Table 11-13   Effects of Acute Hypoxia in Valvular Heart Disease and Cardiomyopathy

Patient	Diagnosis	Age Sex	BSA	Condition	Sa_{O_2}	CI	HR	SI	Pressures (mm Hg)				Tm (sec.)			Blood Volume (mL/M²)	
									PAm	LAm	P_d	BAm	PA-BA	LA-BA	PA-LA	CBV	PBV
P.H.	MS	37 F	1.57	C	92.9	2.56	65	39	10	6	8.0	88	12.8	7.3	5.5	546	234
				H	69.5	3.11	76	41	14	6	10.0	82	10.0	6.4	3.6	516	186
W.H.	MR	44 M	2.02	C	—	3.00	58	52	14	8	11.0	98	13.0	7.1	5.9	650	296
				H	—	3.30	75	44	19	5	12.0	85	10.8	6.4	4.4	615	250
C.T.	MS	29 F	1.86	C	96.7	1.83	80	23	20	13	16.5	94	18.7	10.7	8.0	575	245
	TS			H	81.3	2.08	99	21	26	14	20.0	96	16.3	10.1	6.2	565	215
S.F.	MS	44 M	1.74	C	94.6	2.93	86	34	20	12	16.0	92	10.4	6.0	4.4	510	248
				H	78.8	3.39	97	35	32	24	23.0	100	10.0	5.6	4.4	565	400
E.R.	MR	51 M	1.72	C	96.9	1.73	69	25	22	14	18.0	80	30.2	16.3	13.9	880	214
				H	72.2	1.86	77	24	36	14	25.0	100	23.6	16.7	6.9	730	286
S.C.	MS	54 F	1.52	C	95.7	2.56	100	22	28	16	22.0	100	13.0	6.3	6.7	555	211
				H	84.2	2.54	108	22	30	15	22.5	84	11.4	6.3	5.1	470	258
B.M.	MS	26 M	1.68	C	88.3	1.60	76	21	44	18	31.0	68	21.7	12.0	9.7	580	242
				H	76.6	1.57	87	18	60	24	42.0	64	22.6	13.4	9.2	590	360
C.H.	AR	36 M	1.79	C	93.9	3.04	64	47	9	5	7.0	84	13.4	6.3	7.1	668	240
				H	56.1	4.23	78	54	12	5	8.5	66	8.8	5.4	3.4	624	307
P.L.	AR	27 M	1.88	C	98.6	2.17	98	22	11	2	6.5	77	18.2	9.7	8.5	660	237
				H	77.5	2.84	105	27	14	2	8.0	69	15.0	10.0	5.0	710	278
H.B.	AR	17 F	1.47	C	95.1	2.92	100	29	12	4	8.0	—	13.8	8.1	5.7	674	200
				H	60.8	3.55	98	36	18	4	11.0	—	9.4	6.0	3.4	558	328
M.M.	AS	47 F	1.73	C	93.7	3.51	80	44	14	8	11.0	83	12.4	6.8	5.6	713	328
	AR			H	82.6	4.07	80	51	14	6	10.0	88	10.1	5.3	4.8	690	169
A.F.	AS	39 F	1.61	C	95.4	2.20	71	31	15	9	12.0	82	13.4	8.8	4.6	492	178
				H	73.6	2.00	91	22	22	10	16.0	78	12.9	7.6	5.3	430	285
A.W.	AR	25 F	1.75	C	93.6	2.42	83	29	16	10	18.0	90	12.1	5.0	7.1	487	213
				H	67.4	3.45	72	40	21	10	15.5	90	8.1	4.4	3.7	462	360
E.M.	AS	30 F	1.58	C	93.7	1.69	60	28	20	13	16.5	86	23.9	10.1	12.8	674	329
	AR			H	—	1.97	59	33	25		17.5	76	17.9	6.9	10.0	588	282
N.S.	AS	50 M	1.78	C	90.0	2.83	71	40	21	11	16.0	81	16.5	10.5	6.0	781	264
				H	54.7	3.69	100	37	29	14	21.5	90	11.1	6.8	4.3	679	378
C.M.	AS	47 M	1.98	C	—	3.06	77	40	30	14	22.0	92	14.4	6.7	7.7	742	306
				H	—	3.22	75	43	32	10	21.0	92	13.5	7.6	5.9	720	286
R.S.	IC	21 M	1.82	C	97.0	4.40	84	52	11	3	7.0	100	8.1	4.2	3.9	592	251
				H	72.0	4.43	85	52	16	2	9.0	100	7.4	4.0	3.4	592	230
R.Sc.	IC	47 M	1.86	C	90.5	3.63	60	60	17	10	13.5	88	9.8	6.0	3.8	594	230
				H	80.8	3.26	66	49	20	10	15.0	92	10.4	7.2	3.2	568	174
Control mean					94.2	2.67	77	45.4	18.6	9.8	14.2	87	15.3	8.2	7.1	632	288
±S.E.					±0.74	±0.18	±3.2	±2.8	±2.04	±1.07	±1.52	±2.1	±1.29	±0.69	±0.66	±104.6	±14.2
Hypoxia mean					72.5	3.03	85	36.1	24.4	10.3	17.1	85	12.7	7.6	5.1	593	238
±S.E.					±2.42	±0.20	±3.3	±2.7	±2.70	±1.52	±1.97	±2.8	±1.10	±0.75	±0.46	±89.1	±10.9
p value					<0.01	<0.05	<0.05	N.S.	<0.01	N.S.	<0.01	N.S.	<0.01	<0.05	<0.05	<0.05	<0.02

Sa_{O_2} = arterial blood oxygen saturation (%)
MR = mitral regurgitation
TS = tricuspid stenosis
Other symbols and abbreviations are identical to those used in Table 11-1

AR = aortic regurgitation
C = control
H = acute hypoxia

EFFECTS OF ACUTE HYPOXIA

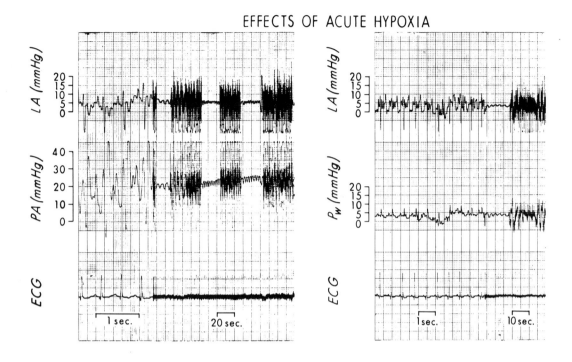

Figure 11-3. In a patient with mild chronic pulmonary disease, a rise in pulmonary arterial pressure was associated with no change in left atrial pressure. The left atrial and pulmonary wedge mean pressures were identical during the inhalation of low oxygen.

The changes in both CBV and PBV were statistically significant and were at variance with the results reported by other workers.[150,151]

In a normal subject, acute hypoxia produced similar responses, i.e., a significant rise in PAm, no change in LAm and a moderate decrease in PBV. These discordant changes in the pulmonary blood pressure and volume again suggest active pulmonary vasoconstriction. During continuous infusion of acetylcholine into the pulmonary artery with the subject breathing low oxygen, PAm decreased and PBV was unchanged (Figure 11-4).

Our studies and the reports of others indicate that acute hypoxia does indeed cause pulmonary vasoconstriction in man. At present, the specific identity of the vascular segment or segments involved is uncertain, although the evidence suggests primary if not exclusive participation by the precapillary elements, the pulmonary arteries and arterioles.[152,153] Recent demonstrations that alveolar gas may diffuse through the walls of pulmonary precapillary vessels emphasize the accessibility of these vessels to conditions in the surrounding pulmonary tissue and support the possibility that they may react to the low alveolar oxygen tension by vasoconstriction.[154,155] A more detailed discussion of vasomotion in the pulmonary vascular bed appears in Chapter 16.

In 4 patients the inhalation of low oxygen was continued for more than 16 minutes. Multiple indicator-dilution

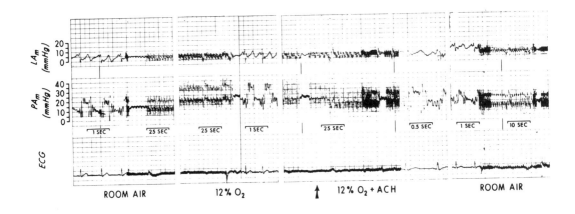

Figure 11-4. In a normal subject, inhalation of 12% oxygen produced a rise in the pulmonary arterial pressure associated with no change in the left atrial pressure. While the subject was breathing low oxygen, continuous infusion of acetylcholine into the pulmonary artery caused a decrease in the pulmonary arterial pressure. When 12% oxygen was changed to room air, the pulmonary arterial pressure returned to normal. The transient rise in left atrial pressure was an artifact, due to inadvertent shift of the baseline.

curves were recorded during this prolonged hypoxia, and 350 ml of blood were sampled in each case (Table 11-14). Toward the end of the study period, the responses of BAm and PAm were entirely different from those observed when the period of acute hypoxia was less than 15 minutes and loss of blood less than 140 ml. A striking decline in BAm occurred, 33 mm Hg or more in 3 of 4 patients. PAm and LAm declined in all patients. CBV decreased in all 4 patients, and PBV in 3. These findings suggest that active pulmonary vasomotion is no longer demonstrable after a prolonged period of hypoxia, particularly after removal of considerable blood. Instead, BAm and PAm decrease comparably. This reduction was not due to exceptionally severe arterial oxygen desaturation inasmuch as the saturation was never less than 74% during the hypoxia period.

Fishman and associates also noted a tendency of the elevated PAm to fall toward initial levels in a number of patients as inhalation of low oxygen was continued.[135] The late reduction in PAm is secondary to systemic hypotension, which may supervene when hypoxia is continued too long. More than 20 years ago, Barcroft and Edholm noted similar changes and even vasodepressor-like responses in man during acute hypoxia combined with phlebotomy.[102] They attributed the changes to peripheral vasodilatation and increased blood flow to the skeletal muscles, resulting in a decrease in venous return and effective CO.

High Oxygen. Many workers have demonstrated that inhalation of 100% oxygen (hyperoxia) may lower elevated PAm and PVR in many patients with cardiopulmonary disease.[114,133,156-163] Others have observed similar reductions even when PAm and PVR were normal.[164-166]

We have reported previously the effects of hyperoxia on the PBV, PAm, LAm and P_d in 8 patients with organic heart disease.[163] PBV declined significantly in 4, accompanied by a decrease or no change in the P_d.

Table 11-15 Effects of Inhalation of 100% Oxygen in Valvular Heart Disease

Patient	Age Sex	BSA	Diagnosis	Condition	CI	HR	SI	Pressures (mm Hg)				Tm (seconds)			Blood Volume (mL/M²)	
								PAm	LAm	P_d	BAm	PA-BA	LA-BA	PA-LA	CBV	PBA
E.W.	24 F	1.67	MS	C	3.12	82	38	32	25	28.5	78	11.04	4.5	6.9	592	359
				O_2	3.05	75	41	30	22	26.0	81	10.4	4.5	5.9	528	300
W.M.	56 M	1.82	MS	C	1.67	84	20	39	36	37.5	120	21.8	12.7	9.1	610	253
				O_2	1.51	84	18	30	29	29.5	104	20.6	12.9	7.7	512	194
A.L.	31 F	1.48	MS	C	1.44	80	18	42	22	32.0	96	14.6	6.4	8.2	350	194
				O_2	1.64	80	20	28	20	24.0	100	14.5	7.4	7.1	396	195
E.V.	41 F	1.72	MS	C	1.96	85	23	60	20	40.0	80	17.5	7.2	10.3	570	337
				O_2	2.10	78	27	48	18	33.0	72	17.2	7.5	9.7	605	339
C.W.	28 M	1.79	MR MS	C	2.43	80	30	60	24	42.0	100	30.3	21.1	9.2	1200	372
				O_2	2.18	80	27	46	26	36.0	96	31.7	21.6	10.6	1150	374
G.M.	59 M	1.62	AS	C	2.79	70	40	12	5	8.5	72	13.8	7.5	6.3	640	293
				O_2	2.77	80	35	13	6	9.5	72	14.3	8.1	6.2	670	286
R.F.	30 M	1.85	AS	C	3.33	86	39	14	10	12.0	80	12.8	6.2	6.6	712	366
				O_2	2.75	85	32	14	12	13.0	84	11.8	6.8	5.0	542	229
A.W.	25 F	1.75	AS	C	2.42	75	32	16	10	13.0	90	12.8	7.0	5.8	518	233
				O_2	2.57	64	40	15	10	12.5	88	12.4	6.4	6.0	532	257
B.C.	36 M	1.96	AS	C	3.04	95	32	34	23	28.5	84	14.7	7.9	6.8	745	342
				O_2	2.84	95	30	33	28	30.5	92	16.2	8.6	7.6	770	362
J.S.	62 M	1.90	AS	C	1.64	72	23	42	22	32.0	86	24.2	13.5	10.7	655	293
				O_2	1.50	75	20	44	27	35.0	88	26.0	14.2	11.8	654	295
C.H.	36 M	1.79	AR	C	3.01	70	43	9	5	7.0	84	15.2	8.1	7.1	765	356
				O_2	2.77	60	46	8	4	6.0	84	15.1	8.5	6.6	700	304
H.A.	44 M	1.92	AR	C	2.92	90	33	44	24	34.0	100	25.8	17.8	8.0	1260	376
				O_2	2.52	90	28	40	28	34.0	100	26.7	19.2	7.5	1130	315
Control	mean				2.48	81	30.9	33.7	18.8	26.2	89.2	17.9	10.0	7.9	718	315
	±S.E.				±0.19	±2.3	±2.4	±5.1	±2.7	±3.7	±3.8	±1.8	±1.5	±0.5	±76.1	±17.5
100% O_2	mean				2.35	79	30.3	29.1	19.2	24.1	88.4	18.1	10.5	7.6	682	288
	±S.E.				±0.16	±2.8	±2.6	±4.0	±2.7	±3.2	±3.0	±1.9	±1.6	±0.6	±68.0	±17.1
	p value				NS	NS	NS	<0.025	NS	<0.10	NS	NS	<0.01	NS	NS	<0.10

C = Control period
O_2 = During inhalation of 100% O_2
The symbols and abbreviations are identical to those used in Tables 11-1 and 11-6

In Table 11-15 are data from 12 patients with valvular heart disease before and during inhalation of 100% oxygen, including 7 of the 8 patients reported previously. The average PAm, P_d, CBV and PBV all decreased. The differences between the mean values in the control period and in the period of breathing 100% oxygen were not statistically significant for P_d and CBV, but the difference was statistically significant (p<0.02) for PAm. Consistent with our previous results, 5 patients showed a significant reduction in PBV, accompanied by a decrease or no change in the PAm and P_d. These pressures declined distinctly in 3 patients without an appreciable change in the volumes. Neither the P_d nor the PBV were affected in the remaining 4, and changes in the LAm were variable.

The present studies confirm our previous report that hyperoxia probably causes reflex systemic venodilatation in some patients with passive redistribution of blood from the pulmonary to the systemic compartment. Such an explanation could account for the absence of hyperoxic effects on PAm in isolated lung preparations.[167,168] Moreover, it would also help explain the additive effects of acetylcholine and hyperoxia observed in cardiac patients,[162] acetylcholine abolishing heightened pulmonary vascular tone and hyperoxia reducing the PBV.

Carbon Dioxide. The reported effects of breathing air enriched with carbon dioxide (CO_2) on the pulmonary circulation have been inconsistent and in animals most investigators have found rise in PAm similar to that observed during inhalation of low oxygen.[114,118,128,130,167-173] Recent workers have suggested that the pulmonary vasoconstrictor effect of hypercapnia is due to the acidosis produced.[145,146,174]

Table 11-16   Effects of CO_2 Inhalation on the Pulmonary Circulatory Dynamics in Mitral Valve Disease (after Paul et al.)

Patient No.	Condition	CO	HR	SV	Pressures (mm Hg)			PVR	PBV
					PAm	LAm	BAm		
4	R	5.40	68	79	15	8	97	1.30	580
	CO_2	5.62	72	78	16	8	81	1.42	620
6	R	2.69	123	24	17	10	112	2.60	185
	CO_2	3.06	106	31	17	8	109	2.94	391
7	R	3.47	87	40	28	20	109	2.31	293
	CO_2	3.94	88	45	33	23	122	2.54	496
8	R	4.76	88	54	30	22	100	1.68	553
	CO_2	6.22	95	65	34	24	103	1.61	564
9	R	3.77	50	75	12	5	72	1.86	445
	CO_2	4.53	57	79	17	8	88	1.99	472
10	R	4.57	74	62	39	22	93	3.72	328
	H	5.14	76	68	35	21	94	2.72	463
	CO_2	5.30	98	54	44	24	96	3.77	147
11	R	5.41	65	83	32	21	32	2.03	659
	H	5.26	59	89	28	20	28	1.52	733
	CO_2	6.68	70	95	41	23	41	2.69	589
14	R	4.50	63	71	31	23	83	1.78	741
	H	4.93	68	73	31	22	86	1.83	954
	CO_2	6.04	104	58	59	42	100	2.81	1008

R = Room air
H = Voluntary hyperventilation
CO = Cardiac output (L/min)
HR = Heart rate (beats/min)
SV = Stroke volume (ml/beat)

PAm = Pulmonary arterial mean
LAm = Left atrial mean
BAm = Systemic arterial mean
PVR = Pulmonary vascular resistance (unit)
PBV = Pulmonary blood volume (ml)

In normal subjects inhalation of 5% CO_2 caused no increase in pulmonary blood flow or arterial pressure.[133,175] On the other hand, Fishman and associates found that inhalation of 3 to 5% CO_2 raised the PAm in patients with chronic pulmonary disease, an effect which was attributed to an increase in pulmonary blood flow.[175] The increase in pulmonary blood flow might have resulted from increased work of breathing, exaggerated ventilatory drive, and/or an obscure effect of carbon dioxide on the myocardium. Others have attributed the rise in cardiac output during CO_2 inhalation to release of catecholamines.[176]

Shephard reported an elevation of pulmonary arterial pressure in patients with congenital heart disease during inhalation of 5% CO_2.[177]

Paul and co-workers studied the effects of CO_2 breathing on the pulmonary circulation in 14 patients with mitral valve disease.[178] They found an increase in PAm (24% higher than control), LAm (31% higher than control), CO (16% more than control), and PVR (13% above control). In the 5 patients in whom the PBV was measured, it was markedly increased in 2 and slightly increased in 3 (Table 11-16). The average increase was 98 ml or 24% more than the average control values. PBV decreased in 2 patients during CO_2 breathing after voluntary hyperventilation. The authors explained the elevation of PAm during inhalation of CO_2 by pulmonary vasoconstriction. They further speculated that the tendency of voluntary hyperventilation to expand the pulmonary vascular bed and that of increased alveolar CO_2 concentration to constrict it might be competitive influences.

The inconsistent effects of CO_2 on pulmonary circulation reported by various workers may be partly explained on the basis of the recent findings by Vile and Shepherd.[179] They demonstrated two opposing actions of CO_2 on isolated perfused lungs of cats: a pulmonary vasodilator action due to direct effect of CO_2 and a vasoconstrictor action caused by the increase in hydrogen ion concentration.

Change of Total Blood Volume

Intravenous Infusion of Blood or Fluid. Early studies indicated that rapid infusion of large amounts of dextrose in water, physiologic saline or dextran to normal subjects and patients with cardiac disease invariably caused significant rises in right atrial pressure (RAm), LAm and PAm.[180-184] The pressure rise presumably resulted from elevation of left and right ventricular end-diastolic pressures. Although CO did not vary consistently, CBV was increased in those normal subjects and in patients in whom it was measured.[181-184]

Frye and Braunwald reported that without ganglionic blockade large autotransfusions of blood removed within 2 weeks were not associated with significant increases in either CO or intrathoracic blood volume in normal subjects.[185] The latter was estimated by injecting an indicator into the right atrium and sampling from a systemic artery. After a constant, continuous infusion of trimethaphane (Arfonad) at a rate ranging from 1.0 to 10.4 mg per minute, sufficient to lower the systemic systolic arterial pressure by approximately 40 mm Hg, autotransfusion resulted in a substantial increase in the intrathoracic blood volume and CO. According to these authors, partial ganglionic blockade diminishes venous tone and allows venodilatation, increasing the capacity of the venous bed. In the presence of diminished venous tone and an expanded systemic venous bed, the hypervolemia induced by blood transfusion would result in a larger fraction of the infused blood entering the thorax with the CO rising accordingly.

Freitas and co-workers reported changes in PBV during the intravenous infusion of 3.5% polyvinyl pyrolidine, a volume expander, in subjects with normal cardiovascular systems and in patients with systemic hypertension.[186] The solution was given at a constant rate of 38 ml/min. Seventeen patients received 1000 ml of the solution, and the PBV increased in 10 and decreased in 7. The average overall change, however, was statistically insignificant. On the other hand, a significant increase in the PAm, LAm and RAm was observed. These workers suggested that the rapidly infused solution was pooled in the peripheral circulation and they attributed the pressure-volume changes in the pulmonary vascular bed to the low distensibility of the system.

Varnauskas and Korsgren studied the effects of Rheomacrodex (a volume expander) infusion on PBV and pulmonary extravascular water volume in patients with valvular heart disease.[187] The infusion was given at 20 ml per minute, and approximately 500 ml of Rheomacrodex was infused into each patient. The PBV was estimated by the double indicator-dilution method and the pulmonary extravascular water volume by a "diffusible" indicator, tritiated water. After Rheomacrodex infusion, CO, SV, RAm, LAm and PAm all increased. No appreciable change in the PBV was observed. Changes in the pulmonary extravascular water volume were inconsistent and not correlated with the elevated LAm.

We studied the effects of rapid infusion of dextran or normal saline solutions in 5 patients, including 4 with

valvular heart disease and 1 with idiopathic cardiomyopathy. The results are summarized in Table 11-17. CI and HR increased consistently and significantly in all patients, but the change in SI was variable. For the entire group, elevation of the LAm, PAm and P_d pressures was statistically significant. Both CBV and PBV also increased significantly.

In order to assess the effects of rapid blood transfusion and removal on pulmonary circulatory dynamics, the following study was undertaken. About 400 ml of blood was removed from each subject 2 days before cardiac catheterization. The blood removed was stored in ACD solution for future autotransfusion. On the day of study, determinations of CO, pulmonary vascular pressures and volume were made during each of the following periods: (a) control, (b) rapid removal of two 200 ml aliquots from an antecubital vein, (c) reinfusion of the 400 ml of blood removed under (b), (d) equilibrium or second control period, (e) rapid infusion of the 300 to 400 ml of blood removed 2 days prior to the study.

The effects of rapid blood transfusion were studied in 2 normal subjects, 4 patients with mitral valve disease and 3 patients with aortic valve disease. The data obtained during periods (d) and (e) are presented in Table 11-18. Changes in the CI, HR and SI were variable. In normal subjects and in patients with valvular heart disease, LAm, PAm and P_d rose consistently. The pressure rise was usually much greater in the patients than in the normal subjects (Figure 11-5). The pressures rose to a maximum during the period of transfusion. A few minutes after completion of the transfusion, when the dilution curves were being inscribed, the pressures were usually a few mm Hg lower than the

Table 11-17 Hemodynamic Effects of Rapid Infusion of Dextran or Normal Saline Solutions in Patients with Cardiac Disease

Patient	Age	Sex	Diagnosis	Periods of Study	Blood Flow			Pressures (mm Hg)				Tm (seconds)			Blood Volume (ml/M²)	
					CI	HR	SI	PAm	LAm	P_d	BAm	PA-BA	LA-BA	PA-LA	CBV	PBV
T.B.	18	F	AS	C	2.21	48	46	16	9	12.5	88	10.5	6.2	4.3	386	152
				D	3.60	74	49	28	17	22.5	90	7.8	3.8	4.0	470	245
B.M.	55	M	MS	C	2.80	56	50	20	13	16.5	96	10.6	6.4	4.2	494	196
				D	3.32	72	46	32	22	26	92	10.7	6.2	4.5	562	248
M.C.	50	F	MS	C	2.90	69	42	20	14	17	72	21.0	12.0	9.0	1020	435
			MR	D	3.61	90	40	32	22	27	76	20.3	11.8	8.1	1118	486
V.G.	35	F	MS	C	2.31	62	37	21	15	18	88	14.5	8.9	5.6	560	214
				S	2.80	66	42	30	28	29	82	12.2	6.7	5.5	573	257
R.M.	59	M	IC	C	1.40	72	20	33	17	25	93	34.6	21.7	12.9	810	298
				D	1.81	76	23	42	19	30.5	87	28.9	17.4	11.5	865	355
Control mean					2.32	61.4	39	22.0	13.6	17.8	87.4	18.2	11.0	7.2	654	259
±S.E.					±0.27	±4.35	±5.2	±2.88	±1.33	±2.03	±4.14	±4.51	±2.86	±1.67	±115	±50.0
Dextran mean					3.03	75.6	40	32.8	21.6	27.0	85.4	16.0	9.2	6.7	718	318
±S.E.					±0.34	±3.97	±4.5	±2.42	±1.86	±1.37	±2.89	±3.84	±2.43	±1.39	±120	±46.7
p value					<0.02	<0.02	N.S.	<0.05	<0.02	<0.02	N.S.	N.S.	N.S.	N.S.	<0.01	<0.01

C = Control period

D = During dextran infusion

S = During saline infusion

Other symbols and abbreviations are identical to those used in Table 11—1

Table 11-18 Effects of Blood Transfusion in Normal Subjects and in Patients with Valvular Heart Disease

Patients	Periods of Study	Blood Flow			Pressures (mm Hg)				Tm (seconds)			Blood Volume (ml/M²)	
		CI	HR	SI	PAm	LAm	P_d	BAm	PA-BA	LA-BA	PA-LA	CBV	PBV
I. Normal Subjects													
J.R.	A	2.37	67	35	9	5	7	80	14.7	7.6	7.1	576	282
	B	2.44	72	34	12	5	8.5	89	14.5	8.2	6.3	590	255
	C	2.40	68	36	12	5	8.5	90	14.9	7.8	7.1	605	288
R.L.	A	2.54	86	30	14	4	9	120	12.1	6.4	5.7	598	241
	B	2.62	72	37	15	7	11	118	12.7	7.9	4.8	621	210
	C	2.54	72	35	19	8	13.5	125	11.5	5.8	4.7	570	242
II. Patients with MVD													
M.D.	A	3.02	94	33	19	15	17	70	13.0	6.2	6.8	652	340
	D	3.64	90	39	27	20	23.5	73	11.9	6.1	5.8	722	355
J.H.	A	2.94	84	35	28	18	23	80	13.4	7.6	5.8	658	284
	D	3.00	86	35	33	26	29.5	75	13.6	7.6	6.0	680	300
J.W.	A	3.00	54	56	31	25	28	84	15.2	6.0	9.2	825	430
	D	3.16	65	49	40	30	35	100	14.6	5.9	8.5	775	445
M.M.	A	1.79	120	15	45	15	30	96	27.6	14.3	13.3	825	400
	D	1.72	120	14	48	30	39	100	27.5	13.5	14.0	790	405
III. Patients with AVD													
E.S.	A	2.20	62	35	15	11	13	109	17.4	10.5	6.9	638	253
	B	2.45	54	45	22	16	19	113	17.9	10.5	7.4	731	302
	C	2.73	59	46	30	22	26	109	15.5	9.1	6.4	706	294
F.L.	A	3.16	88	36	17	10	13.5	81	10.2	5.1	5.1	537	269
	B	3.26	91	35	20	11	15.5	84	9.6	5.5	4.1	524	223
	C	3.33	95	.35	22	12	17	86	9.6	4.8	4.8	536	268
M.P.	A	1.60	70	23	32	14	23	62	21.5	13.8	7.7	574	204
	B	1.78	68	25	37	19	28	71	22.0	14.1	7.9	655	234
	C	1.76	70	25	37	20	28.5	71	20.9	12.8	8.1	614	238

A = Control
B = 200 ml transfused
C = 400 ml transfused
D = 300 ml transfused
MVD = Mitral valve disease
AVD = Aortic valve disease
Other symbols and abbreviations are the same as those used in Table 11-1

maximum values. Neither CBV nor PBV changed.

The amount of blood transfused in our study was relatively small and the results cannot be compared with observations during the intravenous infusion of large amounts of dextran or other isotonic solutions. However, the LAm reached 26 mm Hg or more after the rapid transfusion of 300 ml of blood in 3 of 4 patients with mitral valve disease, and further transfusion seemed inadvisable. This observation is consistent with the development of pulmonary edema in some patients with predominant mitral stenosis following the rapid infusion of a relatively small amount of blood or fluid. The distensibility of the pulmonary vascular bed was severely compromised in these patients, partly because of structural luminal narrowing and functional vasoconstriction and partly because of increased extravascular water volume. Additional fluid would precipitate transudation into the extravascular space.

Acute Blood Loss. Stead, Warren and associates reported the effects of acute blood loss by phlebotomy or pooling of blood in the limbs in normal

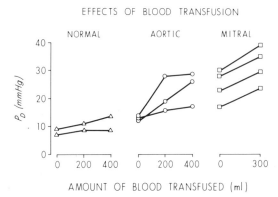

EFFECTS OF BLOOD TRANSFUSION

Figure 11-5. In normal subjects and in patients with aortic or mitral valve disease, rapid infusion of 300 to 400 ml of blood caused a rise in the pulmonary distending pressure. The pressure rise was most noticeable in patients with mitral valve disease and almost imperceptible in normal subjects. The magnitude of pressure rise was directly proportional to the amount of blood infused.

subjects.[188] The pertinent changes included a consistent fall in CO and RAm. Acute circulatory collapse was observed in three instances. The same group of investigators subsequently reported the results of hemodynamic studies of acute blood loss from trauma.[189] When the cardiac index was below 2.6 L/min/M^2, there was generally a reduction in both RAm and BAm. Judson and co-workers reported cardiohemodynamic effects of phlebotomy or venous pooling of blood in patients with or without congestive heart failure.[190] Following phlebotomy or venous pooling of blood, there was a decrease in CO associated with no change in the right ventricular diastolic pressure in patients without failure. On the other hand, in patients with failure an increase in CO and a reduction in the right ventricular diastolic pressure were observed.

We studied the hemodynamic consequences of acute blood removal in 2 normal subjects, 4 patients with mitral valve disease and 4 patients with aortic valve disease. The data obtained during periods (a) and (b) (*vide supra*) are summarized in Table 11-19. Changes in CI and HR were inconsistent. LAm and PAm both declined uniformly (Figure 11-6). The pressure fall was greatest in patients with mitral valve disease and least in normal subjects. It was directly proportional to the amount of blood removed.

CBV increased slightly in the two normal subjects, but PBV remained unchanged. CBV and PBV decreased significantly in two patients (E.S. and F.L.) after removal of 400 ml of blood. In the remaining patients reduction in the CBV and PBV was small and insignificant.

Thus, removal of as little as 200 ml of blood from patients with valvular heart disease may reduce elevated LAm and PAm. When 400 ml of blood is removed from such patients, elevated LAm and PAm may fall to normal.

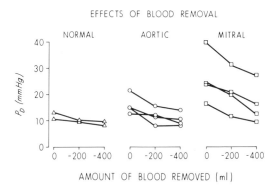

EFFECTS OF BLOOD REMOVAL

Figure 11-6. In normal subjects and in patients with aortic or mitral valve disease, removal of 400 ml of blood resulted in a uniform fall in the pulmonary distending pressure. The pressure fall was most striking in patients with mitral valve disease and least conspicuous in normal subjects. The pressure decline was directly proportional to the amount of blood removed.

Table 11-19   Effects of Blood Removal in Normal Subjects and in Patients with Valvular Heart Disease

Patients	Periods of Study	Blood Flow			Pressures (mm Hg)				Tm (seconds)			Blood Volume (ml/M²)	
		CI	HR	SI	PAm	LAm	P_d	BAm	PA-BA	LA-BA	PA-LA	CBV	PBV
						I. Normal Subjects							
J.C.	A	3.30	90	37	15	11	13	110	11.2	5.9	5.3	615	302
	B	3.06	95	32	12	8	10	110	12.1	7.2	4.9	620	250
	C	3.42	95	36	11	8	9.5	110	12.8	7.6	5.2	725	296
R.L.	A	2.31	104	22	16	5	10.5	118	13.1	7.1	6.0	582	231
	B	2.75	84	33	14	5	9.5	115	12.1	7.1	5.0	648	223
	C	2.76	100	28	13	3	8.0	125	12.7	7.3	5.4	678	230
						II. Patients with MVD							
M.D.	A	2.90	82	35	18	15	16.5	77	13.8	6.8	7.0	680	344
	B	2.70	94	28	13	10	11.5	77	13.8	7.5	5.9	656	288
	C	2.81	97	28	11	8	9.5	50	14.0	6.6	7.4	657	341
J.H.	A	2.86	90	32	28	23	25.5	75	13.6	5.7	7.9	648	377
	B	3.11	90	34	25	20	22.5	75	12.8	5.8	7.0	664	363
	C	2.73	90	30	20	15	17.5	65	14.0	6.0	8.0	638	355
J.W.	A	2.60	58	45	30	18	24	84	15.6	5.9	9.7	680	420
	B	2.78	62	45	27	15	21	84	14.6	6.2	8.4	675	396
	C	2.73	68	40	22	11	16.5	74	14.7	5.3	9.4	674	416
M.M.	A	1.90	120	14	49	31	40	100	27.0	14.4	12.6	855	402
	B	1.66	120	13	40	23	31.5	90	28.6	16.3	12.3	800	341
	C	1.59	120	13	35	20	27.5	84	30.8	16.5	14.3	820	380
						III. Patients with AVD							
F.P.	A	3.56	75	48	14	11	12.5	88	12.9	7.1	4.8	765	345
	B	3.58	63	57	13	11	12	80	13.1	7.2	5.9	780	352
	C	3.37	60	56	10	8	9	80	13.8	8.1	5.7	775	322
E.S.	A	2.41	55	44	18	12	15	108	15.9	9.5	6.4	638	257
	B	2.18	61	36	11	5	8	109	15.9	9.2	6.7	576	248
	C	2.09	62	34	11	5	8	107	15.8	9.6	6.2	550	216
F.L.	A	3.52	88	40	20	10	15	90	9.9	5.1	4.8	581	323
	B	3.31	90	37	16	7	11.5	86	10.8	5.5	5.3	605	294
	C	2.78	95	29	15	6	10.5	86	11.3	6.5	4.8	522	223
M.P.	A	1.58	74	21	29	12	21.5	71	20.6	12.5	8.1	537	216
	B	1.44	80	18	22	9	15.5	68	20.1	13.8	6.3	480	151
	C	1.44	74	19	21	7	14	62	21.6	13.2	8.4	514	201

A = Control
B = 200 ml withdrawn
C = 400 ml withdrawn
Other symbols and abbreviations are the same as those used in Tables 11-1 and 11-18

In patients with valvular heart disease, particularly those with predominant mitral stenosis, even a small reduction in the total blood volume and PBV may significantly improve the pressure-volume ratio in the pulmonary vascular bed and cause a disproportionately large fall in the pulmonary vascular pressure.[191]

Early in our study we removed 200 ml of blood rapidly in three consecutive periods from a patient with aortic valvular disease and a low CI. After the total of 600 ml had been removed, BAm and PAm both fell precipitously and CO dropped further, resulting in a transient convulsive seizure. The depleted blood volume was replaced immediately and the patient recovered from the episode uneventfully (Figure 11-7). Since this unpleasant incident, we have limited the blood removed to not more than 400 ml, and no additional untoward effects have been observed.

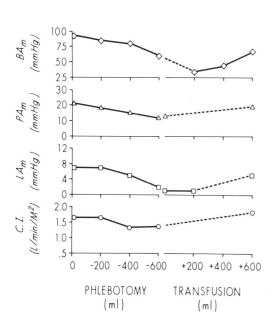

Figure 11-7. In a patient with aortic valve disease and low cardiac index, removal of 600 ml of blood caused a precipitous fall in both systemic and pulmonary arterial pressures. The left atrial mean pressure fell almost to zero. Cardiac index declined further, resulting in a transient convulsive seizure. Following immediate replacement of the blood, the cardiac index, systemic and pulmonary arterial pressures were increased. The patient recovered uneventfully.

High Altitude*

At high altitude, altered cardiac functions have been reported including tachycardia, decreased SV, reduced CO and lowered BAm. Pulmonary hypertension in high altitude residents was first suggested by Hurtado in 1930.[192] In 1947 Rotta described radiologic evidence of pulmonary arterial enlargement.[193]

*I am indebted to Dr. Herbert N. Hultgren, Professor of Medicine, Stanford University School of Medicine, for pertinent information and for many references included in the review, *Circulatory Adaptation to High Altitude*, written by him and Dr. Robert F. Grover, published in the Annual Review in Medicine, *19*, 119, 1968.

Hemodynamic studies, including the measurement of PAm, in 13 healthy residents at high altitude (14,900 ft) was first reported in 1956 by Rotta and associates.[194] Six were adult males born at sea level who had resided for 1 year at high altitude, and 7 were adult males who had lived permanently at high altitude. The PAm in these two groups was 18 and 24 mm Hg respectively, in contrast to the value of 12 mm Hg in 7 residents at sea level. Other investigators have subsequently reported similar findings in natives living at high altitude.[195,196] Despite moderate elevation of the PAm, the Pw was usually normal. The elevated PAm reflected an increase in PVR which was believed to be partly structural and partly functional. Anatomic studies demonstrated thickening and medial hypertrophy of pulmonary arterioles in both man and animals living at high altitude.[197,198] Functionally, sustained vasoconstriction was probably secondary to low alveolar oxygen tension. The postulation of functional vasoconstriction was supported by reduction of PAm during inhalation of 100% oxygen or following the administration of vasoactive drugs such as tolazoline, isoproterenol and acetylcholine.[199-204]

In the high-altitude natives, acute hypoxia, on the other hand, caused a marked rise in the PAm accompanied by a slight increase in CO and no alteration in Pw.[203,205,206] These changes indicated that the pulmonary vasoconstriction was almost entirely confined to the arteries and arterioles.

Employing Newman's slope method, the reliability of which has been questioned, Monge and co-workers reported a significant increase in the CBV of natives living at high altitude.[207] The mean for 10 male natives was 670 ml/M² in contrast to 380 ml/M² in 15 women living at sea level. The ratio of CBV to total blood volume in natives at high altitude was 19.4%, and at sea level 15.2%.

Roy and co-workers recently reported changes in the pulmonary circulatory dynamics of 11 healthy male volunteers before and after 64 to 114 weeks of intermittent stay at an altitude of 14,500 feet.[208] An initial study was conducted with the subjects at sea level, and a second study was done within 46 to 120 hours after their departure from the high altitude. The results are summarized in Table 11-20. After the high altitude stay, CI increased an average of 66% and SI 77%. Increase in LAm and PAm was modest, 16 and 17% respectively. The average CBV initially at sea level was 709 ml/M², increasing to 1361 ml/M² after high altitude. The corresponding values for PBV were 259 and 427 ml/m² Thus,

the average increment of CBV was 97% and of the PBV 76%. No increase in PBV was apparent after less than 25 weeks of stay at high altitude, but it increased progressively thereafter. The significant increase in pulmonary blood flow and volume with little or no change in the pulmonary vascular pressures was interpreted as a form of successful adaptation to high altitude hypoxia. It should be emphasized that the second studies were made at sea level 46 hours or more after the subjects departed from high altitude, so that the changes measured might have been significantly less than at high altitude.

Some workers have recently reported the occurrence of so-called high altitude pulmonary edema in healthy but unacclimatized persons exposed to an altitude of over 9000 feet.[209-211] There is no evidence of underlying

Table 11-20 Effects of High Altitude on Pulmonary Circulatory Dynamics (Roy, Bhatia and Gadhoke)

| Subjects | Condition | CI | HR | SI | Pressures (mm Hg) | | Blood Volume (ml/M²) | |
					PAm	LAm	CBV	PBV
1	A	1.9	54	35	12	7	696	310
	B	2.2	54	41	12	5	827	319
2	A	3.3	72	46	15	6	733	330
	B	4.0	54	74	18	6	1260	227
3	A	2.5	60	42	14	6	612	236
	B	5.7	66	86	12	6	1710	314
4	A	3.2	75	43	14	7	746	218
	B	4.4	72	61	17	8	1195	352
5	A	3.4	72	47	11	6	938	352
	B	5.1	60	85	16	8	1411	621
6	A	3.2	72	44	11	4	778	272
	B	2.9	54	54	15	10	1218	435
7	A	3.1	66	47	15	5	555	131
	B	5.0	78	64	18	10	1295	215
8	A	3.0	75	40	15	4	615	175
	B	5.6	72	78	15	6	1497	471
9	A	3.6	90	40	12	5	887	310
	B	6.3	75	87	17	6	1795	514
10	A	2.1	72	29	15	8	630	263
	B	6.0	66	91	16	7	1804	764
11	A	2.7	72	38	16	7	610	179
	B	2.8	48	58	18	10	961	462
Average	A	2.9	71	41	13.6	6	709	259
	B	4.5	62	71	16.0	7	1361	427
% change		+60	−10	+77	+17	+16	+97	+76

A = at sea level; B = at high altitude (14,500 feet)
Other symbols and abbreviations are identical to those used in Table 11-1

cardiac or pulmonary disease in subjects who have had repeated attacks of high altitude pulmonary edema. Hemodynamic studies have demonstrated elevation of PAm but normal Pw or LAm.[210],[211] The mechanism by which pulmonary edema is produced remains obscure. There is some evidence to suggest that the underlying mechanism may be similar to that of pulmonary edema observed in severe pulmonary embolism.[212] In both conditions pulmonary hypertension is produced as a result of obstruction to a major portion of the pulmonary vascular bed. The areas which are not obstructed may be subjected to abnormally high pulmonary arterial pressure and flow. This high pressure may be transmitted directly through short vessels to the pulmonary capillaries, where transudation of fluid into the alveoli may take place when the hydrostatic pressure greatly exceeds the plasma osmotic pressure. Inhalation of 100% oxygen results in prompt reduction of PAm and relief of symptoms.

Change in Acid-Base Balance

In 1958 Liljestrand demonstrated pulmonary vasoconstriction in the presence of increased hydrogen-ion concentration in the circulating blood and postulated that the pressor effect of hypoxia might be secondary to acidosis resulting from local release of lactic acid.[144] Subsequently, other investigators have explored the vasomotor effects of various hydrogen-ion concentrations on the pulmonary circulation.[145-149,213]

In 1961-62 Bergofsky and co-workers reported the effects of acute alkalosis and acidosis on pulmonary hemodynamics.[145],[214] The pulmonary arterial pressor response to acute hypoxia in man was not influenced by the administration of either sodium bicarbonate or Tris buffer. Neither extracellular nor intracellular acidosis appeared to affect this response. On the other hand, a consistent rise in PAm was observed in anesthetized dogs during acute acidosis induced by the infusion of lactic acid or hydrochloric acid, or the inhalation of 5% carbon dioxide. Since the pulmonary blood flow and left ventricular diastolic pressure were unchanged, the rise in PAm was attributed to pulmonary vasoconstriction. The data further suggested that the hydrogen ion rather than its associated anion was responsible for the pulmonary vasopressor response in acute acidosis.

Several years later Enson and colleagues studied the relation between arterial blood oxyhemoglobin saturation and PAm.[146] In a series of 43 patients with chronic pulmonary disease, PAm correlated with both oxygen saturation and hydrogen-ion concentration significantly better than with either of the two variables considered singly. At high pH, the PAm was relatively insensitive to hypoxemia, and at low pH the PAm was extremely sensitive to hypoxemia.

Guintini and co-workers reported a parallel increase of approximately 30% in CO and PBV during infusion of sodium bicarbonate in 4 patients with normal cardiovascular system.[215] Similar changes were noted during infusion of Tris buffer in 8 patients with chronic bronchitis and emphysema, with or without cor pulmonale.[215] The pertinent data are presented in Tables 11-21 A and B.

Recently, Rudolph and Yuan demonstrated the importance of the relationship between hypoxia and hydrogen-ion concentration in the PVR response in newborn calves.[148] In general, the lower the pH, the greater was the

Table 11-21A Effects of Infusion of Sodium Bicarbonate on Pulmonary Bood Volume (after Giuntini et al.)

Patients	Diagnosis	BSA	Condition	CI	HR	SI	PBV
1	Pul. tbc.	1.80	A	3.98	93	43	290
			B(1)	4.44	93	48	339
2	Pul. tbc.	1.53	A	3.14	69	46	208
			B(2)	3.54	75	47	243
3	Broncho. ca.	1.98	A	4.38	80	55	336
			B(3)	5.31	81	65	354
4	Pleural thickening	1.71	A	4.13	87	47	253
			B(3)	4.62	83	55	287
Average			A	3.91	82	48	272
			B	4.48	83	58	306

Pul. tbc.   = pulmonary tuberculosis, far advanced;
Bronch. ca. = bronchogenic carcinoma;
A   = control period;
B   = during infusion of sodium bicarbonate;
(1)   = one determination (3rd minute);
(2)   = average of four determinations (between 1st and 12th minutes);
(3)   = average of three determinations (between 4th and 12th minutes).
Other symbols and abbreviations are identical to those used in Table 11-1

Table 11-21B Effects of Infusion of Tris on Pulmonary Blood Volume (after Giuntini et al.)

Patients	BSA	Condition	CI	HR	SI	PBV
5	1.59	A	2.68	63	42	244
		B(11)	4.09	75	53	299
6	1.54	A	2.88	103	28	228
		B(9)	4.01	114	35	277
7	1.68	A	2.23	77	28	252
		B(11)	3.01	85	35	300
8	1.75	A	2.70	71	38	269
		B(4)	3.58	74	48	387
9	1.88	A	2.80	59	48	312
		B(4)	3.16	58	54	424
10	1.57	A	2.41	77	31	293
		B(12)	3.08	80	38	345
11	1.73	A	2.83	84	34	313
		B(12)	3.72	95	39	411
12	2.03	A	4.30	63	68	392
		B(12)	6.01	78	77	444
Average		A	2.98	75	39	288
		B	3.83	82	47	373

Patients 5-8 had a diagnosis of chronic bronchitis and emphysema;
Patients 9-12 had a diagnosis of cor pulmonale;
A = control period;
B = during infusion of Tris; the figures in the parentheses denote the minutes of infusion
    when the studies were repeated.
Other symbols and abbreviations are identical to those used in Table 11-1

PVR response to reduction of oxygen tension. Lloyd, using dog preparations, also showed that administration of alkali induced pulmonary vasodilatation in the presence of severe hypoxia.[147]

In 1967 Harvey and associates reported the effects of acute increase in blood hydrogen-ion concentration on pulmonary hemodynamics in 15 patients with obstructive lung disease.[149] PAm rose when the blood hydrogen-ion concentration increased. The pressor response was attributed to pulmonary arterial vasoconstriction and was independent of changes in CO, PBV and left veno-atrial pressure. It was not related to an increase in ventilation, because PAm fell as voluntary hyperventilation was increased to a degree comparable to that which occurred during the infusion of acid.

All these studies appear to indicate that acute acidosis induces pulmonary vasoconstriction resulting in a reduction in PBV, while acute alkalosis is associated with pulmonary vasodilatation and augmented PBV, and that acute acidosis enhances the pulmonary vascular response to hypoxia while acute alkalosis diminishes that response.

Temporary Occlusion of a Pulmonary Artery

In 1951 Carlens and associates reported a method for producing temporary unilateral pulmonary arterial occlusion in dogs and in man.[216] By means of single-lumen, balloon-tipped catheter in the initial study and a double-lumen catheter in subsequent investigations, they were able to produce complete and safe unilateral occlusion. Since then, other workers using similar techniques have presented findings in patients studied prior to thoracic surgery.[217,218] In 1957 Brofman and co-workers reported the results of complete occlusion of a pulmonary artery in a series of more than 100 patients.[219] Temporary occlusion produced no symptoms and was well tolerated. No significant change was noted in the electrocardiogram, BAm, arterial blood oxygen saturation, CO and oxygen uptake. During occlusion the ratio of minute oxygen uptake to minute ventilation remained relatively constant despite the fact that the occluded lung continued to ventilate without exchanging oxygen. The oxygen uptake of the unoccluded lung per unit of ventilation rose as much as twice the control value. With twice the control pulmonary flow perfusing one lung, the average PAm rose 30%, from 17 to 23 mm Hg. The systolic pressure rise was greater than the diastolic. Distal to the occlusion, the PAm fell to an average of 8 mm Hg, similar to the Pw.

In 1958 Charms and associates reported a study of unilateral pulmonary arterial occlusion in 28 patients with chronic pulmonary disease.[220] The control PAm varied from normal to three times normal. Approximate doubling of unilateral pulmonary blood flow was attended by an inconsistent increase in the PAm, not related to the control PAm. The data suggested that pulmonary hypertension in chronic pulmonary disease must often have causes other than organic arteriolar disease, such as increased intrapleural and intrapulmonic pressures.

Temporary occlusion of a pulmonary artery in a normal subject must create a considerable increase in physiologic dead space if alveolar ventilation continues on the occlusion side. Under these circumstances, total ventilation should increase about 80% to maintain normal arterial oxygen and CO_2 tensions. No investigators have reported such an increase in total ventilation.[291,221] If tidal volume, respiratory rate and oxygen uptake remain the same, the findings could be explained only if some or all of the ventilation of the non-perfused lung was shifted to the perfused lung.

Some workers have found no significant shift of ventilation during temporary unilateral pulmonary arterial occlusion,[216,221-223] but others have reported a redistribution of ventilation from the non-perfused lung to the perfused lung in both dogs and man.[224-226] Redistribution was explained by local

bronchoconstriction and regional atelectasis induced by low alveolar CO_2
tension in the non-perfused lung resulting from decreased elimination of
CO_2.[226] Redistribution may be prevented by adding CO_2 to the gas
inspired by the non-perfused lung,
sufficient to maintain normal alveolar
CO_2 tension.[224-227]

Finley and associates reported that
minimal surface tension of lung extracts
increased within 15 minutes after unilateral pulmonary arterial occlusion. [228-229]
Some workers found a generalized increase in alveolar surface forces after
occlusion,[230-231] but others have failed to
confirm this finding.[232]

McQuire and associates used the
mean transit time method to estimate
the change in PBV in 9 patients during
temporary unilateral pulmonary arterial occlusion.[233] PBV declined in all
but 1 case. The average fall was 26%.
The fact that the volume decreased
less than 50% indicates that the volume
of the unoccluded lung must have
increased. Their results are summarized
in Table 11-22. Aramendia and co-
workers measured the PBV in a series
of 11 dogs after ligation of the left
pulmonary artery.[234] Blood ordinarily

circulating through the occluded lung
was shunted into the remainder of the
pulmonary vascular bed and the total
PBV did not change significantly. This
adaptation took place with only slight
modifications in the circulation time
and the pressure of the system. The
authors suggested that increased flow
through the unoccluded lung caused
new or otherwise closed vascular
channels to open.

Pulmonary Embolization

Several excellent clinical reviews
on pulmonary embolism and infarction
have recently appeared.[235-238] According
to Dexter, pulmonary thromboembolism is currently the leading lethal
form of pulmonary disease at autopsy
in adults in a general hospital.[239] The
major hemodynamic consequences are
increased PAm proximal to the obstruction and reduction in pulmonary
blood flow.

Fatal pulmonary thromboembolism
in man is always massive and occludes
a large segment of the pulmonary
vasculature. In most cases thromboemboli occlude a multitude of small
muscular arteries of 0.1 to 1 mm di-

Table 11-22   Effects of Unilateral Occlusion upon Pulmonary Blood Volume in Man
(after McQuire, Dock, Hyland, Harrison, Haynes and Dexter)

Patient		Pulmonary Blood Volume (ml/M^2)			
		Before Occlusion	During Occlusion	Change	
				ml/M^2	%
1		244	179	−65	−27
2		168	145	−23	−14
3		153	119	−34	−22
4		273	173	−100	−37
5		237	199	−38	−16
6		388			
	RPA		243	−145	−37
	LPA		261	−127	−33
7		320	167	−153	−48
8		198	137	−61	−31
9		193	200	+ 7	+ 4
mean		256	182	−74	−26

RPA = right pulmonary artery
LPA = left pulmonary artery

ameter, a few large elastic arteries, and, rarely, arterioles.

The average arterial volume of embolized lung was only about one third normal in 36 typical fatal cases. The average normal pulmonary arterial volume in the right lung was measured as 63 ml/M^2, and in the left lung 56 ml/M^2. In patients with fatal pulmonary embolism, the same respective volumes were 21 and 22 ml/M^2.[239]

The clinical picture of pulmonary embolism has been well described, and the symptoms may be grouped in the following categories: (a) tachypnea, hyperventilation and cyanosis; (b) acute cor pulmonale with pulmonary hypertension and right ventricular failure; (c) circulatory collapse with hypotension and shock; (d) reduced coronary blood flow and angina; and (e) left ventricular failure and pulmonary edema. Pulmonary infarction following embolism may be manifested by pleuritic chest pain, hemoptysis, cough, fever and radiologic changes.

Ligation of one main branch of the pulmonary artery in dogs and in man causes little or no overall circulatory change. The remaining lung is able to accommodate the entire pulmonary blood flow with little elevation of the PAm. If the equivalent of more than 50 to 60% of the cross-sectional area of the main pulmonary artery is occluded by the embolization, however, circulatory and respiratory changes are likely.

Limited data from our laboratory have indicated that PBV is usually subnormal in thromboembolic pulmonary hypertension in man (Chapter 8).

Parker and Smith divided experimental pulmonary embolization into three categories, according to its extent.[236] In massive pulmonary embolization causing near total pulmonary arterial occlusion, death is usually rapid. In medium-sized pulmonary embolization, with or without infarction, the outcome may be favorable. Expanded bronchial circulation nourishes the lung tissue, adequately preventing infarction. If bronchial arterial flow is impaired by severe congestion or infection, however, pulmonary infarction may occur despite the augmented accessory vasculature in the involved parenchyma. With miliary pulmonary embolization, widespread reflex pulmonary arteriolar vasoconstriction causing marked pulmonary hypertension has been reported by a number of workers.[240-242] The vasoconstriction was probably mediated through sympathetic impulses because the abrupt pulmonary hypertensive response was absent after prior partial sympathectomy or autonomic blockade. Others, however, have expressed doubt that reflex pulmonary vascular constriction could occur from miliary embolization of the lungs.[243,244]

Hyman and co-workers reported the effects of acute pulmonary embolization produced by administration of macerated autogenous clot in dogs before and after administration of various pharmacologic agents.[242] The pertinent results are reproduced in Table 11-23. Without pharmacologic intervention, pulmonary embolization caused a marked rise in the PAm, a slight decline in the pulmonary venous pressure and appreciable reduction in the pulmonary-left atrial blood volume. In addition to the mechanical effects involved, these changes were considered manifestations of active pulmonary vasoconstriction. Administration of hexamethonium, atropine, methysergide (a serotonin antagonist), and norepinephrine did not significantly influence changes in the pulmonary vascular pressures or in the pulmonary-left atrial blood volume. Isoproterenol, on the other hand, produced active pulmo-

Table 11-23   Effects of Acute Pulmonary Embolism on Pulmonary Vascular Pressures
and Pulmonary Blood Volume Before and After Administration of Various
Kinds of Pharmacologic Agents (after Hyman, Myers and Meyer)

Periods of Study	No. of Dogs	PAm A	PAm B (3)	(10)	(20)	(40)	PVm A	PVm B (3)	(10)	(20)	(40)	PBV A	PBV B (3)	(10)	(20)	(40)
Control	25	15.6	34.0	29.0	24.0	21.0	3.4	1.6	2.9	2.6	2.3	10.4	6.6	6.6	6.8	6.9
Hexamethonium	16	15.0	24.0	20.0	18.0	16.8	4.0	−2.4	−2.0	−2.5	−2.1	10.0	5.4	5.6	5.7	5.6
Atropine	10	18.6	34.8	28.4	25.2	22.8	2.3	0.9	0.8	0.8	0.8	13.0	11.2	11.7	11.8	11.1
Norepinephrine	13	17.0	32.5	29.0	25.5	23.4	3.5	1.7	2.7	2.4	2.4	10.5	11.3	11.4	12.3	12.0
Methysergide	15	12.6	27.0	21.6	21.0	20.0	2.8	−0.5	−0.4	−0.2	−0.4	11.5	10.2	10.9	11.5	11.0
Isoproterenol	14	15.1	27.2	24.4	20.5	18.8	1.7	0.8	1.0	1.2	1.3	10.4	12.6	12.7	13.3	12.9

PAm = pulmonary arterial mean pressures (mm Hg);
PVm = large pulmonary venous mean pressure (mm Hg);
PBV = pulmonary blood volume including a portion of left atrial volume (ml/kg);
A   = before pulmonary embolism;
B   = after pulmonary embolism, the figures in parentheses denoting the minutes

nary vasodilatation, manifested by an increase in the pulmonary-left atrial blood volume and a decrease in PAm.

Some years ago, Comroe and coworkers suggested that blood clot lodged in the lung might liberate serotonin from platelets and thus produce widespread pulmonary vasoconstriction.[245] Along the same line, Thomas and associates released autogenous venous thrombi into dog lungs and demonstrated bronchoconstriction accompanied by a rapid rise in PVR and a fall in lung compliance.[246] Bronchoconstriction was completely prevented by the administration of heparin or by a serotonin antagonist. The authors suggested that bronchoconstriction in the dog caused by autogenous pulmonary emboli resulted from thrombi-induced serotonin release and that heparin prevented the reaction by its antithrombic action. Sanders and associates, however, found that the amount of serotonin in human and dog blood was insufficient to account for the pulmonary hypertension which followed pulmonary embolism.[247]

We studied the effects of acute pulmonary embolization produced by plastic spheres on pulmonary blood flow, pressures and volume in dogs

(Table 11-24).* PAm always rose sharply in the initial phase. Ten to 40 minutes after pulmonary embolization, however, the PAm usually declined gradually, sometimes almost approaching the control level. Both RAm and LAm were unchanged in all cases. PBV was determined initially by the mean transit time method, with sequential injections of indicator into the main pulmonary artery and left atrium and sampling from a femoral artery through a cuvette densitometer. A substantial reduction in the PBV was observed in every case. Subsequently, pulmonary-left heart volume was measured after injection of the indicator into the pulmonary artery and sampling at the aortic root. The direction and magnitude of the change in pulmonary-left heart volume was almost identical to that observed for PBV.

Other Conditions

Change in Temperature. DePasquale and associates studied the effects of temperature change in dogs.[248] The pulmonary-left atrial blood volume was

*I am indebted to Mr. Russell Luepker and Mr. James LoGerfo for their participation in this study during their summer student fellowships.

Table 11-24 Effects of Acute Pulmonary Embolization on Pulmonary Blood Volume in Dogs

Dog No.	Weight	Condition	CO (L/min)	Pressures (mm Hg) PAm	RAm	Tm (PA-LA)	PBV (ml) Total	Per Kg	Per Cent Change After Embolization Tm(PA-LA)	PBV
1	15	B	0.76	13.3	4.5	11.9	150	10.0	−14	− 2
		A	0.85	24.1	5.0	10.3	146	9.7		
2	17	B	1.15	13.5	5.0	9.6	183	10.8	−17	−25
		A	1.04	21.2	6.0	8.0	138	8.1		
3	18	B	1.08	15.5	5.8	9.5	168	9.4	−12	−20
		A	0.98	23.8	6.0	8.3	135	7.5		
4	14	B	1.01	20.5	4.8	8.7	147	10.5	−20	−18
		A	1.04	34.5	5.0	7.0	121	8.6		

B   = before embolization;
A   = after embolization;
CO   = cardiac output;
RAm = right atrial mean pressure.
Other symbols and abbreviations are identical to those used in Table 11-1

determined by injecting indicator into the pulmonary artery and sampling from the left atrium. When the surrounding temperature was decreased to 14°C, the pulmonary venous pressure rose, and pulmonary-left atrial blood volume declined slightly or did not change. When the surrounding temperature was increased to 40°C, the pulmonary venous pressure declined and pulmonary-left atrial volume increased. The authors felt that cold caused active constriction of the pulmonary veins, partly due to a direct effect of cold blood on the vessel wall. In addition, increased blood viscosity in the cold may reduce the rate of blood flow and increase the hematocrit. On the other hand, the pulmonary veins responded to heat in the same manner as the peripheral veins, that is, by vasodilatation and a decrease in tone.

Reactive Hyperemia in Legs. Korsgren and associates studied the PBV in 10 patients with valvular heart disease during reactive hyperemia in the legs.[94] Simultaneous injections of one indicator into the main pulmonary artery and another indicator into the left atrium were followed by collection of arterial blood from the brachial artery and from the femoral artery at rest and during reactive hyperemia.

No consistent difference was found between PBV calculated from the brachial arterial curves and from the femoral arterial curves during active hyperemia. Thus, changes in peripheral flow distribution did not influence the validity and accuracy of the double indicator method for determination of PBV. Furthermore, reactive hyperemia in the legs did not in itself cause a significant change in PBV in patients with valvular heart disease.

Pulmonary Arterial Constrictor Substance (PACS). In an exciting recent report, Robin and associates described the hemodynamic effects of an active humoral agent, pulmonary arterial constrictor substance (PACS), obtained *in vivo* by repeated saline solution washings of the lungs of young calves.[249] This material produced precapillary pulmonary hypertension and a marked increase in PVR in dogs or calves when injected into either the right atrium or the femoral artery. CO, HR, BAm and arterial blood oxygen tension were not affected.

Pulmonary hypertension following PACS injection was considered to be a consequence of pulmonary vasoconstriction rather than mechanical occlusion of pulmonary vessels. The site of constriction was probably the pulmonary arterioles, inasmuch as the Pw was unchanged following PACS injection. The diameter of the main pulmonary artery and its proximal branches was markedly increased roentgenographically. Changes in PBV or Vc have not been studied, but a decrease in PBV would be expected. PACS differs chemically and pharmacologically from other substances previously investigated for pulmonary pressor

activity, such as histamine, serotonin, bradykinin, ATP, epinephrine and norepinephrine.

The possibility is recognized that release of PACS might predispose to local hypoxia, resulting in vasoconstriction of the small precapillary pulmonary arterioles. The precise role of PACS in the regulation of the pulmonary circulation and its relation to hypoxia will require further investigation. Isolation and chemical characterization of the specific agent concerned will be especially important.

REFERENCES

1. Gauer, O.H., and Thron, H.L.: Postural changes in circulation. *In* W.F. Hamilton and P. Dow (eds), *Handbook of Physiology*, Section 2, Circulation, vol. 3, Chapter 67, p. 2409, Washington, D.C., American Physiological Society, 1965.

2. Reeves, J.T., Grover, R.F., Blount, S.G., and Filley, G.F.: Cardic output response to standing and treadmill walking. J. Appl. Physiol., *16*, 283, 1961.

3. Bevegard, S., Holmgren, A., and Josson, B.: The effect of body position on the circulation at rest and during exercise, with special reference to the influence on the stroke volume. Acta Physiol. Scand., *49*, 279, 1960.

4. McMichael, J., and Sharpey-Schafer, E.P.: Cardiac output in man by a direct Fick method. Effects of posture, venous pressure change, atropine, and adrenaline. Brit. Heart J., *6*, 33, 1944.

5. Stead, E.A., Warren, J.V., Merrill, A.J., and Brannon, E.S.: The cardiac output in male subjects as measured by the technique of right atrial catheterization. Normal values with observations on the effect of anxiety and tilting. J. Clin. Invest., *24*, 326, 1945.

6. Lagerlöf, H., Eliasch, H., Werkö, L., and Berglund, E.: Orthostatic changes of pulmonary and peripheral circulation in man. Preliminary report. Scand. J. Clin. Lab. Invest., *3*, 85, 1951.

7. Donald, K.W., Bishop, J.M., Cumming, G., and Wade, O.L.: The effect of nursing positions on the cardiac output in man. Clin. Sci., *12*, 199, 1953.

8. Weissler, A.M., Leonard, J.J., and Warren, J.V.: Effects of posture and atropine on the cardiac output. J. Clin. Invest., *36*, 1656, 1957.

9. Sancetta, S.M.: Acute hemodynamic effects of total head-down body tilt and hexamethonium in normal and pulmonary emphysematous subjects. J. Lab. & Clin. Med., *49*, 684, 1957.

10. Martin, C.J., Cline, F., and Marshall, H.: Lobar alveolar gas concentration: Effect of body position. J. Clin. Invest., *32*, 617, 1953.

11. Mattson, S.B., and Carlens, E.: Lobar ventilation and oxygen uptake in man. Influence of body position. J. Thorac. Surg., *30*, 676, 1955.

12. Riley, R.L., Permutt, S., Said, S., Godfrey, M.P.W., Cheng, T.O., Howell, J.B.L., and Shepard, R.H.: Effect of posture on pulmonary dead space in man. J. Appl. Physiol., *14*, 339, 1959.

13. West, J.B., and Dollery, C.T.: Distribution of blood flow and ventilation-perfusion ratio in the lung, measured with radioactive CO_2. J. Appl. Physiol., *15*, 405, 1960.

14. Dollery, C.T., Dyson, N.A., and Sinclair, J.D.: Regional variations in uptake of radioactive CO_2 in the normal lung. J. Appl. Physiol., *15*, 411, 1960.

15. West, J.B.: Regional differences in gas exchange in the lung of erect man. J. Appl. Physiol., *17*, 893, 1962.

16. Ball, W.C., Stewart, P.B., Newsham, L.G.S., and Bates, D.V.: Regional pulmonary function studies with Xenon.[133] J. Clin. Invest., *41*, 519, 1962.

17. Sjöstrand, T.: The regulation of the blood distribution in man. Acta Physiol. Scand., *26*, 312, 1952.

18. Sjöstrand, T.: Volume and distribution of blood and their significance in regulating the circulation. Physiol. Rev., *33*, 202, 1953.

19. Weissler, A.M., McCraw, B.H., and Warren, J.V.: Pulmonary blood volume determined by a radioactive tracer technique. J. Appl. Physiol., *14*, 531, 1959.

20. Holmgren, A., and Ovenfors, C.O.: Heart volume at rest and during muscular work in the supine and in the sittting position. Acta med. Scand., *167*, 267, 1960.

21. Naimark, A., and Wasserman, K.: The effect of posture on pulmonary capillary blood flow in man. J. Clin. Invest., *41*, 949, 1962.

22. Bondurant, S., Hickam, J.B., and Isley, J.K.: Pulmonary and circulatory effects of acute pulmonary vascular engorgement in normal subjects. J. Clin. Invest., *36*, 59, 1957.

23. Ross, J.C., Ley, G.D Coburn, R.F., Eller, J.L., and Forster, R.E.: Influence of pressure suit inflation on pulmonary diffusing capacity in man. J. Appl. Physiol., *17*, 259, 1962.

24. Daly, W.J., Giammona, S.T., and Ross, J.C.: The pressure-volume relationship of the normal pulmonary capillary bed. J. Clin. Invest., *44*, 1261, 1965.

25. Trimby, R.H., and Nicholson, H.C.: Some observations on the nature of the respiratory waves in arterial blood pressure. Am. J. Physiol., *129*, 289, 1940.

26. Schuler, R.H., Ensor C., Gunning, R.E., Moss, W.G., and Johnson, V.: The differential effects of respiration on the left and right ventricles. Am. J. Physiol., *137*, 620, 1942.

27. Dupee, C., and Johnson, V.: Respiratory changes in pulmonary vascular capacity. Am. J. Physiol., *139*, 95, 1943.

28. Brecher, G.A., and Mixter, G.: Effect of respiratory movements on superior vena cava under normal and abnormal conditions. Am. J. Physiol., *172*, 457, 1953.

29. Mixter, G.: Respiratory augmentation of inferior vena caval flow demonstrated by a low resistance phasic flowmeter. Am. J. Physiol., *172*, 446, 1953.

30. Brecher, G.A., and Hubay, C.A.: Pulmonary blood flow and venous return during spontaneous respiration. Circ. Res., *3*, 210, 1955.

31. Burton, A.C., and Patel, D.J.: Effect on pulmonary vascular resistance of inflation of the rabbit lung. J. Appl. Physiol., *12*, 229, 1958.

32. Lawson, H.D., Bloomfield, R.A., and Cournand, A.: The influence of the respiration on the circulation in man. Am. J. Med., *1*, 315, 1946.

33. Yu, P.N., Lovejoy, F.W., Joos, H.A., Nye, R.E., Beatty, D.C., and Simpson, J.H.: Pulmonary "capillary" pressure in various cardiopulmonary diseases at rest and under stress. Am. Heart J., *49*, 31, 1955.

34. DuBois, A., and Marshall, R.: Measurements of pulmonary capillary blood flow and gas exchange throughout the respiratory cycle in man. J. Clin. Invest., *36*, 1566, 1957.

35. Morkin, E., Collins, J.A., Goldman, H.S., and Fishman, A.P.: Pattern of blood flow in the pulmonary veins of the dog. J. Appl. Physiol., *20*, 1118, 1965.

36. Morgan, B.C., Dillard, D.H., and Guntheroth, W.G.: Effect of cardiac and respiratory cycle on pulmonary vein flow, pressure and diameter. J. Appl. Physiol., *21*, 1276, 1966.

37. Kinnen, E., Stankus, A., and Yu, P.N.: Pulmonary venous blood flow characteristics. Presented at the 20th Annual Conf. on Engr. in Med. & Biol., Boston, Mass., Nov. 13-16, 1967.

38. Hamilton, W.F., Woodbury, R.A., and Harper, H.T.: Arterial, cerebrospinal and venous pressures in man during cough and strain. Am. J. Physiol., *141*, 42, 1944.

39. Sharpey-Schafer, E.P.: Effect of respiratory acts on the circulation. *In* W.F. Hamilton and P. Dow (eds), *Handbook of Physiology*, Section 2, vol. 3. Chapter 52, p. 1875, Washington, D.C., American Physiological Society, 1965.

40. Lee, G., de J., Mathews, M.B., and Sharpey-Schafer, E.P.: The effect of the Valsalva maneuver on the systemic and pulmonary arterial pressure in man. Brit. Heart J., *16*, 311, 1954.

41. Elisberg, E., Singian E., Miller, G., and Katz, L.N.: The effect of the Valsalva maneuver on circulation. III. The influence of heart disease on the expected poststraining overshoot. Circulation, *7*, 880, 1953.

42. McIntosh, H.D., Burnum, J.F., Hickam, J.B., and Warren, J.V.: Circulatory changes produced by the Valsalva maneuver in normal subjects, patients with mitral stenosis, and autonomic nervous system alterations. Circulation, *9*, 511, 1954.

43. Fox, I.J., Crowley, W.P., Grace, J.B., and Wood, E.H.: Effects of the Valsalva maneuver on blood flow in the thoracic aorta in man. J. Appl. Physiol., *21*, 1553, 1966.

44. Meier, P., and Zierler, K.L.: On the theory of the indicator dilution method for measurement of blood flow and volume. J. Appl. Physiol., *6*, 731, 1954.

45. Dow, P.: Estimations of cardiac output and central blood volume by dye dilution. Physiol. Rev., *36*, 77, 1956.

46. Ross, J.C., Lord, T.H., and Ley, G.D.: Effect of pressure-suit inflation on pulmonary-diffusing capacity. J. Appl. Physiol., *15*, 843, 1960.

47. Johnson, R.L., Spicer, W.S., Bishop, J.M., and Forster, R.E.: Pulmonary capillary blood volume, flow and diffusing capacity during exercise. J. Appl. Physiol., *15*, 893, 1960.

48. Maloney, J.V., Affeldt, J.E., Sarnoff, S.J., and Whittenberger, J.L.: Electrophrenic respiration. IX. Comparison of effects of positive pressure breathing and electrophrenic respiration on the circulation during hemorrhagic shock and barbiturate poisoning. Surg., Gynec. & Obst., *92*, 672, 1951.

49. Ankeney, J.L., Hubay, C.A., Hackett, P.R., and Hingson, R.A.: Effect of positive and negative pressure respiration on unilateral pulmonary blood flow in the open chest. Surg., Gynec. & Obst., *98*, 600, 1954.

50. Linde, L.M., Simmons, D.H., and Ellman, E.L.: Pulmonary hemodynamics during positive pressure breathing. J. Appl. Physiol., *16*, 644, 1961.

51. Beecher, H.K., Bennett, H.S., and Basset, D.L.: Circulatory effects of increased pressure in the airway. Anesthesiol., *4*, 612, 1943.

52. Motley H.L., Cournand, A., Eckman, M., and Richards, D.W.: Physiological studies on man with the pneumatic balance resuscitator, "Burns Model." J. Aviat. Med., *17*, 431, 1946.

53. Barach, A.L., Fenn, W.O., Ferris, E.B., and Schmidt, C.F.: The physiology of pressure breathing. J. Aviat. Med., *18*, 73, 1947.

54. Werkö, L.: The influence of positive pressure breathing on the circulation in man. Acta med. Scand. Suppl. 193, 1947.

55. Cournand, A., Motley, H.L., Werkö, L., and Richards, D.W.: Physiological studies of the effects of intermittent positive pressure breathing on cardiac output in man. Am. J. Physiol., *152*, 162, 1953.

56. Braunwald, E., Binion, J.T., Morgan, W.L., and Sarnoff, S.J.: Alterations in central blood volume and cardiac output induced by positive pressure breathing and counteracted by metaraminol (Aramine). Circ. Res., *5*, 670, 1957.

57. Kilburn, K.H., and Sieker, H.O.: Hemodynamic effects of continuous positive and negative pressure breathing in normal man. Circ. Res., *8*, 660, 1960.

58. Roncoroni, A.J., Agrest, A., Roehr, E., and Grzesko, S.: Hemodynamics during mechanical ventilation. Am. Heart J., *64*, 207, 1962.

59. Fenn, W.O., Otis, A.B., Rahn, H., Chadwick, L.E., and Hegnauer, A.H.: Displacement of blood from the lungs by pressure breathing. Am. J. Physiol., *151*, 258, 1947.

60. Hubay, C.A., Brecher, G.A., and Clement, F.L.: Etiological factors affecting pulmonary artery flow with controlled respiration. Surgery, *38*, 215, 1955.

61. Huggett, A., St. G.: Studies on the respiration and circulation of the cat. IV. Heart output during respiratory obstruction. J. Physiol., *59*, 373, 1924.

62. Breecher, G.A.: *Venous Return.* New York, Grune & Stratton, 1956.

63. Holt, J.P.: Effect of positive and negative intrathoracic pressure on cardiac output and venous pressure in the dog. Am. J. Physiol., *142*, 594, 1944.

64. Ernsting, J.: Compliance of the human lungs during positive and negative pressure breathing. J. Physiol., *144*, 14P, 1958.

65. Hickam, J.B., and Cargill, W.H.: Effects of exercise on cardiac output and pulmonary arterial pressure in normal persons and in patients with cardiovascular disease and pulmonary emphysema. J. Clin. Invest., *27*, 10, 1948.

66. Riley, R.L., Himmelstein, A., Motley, H.L., Weiner, H.M., and Cournand, A.: Studies of the pulmonary circulation at rest and during exercise in normal individuals and in patients with chronic pulmonary disease. Am. J. Physiol., *152*, 372, 1948.

67. Dexter, L., Whittenberger, J.L., Haynes, F.W., Goodale, W.T., Gorlin, R., and Sawyer, C.G.: Effect of exercise on circulatory dynamics of normal individuals. J. Appl. Physiol., *3*, 439, 1951.

68. Donald, K.W., Bishop, J.M., and Wade, O.L.: A study of minute-to-minute changes of arterio-venous oxygen content difference, oxygen uptake and cardiac output and rate of achievement of a steady state during exercise in rheumatic heart disease. J. Clin. Invest., *33*, 1146, 1954.

69. Donald, K.W., Bishop, J.M., Cummings, G., and Wade, O.L.: The effect of exercise on the cardiac output and circulatory dynamics of normal subjects. Clin. Sci., *14*, 37, 1955.

70. Sancetta, S.M., Rakita, L., Heckman, G., and Janouskovec, H.: Response of pulmonary artery pressure and total pulmonary resistance of untrained convalescent man to prolonged steady state exercise. J. Clin. Invest., *36*, 1138, 1957.

71. Slonim, N.B., Ravin, A., Balchum, O.J., and Dressler, S.H.: The effect of mild exercise in the supine position on the pulmonary arterial pressure of five normal human subjects. J. Clin. Invest., *33*, 1022, 1954.

72. Barrett-Boyes, B.G., and Wood, E.H.: Hemo-dynamic response of healthy subjects to exercise in the supine position while breathing oxygen. J. Appl. Physiol., *11*, 129, 1957.

73. Harris, P., and Heath, D.: *The Human Pulmonary Circulation*, Baltimore, Williams & Wilkins Co., 1962, p. 106.

74. Wang, Y., Marshall, R.J., and Shepherd, J.T.: The effect of changes in posture and of graded exercise on stroke volume in man. J. Clin. Invest., *39*, 1051, 1960.

75. Mitchell, J.H. Sproule, B.J., and Chapman, C.B.: Factors influencing respiration during heavy exercise. J. Clin. Invest., *37*, 1693, 1958.

76. Roncoroni, A.J., Aramendia, P., Gonzalez, R.. and Taquini, A.C.: "Central" blood volume in exercise in normal subjects. Acta Physiol. Latinoam, *9*, 55, 1959.

77. Braunwald, E., and Kelly, E.R.: The effects of exercise on central blood volume in man. J. Clin. Invest., *39*, 413, 1960.

78. Levinson, G.E., Pacifico. A.D., and Frank, M.J.: Studies of cardiopulmonary blood volume. Measurement of total cardiopulmonary blood volume in normal human subjects at rest and during exercise. Circulation, *33*, 347, 1966.

79. Marshall, R.J., and Shepherd, J.T.: Interpretation of changes in "central blood volume" and slope volume during exercise in man. J. Clin. Invest., *40*, 375, 1961.

80. McIntosh, H.D., Gleason, W.L., Miller, D.E., and Bacos, J.M.: A major pitfall in the interpretation of "central blood volume." Circ. Res., *9*, 1223, 1961.

81. Moir, T.W., and Gott, F.S.: The central circulating blood volume in normal subjects and patients with mitral stenosis. Am. Heart J., *61*, 740, 1961.

82. Chaffee, W.R., Smulyan, H., Keighley, J.F., and Eich, R.H.: The effect of exercise on pulmonary blood volume. Am. Heart J., *66*, 657, 1963.

83. Gorlin, R., Sawyer, C.G., Haynes, F.W., Goodale, W.T., and Dexter, L.: Effects of exercise on circulatory dynamics in mitral stenosis. Am. Heart J., *41*, 192, 1951.

84. Ferrer, M., Harvey, R.M., Cathcart, R.T., Cournand, A., and Richards, D.W.: Hemodynamic studies in rheumatic heart disease. Circulation, *6*, 688, 1952.

85. Ball, J.D., Kopelman, H., and Witham, A.C.: Circulatory changes in mitral stenosis at rest and with exercise. Brit. Heart J., *14*, 363, 1952.

86. Gorlin, R., McMillan, I.K.R., Medd, W.E., Matthews, M.B., and Daley, R.: Dynamics of the circulation in aortic valvular disease. Am. J. Med., *18*, 855, 1955.

87. Sancetta, S.M,. and Kleinerman, J.: Effect of mild, steady state exercise on total pulmonary resistance of normal subjects and those with isolated aortic valvular lesions. Am. Heart J., *53*, 404, 1957.

88. Taylor, S.H., Donald, K.W., and Bishop, J.M.: Circulatory studies in hypertensive patients at rest and during exercise with a note on the Starling relationship in the left ventricle in essential hypertension. Clin. Sci., *16*, 351, 1957.

89. Bruce, R.A., Cobb, L.A., Morledge, J.H., and Katsura, S.: Effects of posture, upright exercise, and myocardial stimulation on cardiac output in patients with diseases affecting diastolic filling and effective systolic ejection of the left ventricle. Am. Heart J., *61*, 476, 1961.

90. Harvey, R.M., Smith, W.M., Parker, J.O., and Ferrer, M.I.: The response of the abnormal heart to exercise. Circulation, *26*, 341, 1962.

91. Dexter, L., Lewis, B.M., Houssay, H.E.J., and Haynes, F.W.: Dynamics of both right and left ventricles at rest and during exercise in patients with heart failure. Tr. Ass. Am. Phys., *66*, 266, 1953.

92. Oakley, C., Glick, G., Luria, M.N., Schreiner, B.F., and Yu, P.N.: Some regulatory mechanisms of the human pulmonary vascular bed. Circulation, *16*, 917, 1962.

93. Schreiner, B.F., Murphy, G.W., Glick, G., and Yu, P.N.: Effect of exercise on the pulmonary blood volume in patients with acquired heart disease. Circulation, *27*, 559, 1963.

94. Korsgren, M., Kallay, K., and Varnauskas, E.: Pulmonary and "central" blood volume during reactive hyperaemia in the legs. Clin. Sci., *32*, 415, 1967.

95. Korsgren, M., Leupker, R., Liander, B., and Varnauskas, E.: Pulmonary intra-and extravascular fluid volume changes with exercise. Submitted for publication.

96. Engel, G.L.: *Fainting-Physiological and Psychological Considerations.* Springfield, Charles C Thomas, 1962.

97. Lewis, T.: Vasovagal syncope and the carotid sinus mechanism. Brit Med. J., *1*, 873, 1932.

98. Weissler, A.M., Warren, J.V., Estes, E.H., McIntosh, H.D., and Leonard, J.J.: Vasodepressor syncope. Factors influencing cardiac output. Circulation, *15*, 875, 1957.

99. Weissler, A.M., and Warren, J.V.: Vasodepressor syncope. Am. Heart J., *57*, 786, 1959.

100. Wayne, H.H.: Syncope. Physiologic considerations and an analysis of the clinical

characteristics in 510 patients. Am. J. Med., *30*, 418, 1961.

101. Greene, M.A., Boltox, A.J., and Ulberg, R.J.: Cardiovascular dynamics of vasovagal reactions in man. Circ. Res., *9*, 12, 1961.

102. Barcroft, H., and Edholm, O.G.: On the vasodilatation in human skeletal muscle during post-haemorrhagic fainting. J.Physiol., *104*, 161, 1945.

103. Glick, G., and Yu, P.N.: Hemodynamic changes during spontaneous vasovagal reactions. Am. J. Med., *34*, 42, 1963.

104. Sarnoff, S.J., Brockman, S.K., Gilmore, J.P., Linden, R.J., and Mitchell, J.H.: Regulation of ventricular contraction. Influence of cardiac sympathetic and vagal nerve stimulation on atrial and ventricular dynamics. Circ. Res., *8*, 1108, 1960.

105. Landis, E.M., and Hortenstine, J.C.: Functional significance of venous blood pressure. Physiol. Rev., *30*, 1, 1950.

106. Rashkind, W.J., Lewis, D.H., Henderson, J.B., Heiman, D.F., and Dietrick, R.B.: Venous return as affected by cardiac output and total peripheral resistance. Am. J. Physiol., *175*, 415, 1953.

107. Duggan, J.J., Love, V.L., and Lyons, R.H.: A study of reflex venomotor reactions in man. Circulation, *7*, 869, 1953.

108. Page, E.B., Hickam, J.B., Sieker, H.O., McIntosh,, H.D., and Pryor, W.W.: Reflex venomotor activity in normal persons and in patients with postural hypotension. Circulation, *11*, 262, 1955.

109. Burch, G.E., and Murtadha, M.: A study of the venomotor tone in a short intact venous segment of the forearm of man. Am. Heart J., *51*, 807, 1956.

110. Bartelstone, H.J.: Role of the veins in venous return. Circ. Res., *8*, 1059, 1960.

111. Sharpey-Schafer, E.P.: Venous tone. Brit. Med. J., *2*, 1589, 1961.

112. Aviado, D.M., and Schmidt, C.F.: Reflexes from stretch receptors in blood vessels, heart and lungs. Physiol. Rev., *35*, 247, 1955.

113. Löfving, B.: Cardiovascular adjustments induced from the rostral cingulate gyrus with special reference to sympatho-inhibitory mechanisms. Acta Physiol. Scand., *53*, Suppl. 184, 1961.

114. Fishman, A.P.: Respiratory gases in the regulation of the pulmonary circulation. Physiol. Rev., *41*, 214, 1961.

115. _____: Dynamics of the pulmonary circulation. *In* W.F. Hamilton and P. Dow (eds), *Handbook of Physiology*, Section 2,

Vol. 2, Chapter 48, pp. 1667-1743. Washington, D.C., American Physiological Society, 1963.

116. Aviado, D.M.: *The Lung Circulation*, Vol. 1, Oxford, London, New York, Pergamon Press, 1965, pp. 3-119,

117. Hatcher, J.D., and Jennings, D.B.(eds): *Proceedings of International Symposium on the Cardiovascular and Respiratory Effects of Hypoxia*. New York, Hafner Publishing Co., Inc., 1966.

118. Von Euler, U.S. and Liljestrand, G.: Observations on the pulmonary arterial blood pressure in the cat. Acta Physiol. Scand., *12*, 301, 1946.

119. Liljestrand, G.: Regulation of pulmonary arterial blood pressure. Arch. Int. Med., *81*, 162, 1948.

120. Dirken, M.N.J., and Hemmstra, H.: Alveolar oxygen tension and lung circulation. Quart. J. Exp. Physiol., *34*, 193, 1948.

121. Atwell, R.J., Hickam, J.B., Pryor, W.W., and Page, E.B.: Reduction of blood flow through the hypoxic lung. Am. J. Physiol., *166*, 37, 1951.

122. Duke, H.N.: The site of action of anoxia on the pulmonary blood vessels of the cat. J. Physiol., *125*, 373, 1954.

123. Aviado, D.M., Cerlitti, A., Alanis, J., Bulle, P.H., and Schmidt, C.F.: Effects of anoxia on pressure, resistance and blood (P^{32}) volume of pulmonary vessels. Am. J. Physiol., *169*, 460, 1952.

124. Lewis, B.M., and Gorlin, R.: Effects of hypoxia on pulmonary circulation of the dog. Am. J. Physiol., *170*, 574, 1952.

125. Rahn, H., and Bahnson, H.T.: Effect of unilateral hypoxia on gas exchange and calculated pulmonary blood flow in each lung. J. Appl. Physiol., *6*, 105, 1953.

126. Nahas, G.G., Visscher, M.B., Mather, G.W., Haddy, F.J., and Warner, H.R.: Influence of hypoxia on the pulmonary circulation of nonnarcotized dogs. J. Appl. Physiol., *6*, 467, 1953.

127. Hurlmann, A., and Wiggers, C.J.: The effects of progressive general anoxia on the pulmonary circulation. Circ. Res., *1*, 230, 1953.

128. Stroud, R.C., and Rahn, H.: Effect of O_2 and CO_2 tensions upon the resistance of pulmonary blood vessels. Am. J. Physiol., *172*, 211, 1953.

129. Stroud, R.C., and Conn, H.L.: Pulmonary vascular effects of moderate and severe hypoxia in the dog. Am. J. Physiol., *179*, 119, 1954.

130. Borst, H.G., Whittenberger, J.L., Berglund, E., and McGregor, M.: Effects of unilateral hypoxia and hypercapnia on pulmonary blood

flow distribution in the dog. Am. J. Physiol., *191*, 446, 1957.

131. Rivera-Estrada, C., Saltzman, P.W., Singer, D., and Katz, L.N.: Action of hypoxia on pulmonary vasculature. Circ. Res., *6*, 10, 1958.

132. Motley, H.L., Cournand, A., Werkö, L., Himmelstein, A., and Dresdale, D.: The influence of short periods of induced acute anoxia upon pulmonary artery pressures in man. Am. J. Physiol., *150*, 315, 1947.

133. Westcott, R.N., Fowler, N.O., Scott, R.C., Hauenstein, V.D., and McQuire, J.: Anoxia and pulmonary vascular resistance. J. Clin. Invest., *30*, 957, 1951.

134. Doyle, J.T., Wilson, J.S., and Warren, J.V.: The pulmonary vascular responses to short-term hypoxia in human subjects. Circulation, *5*, 263, 1952.

135. Fishman, A.P., McClement, J., Himmelstein, A., and Cournand, A.: Effects of acute anoxia on the circulation and respiration in patients with chronic pulmonary disease studied during the "steady state." J. Clin. Invest., *31*, 770, 1952.

136. Siebens, A.A., Smith, R.E., and Storey, C.F.: Effect of hypoxia on pulmonary vessels in man. Am. J. Physiol., *180*, 428, 1955.

137. Yu, P.N., Beatty, D.C., Lovejoy, F.W., Nye, R.E., and Joos, H.A.: Hemodynamic effects of acute hypoxia in patients with mitral stenosis. Am. Heart J., *52*, 683, 1956.

138. Fishman, A.P., Fritts, H.W., and Cournand, A.: Effects of acute hypoxia and exercise in the pulmonary circulation. Circulation, *22*, 204, 1960.

139. Yu, P.N., Glick, G., Schreiner, B.F., and Murphy, G.W.: Effects of acute hypoxia on the pulmonary vascular bed of patients with acquired heart disease. Circulation, *27*, 541, 1963.

140. Himmelstein, A., Harris, P., Fritts, H.W., and Cournand, A.: Effect of severe unilateral hypoxia on the partition on pulmonary blood flow in man. J. Thorac. Surg., *36*, 369, 1958.

141. Defares, J.G., Laudin, G., Arborelius, M., Stromblad, R., and Svanberg, L.: Effect of unilateral hypoxia on pulmonary blood flow distribution in normal subjects. J. Appl. Physiol., *15*, 169, 1960.

142. Fritts, H.W., Harris, P., Clauss, R.H., Odell, J.E., and Cournand, A.: Effect of acetylcholine on the human pulmonary circulation under normal and hypoxic conditions. J. Clin. Invest., *37*, 99, 1958.

143. Goldring, R.M., Turino, G.M., Cohen, G., Jameson, A.G., Bass, B.G., and Fishman, A.F.: The catecholamines in the pulmonary arterial pressor response to acute hypoxia. J. Clin. Invest., *41*, 1211, 1962.

144. Liljestrand, G.: Chemical control of the distribution of the pulmonary blood flow. Acta Physiol. Scand., *44*, 216, 1958.

145. Bergofsky, E.H., Lehr, D.E., and Fishman, A.P.: The effect of changes in hydrogen ion concentration on the pulmonary circulation. J. Clin. Invest., *41*, 1492, 1962.

146. Enson, Y., Giuntini, C., Lewis, M.L., Morris, T.Q., Ferrer, M.I., and Harvey, R.M.: The influence of hydrogen ion concentration and hypoxia on the pulmonary circulation. J. Clin. Invest., *43*, 1146, 1964.

147. Lloyd, T.C.: Influence of blood pH on hypoxic pulmonary vasoconstriction. J. Appl. Physiol., *21*, 358, 1966.

148. Rudolph, A.M., and Yuan, S.: Response of the pulmonary vasculature to hypoxia and H^+ ion concentration changes. J. Clin. Invest., *45*, 399, 1966.

149. Harvey, R.M., Enson, Y., Betti, R., Lewis, M.L., Rochester, D.F., and Ferrer, M.I.: Further observations on the effect of hydrogen ion on the pulmonary circulation. Circulation, *35*, 1019, 1967.

150. Honig, C.R., and Tenney, S.M.: Determinants of the circulatory response to hypoxia and hypercapnia. Am. Heart J., *53*, 687, 1957.

151. Fritts, H.W., Odell, J.E., Harris, P., Braunwald, E., and Fishman, A.P.: Effects of acute hypoxia on the volume of blood in the thorax. Circulation, *22*, 216, 1960.

152. Kato, M., and Staub, N.: Response of small pulmonary arteries to unilobar hypoxia and hypercapnia. Circ. Res., *19*, 426, 1966.

153. Sackner, M.A., Will, D.H., and DuBois, A.B.: The site of pulmonary vasomotor activity during hypoxia or serotonin administration. J. Clin. Invest., *45*, 112, 1966.

154. Jameson, A.G.: Diffusion of gases from alveolus to precapillary arteries. Science, *139*, 826, 1963.

155. Sobol, B.J., Bottex, G., Emirgil, C., and Gissen, H.: Gaseous diffusion from alveoli to pulmonary vessels of considerable size. Circ. Res., *13*, 71, 1963.

156. Dressler, S.H., Slonim, N.B., Balchum, O.J., Bronfin, G.J., and Ravin, A.: The effect of breathing 100% oxygen on the pulmonary arterial pressure in patients with pulmonary tuberculosis and mitral stenosis. J. Clin. Invest., *31*, 807, 1952.

157. McGregor, M., Bothwell, T.H., Zion, M.M., and Bradlow, B.A.: The effects of oxygen breathing on the pulmonary circulation in mitral stenosis. Am. Heart J., *46*, 187, 1953.

158. Wilson, R.H., Hoseth, W., and Dampsey, M.E.: The effects of breathing 99.6% oxygen on pulmonary vascular resistance and cardiac output in patients with pulmonary emphysema and chronic anoxia. Ann. Int. Med., *42*, 629, 1955.

159. Tartulier, M., Deyrieux, F., Anterion, H., and Taurniaire, A.: L'inhalation d'un mélange O_2 95% +CO_2 5% chez les emphysémateux au space du coeur pulmonaire chronique. Son effet sur la ventilation et la circulation pulmonaires. Arch Mal. Coeur, *51*, 1164, 1958.

160. Swan, H.J.C., Burchell, H.B., and Wood, E.H.: Effect of oxygen on pulmonary vascular resistance in patients with pulmonary hypertension associated with atrial septal defect. Circulation, *20*, 66, 1959.

161. Bateman, M., Davidson, L.A.G., Donald, K.W., and Harris, P.: A comparison of the effect of acetylcholine and 100 per cent oxygen on the pulmonary circulation in patients with mitral stenosis. Clin. Sci., *22*, 223, 1962.

162. Goldring, R.M., Turino, G.M., Andersen, D.H., and Fishman, A.P.: Cor pulmonale in cystic fibrosis of the pancreas. Circulation, *24*, 942, 1961.

163. Glick, G., Schreiner, B.F., Murphy, G.W., and Yu, P.N.: Effects of inhalation of 100 per cent oxygen on the pulmonary blood volume in patients with organic heart disease. Circulation, *27*, 554, 1963.

164. McGregor, M.: Oxygen tension and the regulation of pulmonary blood flow. *In* J.D. Hatcher and D.B. Jennings (eds), *Proceedings International Symposium Cardiovascular and Respiratory Effects of Hypoxia*, p. 287, New York, Hafner Publishing, Co., Inc., 1966.

165. Storstein, O.: The effect of pure oxygen breathing on the circulation in anoxemia. Acta Med. Scand. (Suppl) 269, 1952.

166. Barratt-Boyes, B.G., and Wood, E.H.: Cardiac output and related measurements and pressure values in the right heart and associated vessels, together with an analysis of the hemodynamic response to the inhalation of high oxygen mixtures in healthy subjects. J. Lab. & Clin. Med., *51*, 72, 1958.

167. Nisell, O.: The action of oxygen and carbon dioxide on the bronchioles and isolated perfused lungs. Acta Physiol. Scand., *21*, Suppl. 73, 1950.

168. Duke, H.N.: Pulmonary vasomotor responses of isolated perfused cat lungs to anoxia and hypercapnia. Quart. J. Exp. Physiol., *36*, 75, 1951.

169. Duke, H.N.: The action of carbon dioxide on isolated perfused dog lungs. Quart. J. Exp. Physiol., *35*, 25, 1949.

170. Hebb, C.O., and Mimmo-Smith, R.H.: Pulmonary vasoconstriction in response to inhalation of CO_2 in the isolated perfused lungs of Macacus Rhesus. Quart. J. Exp. Physiol., *34*, 159, 1948.

171. Bean, J.W., Mayo, W.P., O'Donnell, F., and Gray, G.W.: Vascular response in dog lung induced by alterations in pulmonary arterial CO_2 tension and by acetylcholine. Am. J. Physiol., *166*, 723, 1951.

172. Manfredi, F., and Sieker, H.O.: The effect of carbon dioxide on the pulmonary circulation. J. Clin. Invest., *39*, 295, 1960.

173. Hyde, R.W., Lawson, W.H., and Forster, R.E.: Influence of carbon dioxide on pulmonary vasculature. J. Appl. Physiol., *19*, 734, 1964.

174. Barer, G.R., Howard, P., and McCurrie, J.R.: Effect of carbon dioxide and changes in blood pH on pulmonary vascular resistance in cats. Clin. Sci., *32*, 361, 1967.

175. Fishman, A.P., Fritts, H.W., and Cournand, A.: Effects of breathing carbon dioxide upon the pulmonary circulation. Circulation, *22*, 220, 1960.

176. Sechzer, P.H., Egbert, L.D., Linde, H.W., Cooper, D.Y., Dripps, R.D., and Price, H.L.: Effect of CO_2 inhalation on arterial pressure, ECG and plasma catecholamines and 17-OH corticosteroids in normal man. J. Appl. Physiol., *15*, 454, 1960.

177. Shephard, R.J.: The effect of carbon dioxide on the pulmonary circulation in congenital heart disease. Brit. Heart J., *16*, 451, 1954.

178. Paul, G., Varnauskas, E., Forsberg, S.A., Sannerstedt, R., and Widimsky, J.: Effect of carbon dioxide breathing upon the pulmonary circulation in patients with mitral valve disease. Clin. Sci., *26*, 111, 1964.

179. Viles, P.H., and Shepherd, J.T.: Evidence for a dilator action of carbon dioxide on the pulmonary vessels of the cat. Circ. Res., *22*, 325, 1968,

180. Warren, J.V., Brannon, E.S., Weens, H.S., and Stead, E.A.: Effect of increasing the blood volume and right atrial pressure on the circulation of normal subjects by intravenous infusions. Am. J. Med., *4*, 193, 1948.

181. Witham, A.C., Fleming, J.W., and Bloom, W.L.: The effect of intravenous administration of dextran on cardiac output and other circulatory dynamics. J. Clin. Invest., *30*, 897, 1951.

182. Fleming, J.W., and Bloom, W.L.: Further observations on the hemodynamic effect of plasma volume expansion by dextran. J. Clin. Invest., *36*, 1233, 1957.

183. Doyle, J.T., Wilson, J.S., Estes, E.H., and Warren, J.V.: The effect of intravenous infusion of physiologic saline solution on the pulmonary arterial and pulmonary capillary pressures in man. J. Clin. Invest., 30, 345, 1951.

184. Schnabel, T.G., Eliasch, H., Thomasson, B., and Werkö, L.: The effect of experimentally induced hypervolemia on cardiac function in normal subjects and patients with mitral stenosis. J. Clin. Invest., 38, 117, 1959.

185. Frye, R.L., and Braunwald, E.: Studies on Starling's law of the heart. I. The circulatory response to acute hypervolemia and its modification by ganglionic blockade. J. Clin. Invest., 39, 1043, 1960.

186. Freitas, F.M., de, Faraco, E.Z., Azevedo, D.F.., de, Zaduchliver, J., and Lewin, I.: Behavior of normal pulmonary circulation during changes of total blood volume in man. J. Clin. Invest., 44, 366, 1965.

187. Varnauskas, E., and Korsgren, M.: The effect of plasma expansion by Rheomacrodex on pulmonary blood volume and pulmonary water space. Presented at the European Society for Clinical Investigation, Holland, April 27-29, 1967.

188. Warren J.V., Brannon, E.S., Stead, E.A., and Merrill, A.J.: The effect of venesection and the pooling of blood in the extremities on the atrial pressure and cardiac output in normal subjects with observations on acute circulatory collapse in three instances. J. Clin. Invest., 24, 337, 1945.

189. Brannon, E.S., Stead, E.A., Warren, J.V., and Merrill, A.J.: Hemodynamics of acute hemorrhage in man. Am. Heart J., 31, 407. 1946.

190. Judson, W.E., Hollander, W., Hatcher, J.D., Halperin, M.H., and Friedman, I.H.: The cardiohemodynamic effects of venous congestion of the legs or of phlebotomy in patients with or without congestive heart failure. J. Clin. Invest., 34, 614, 1955.

191. Yu, P.N., Murphy, G.W., Schreiner, B.F., and James, D.H.: Distensibility characterisics of the human pulmonary vascular bed. Study of the pressure-volume response to exercise in patients with or without heart disease. Circulation, 35, 710, 1967.

192. Hultgren, H., and Glover, R.F.: Circulation adaptation to high altitude. Ann. Rev. Med., 19, 119, 1968.

193. Rotta, A.: Physiologic condition of the heart in the natives of high altitude. Am. Heart J., 33, 669, 1947.

194. Rotta, A., Canepa, A., Hurtado, A., Velasquez, T., and Chavez, R.: Pulmonary circulation at sea level and at high altitudes. J. Appl. Physiol., 9, 328, 1956.

195. Penaloza, D., Sime, F., Banchero, N., and Gamboa, R.: Pulmonary hypertension in healthy man born and living at high altitudes. Med. Thorac., 19, 257, 1962.

196. Vogel, J.H.K., Weaver, W.F., Rose, R.L., Blount, S.G., and Grove, R.F.: Pulmonary hypertension on exertion in normal man living at 10,150 feet (Leadville, Colorado). Med. Thorac., 19, 461, 1962.

197. Naeye, R.L.: Hypoxemia and pulmonary hypertension. Arch. Pathol., 71, 447, 1961.

198. Arias-Stella, J., and Saldana, M.: The terminal portion of the pulmonary arterial tree in people native to high altitudes. Circulation, 28, 915, 1963.

199. Grover, R.F., Reeves, J.T., Will, D.H., and Blount, S.G.: Pulmonary vasoconstriction in steers at high altitude. J. Appl. Physiol., 18, 567, 1963.

200. Hultgren, H., Kelly, J. and Miller, H.: Effect of oxygen upon pulmonary circulation in acclimatized man at high altitude. J. Appl. Physiol., 20, 239, 1965.

201. Grover, R.F., Vogel, J.H.K., Voigt, G.C., and Blount, S.G.: Reversal of high altitude pulmonary hypertension. Am. J. Cardiol., 18, 928, 1966.

202. Penaloza, D.: Life at high altitudes. Proc. Conf. of American Health Organization, Washington, D.C., 1966, p. 27.

203. Tenney, S.M.: Physiological adaptations to life at high altitude. Mod. Concept Cardiovasc. Dis., 31, 713, 1962.

204. Vogel, J.H.K., Cameron, D., and Jamieson, G.: Chronic pharmacologic treatment of experimental hypoxic pulmonary hypertension. Am. Heart J., 72, 50, 1966.

205. Grover, R.F.: Pulmonary circulation in animals and man at high altitudes. Ann. N.Y. Acad. Sci., 127, 632, 1965.

206. Hultgren, H., Janis, B., Marticorena, E., and Miller, H.: Diminished cardiovascular response to acute hypoxia at high altitude. Circulation, 36, Suppl. II, 146, 1967.

207. Monge C.C., Cazorla, A.T., Whittembury, G.M., Sakata, Y.B., and Rizo-Patron, C.: A description of the circulatory dynamics in the heart and lungs of people at sea level and at high altitude by means of dye dilution technique. Acta Physiol. Latinoam, 5, 198, 1955.

208. Roy, S.B., Bhatia, M.L., and Gadhoke, S.: Response of pulmonary blood volume to 64 to 114 weeks of intermittent stay at high altitudes. Am. Heart J., 74, 192, 1967.

209. Fred, H.L., Schmidt, A.M., Bates, T., and Hecht, H.H.: Acute pulmonary edema of high altitude, clinical and physiologic observations. Circulation, *25*, 929, 1962.

210. Hultgren, H.N., Lopez, C.E., Lundberg, E., and Miller, H.: Physiologic studies of pulmonary edema at high altitude. Circulation, *29*, 393, 1964.

211. Menon, N.D.: High-altitude pulmonary edema. A clinical study. New Engl. J. Med., *273*, 66, 1965.

212. Kovacs, G.S., Hill, J.D., Aberg, T., Blesovsky, A., and Gerbode, F.: Pathogenesis of arterial hypoxemia in pulmonary embolism. Arch. Surg., *93*, 813, 1966.

213. Downing, S.E., Talner, N.S., and Gardner, T.H.: Cardiovascular responses to metabolic acidosis. Am. J. Physiol., *208*, 237, 1965.

214. Bergofsky, E.H., Lehr, D.E., Tuller, M.A., Rigatto, M., and Fishman, A.P.: The effects of acute alkalosis and acidosis on the pulmonary circulation. Ann. N.Y. Acad. Sci., *92*, 627, 1961.

215. Giuntini, C., Lewis, M.L., Sales-Luis, A., and Harvey, R.M.: A study of the pulmonary blood volume in man by quantitative radiocardiography. J. Clin. Invest., *42*, 1589, 1963.

216. Carlens, E., Hansen, H.E., and Nordenstrom, B.: Temporary unilateral occlusion of the pulmonary artery. J. Thorac. Surg., *22*, 527, 1951.

217. Nemir, P., Stone, H.H., Macknell, T.N., and Hawthorne, H.R.: Studies on pulmonary embolism utilizing the method of controlled unilateral pulmonary artery occlusion. Surg. Forum, *5*, 210, 1954.

218. Sloan, H., Morris, J.D., Figley, M., and Lee, R.: Temporary unilateral occlusion of the pulmonary artery in the preoperative evaluation of thoracic patients. J. Thorac. Surg., *30*, 591, 1955.

219. Brofman, B.L., Charms, B.L., Kohn, P.M., Elder, J., Newman, R., and Rizika, M.: Unilateral pulmonary artery occlusion in man. J. Thorac. Surg., *34*, 206, 1957.

220. Charms, B.L., Brofman, B.L., Elder, J.C., and Kohn, P.M.: Unilateral pulmonary artery occlusion in man. II. Studies in patients with chronic pulmonary disease. J. Thorac. Surg., *35*, 316, 1958.

221. Söderholm, B.: The hemodynamics of the lesser circulation in pulmonary tuberculosis. Effect of exercise, temporary unilateral pulmonary artery occlusion and operation. Scand. J. Clin. Lab. Invest., *9*, Suppl. 26, 1957.

222. Folkow, B., and Pappenheimer, J.R.: Components of the respiratory dead space and their variation with pressure breathing and with bronchoactive drugs. J. Appl. Physiol., *8*, 102, 1955.

223. Julian, D.G., Travis, D.M., Robin, E.D., and Crump, C.H.: Effect of pulmonary artery occlusion upon end-tidal CO_2 tension. J. Appl. Physiol., *15*, 87, 1960.

224. Nisell, O.I.: Some aspects of the pulmonary circulation and ventilation. Int. Arch. Allergy, *3*, 142, 1952.

225. Severinghaus, J.W., Swenson, E.W., Finley, T.N., Lategola, M.T., and Williams, J.: Unilateral hypoventilation produced in dogs by occluding one pulmonary artery. J. Appl. Physiol., *16*, 53, 1961.

226. Swenson, E.W., Finley, T.N., and Guzman, S.V.: Unilateral hypoventilation in man during temporary occlusion of one pulmonary artery. J. Clin. Invest., *40*, 828, 1961.

227. Venrath, H., Rotthoff, R., Valentin, H., and Bolt, W.: Bronchospirographische Untersungen bei Durchblutungsstörungen im kleinen Kreislauf. Beitr. Klin. Tuberk., *107*, 291, 1952.

228. Finley, T.N., Swenson, E.W., Clements, J.A., Gardner, R.E. Wright, R.R., and Severinghaus, J.W.: Changes in mechanical properties, appearance and surface activity of extracts of one lung following occlusion of its pulmonary artery in the dog. Physiologist, *3*, 56, 1960.

229. Finley, T.N., Tooley, W.H., Swenson, E.W., Gardner, R.E., and Clements, J.A.: Pulmonary surface tension in experimental atelectasis. Am. Rev. Resp. Dis., *89*, 372, 1964.

230. Chernick, V., Hodson, W.A., and Greenfield, L.J.: Effect of chronic pulmonary artery ligation on pulmonary mechnics and surfactant. J. Appl. Physiol., *21*, 1315, 1966.

231. Giammona, S.T., Mandelbaum, I., Foy, J., and Bondurant, S.: Effects of pulmonary artery ligation on pulmonary surfactant and pressure-volume characteristics of dog lung. Circ. Res., *18*, 683, 1966.

232. Edmunds, L.H., and Huber, G.L.: Pulmonary artery occlusion. I. Volume-pressure relationships and alveolar bubble stability. J. Appl. Physiol., *22*, 990, 1967.

233. McQuire, L.B., Dock, D.S., Hyland, J.W., Harrison, D.C., Haynes, F.W., and Dexter, L.: Evaluation of slope method for measuring pulmonary blood volume in man. J. Appl. Physiol., *17*, 497, 1962.

234. Aramendia, P., Fermoso, J.D., and Taquini, A.C.: Pulmonary blood volume in experimental unilateral pulmonary artery occlusion. Circ. Res., *9*, 44, 1961.

235. Wolff, L.: Pulmonary embolism. Circulation, *6*, 768, 1952.

236. Parker, B.M., and Smith, J.R.: Pulmonary embolism and infarction. Am. J. Med., *24*, 402, 1958.

237. Krause, S., and Silverblatt, M.: Pulmonary embolism. A review with special emphasis on clinical and electrocardiographic diagnosis. Arch. Int. Med., *96*, 19, 1955.

238. Dexter, L., Dock, D.S., McQuire, L.B., Hyland, J.W., and Haynes, F.W.: Pulmonary embolism. Med. Clin. N. Am., *44*, 1251, 1960.

239. Dexter, L.: Thromboemboli as a cause of cor pulmonale. Bull. N.Y. Acad. Med., *41*, 981, 1965.

240. Price, K.C., Hata, D., and Smith, J.R.: Pulmonary vasomotion resulting from miliary embolism of lungs. Am. J. Physiol., *182*, 183, 1955.

241. Bernthal, T., Horres, A.D., and Taylor, J.T.: Pulmonary vascular obstruction in graded tachypneagenic diffuse embolism. Am. J. Physiol., *200*, 279, 1961.

242. Hyman, A.L., Myers, W.D., and Meyer, A.: The effect of acute pulmonary embolus upon cardiopulmonary hemodynamics. Am. Heart J., *67*, 313, 1963.

243. Griffin, G.D.J., and Essex, H.E.: Experimental embolism of the pulmonary arterioles and capillaries. Surgery, *26*, 707, 1949.

244. Daley, R., Wade, J.D., Maraist, F., and Bing, R.J.: Pulmonary hypertension in dogs induced by injection of Lycopodium spores into the pulmonary, artery, with special reference to the absence of vasomotor reflexes. Am. J. Physiol., *164*, 380, 1951.

245. Comroe, J.H., Van Lingen, B., Stroud, R.C., and Roncoroni, A.: Reflex and direct cardio-pulmonary effects of 5-OH-tryptamine (Serotonin); their possible role in pulmonary embolism and coronary thrombosis. Am. J. Physiol., *173*, 379, 1953.

246. Thomas, D., Stein, M., Tanabe, G., Rege, V., and Wessler, S.: Mechanism of broncho-constriction produced by thromboemboli in dogs. Am. J. Physiol., *206*, 1207, 1964.

247. Sanders, R., Waalkes, T.P., Gilbert, G.W., and Terry, L.L.: Serotonin (5-hydroxytryptamine) and pulmonary thromboembolism. Surg., Gynec. & Obst., *109*, 455, 1959.

248. DePasquale, N.P., Burch, G.E., and Hyman, A.L.: Pulmonary venous responses to immersion hyperthermia and hypothermia. Am. Heart J., *70*, 486, 1965.

249. Robin, E.D., Cross, C.E., Millen, J.E., and Murdaugh, H.V.: Humoral agent from calf-lung producing pulmonary arterial vasoconstriction. Science, *156*, 827, 1967.

Chapter 12

Effects of Pharmacologic Agents on Pulmonary Blood Volume

Pharmacologic studies of the pulmonary circulation are important because they may provide information concerning (a) the regulation of the pulmonary circulation, (b) the effectiveness of proposed therapy for pulmonary hypertension, (c) factors responsible for maintaining pulmonary hypertension in patients with cardiopulmonary disease, and (d) relationships between pulmonary circulatory dynamics and myocardial function.[1]

All drugs which act on the pulmonary circulation affect the heart and the systemic circulation; a drug acting exclusively on the pulmonary vessels has not yet been found. Further, the effects of a pharmacologic agent in animals may not be applicable to human subjects. Finally, the effects in patients with diseased pulmonary vessels may not always be expected in normal subjects.

Limitations in the methodology and techniques used for assessing the effects of pharmacologic agents on the pulmonary circulation may include (a) uncertainty regarding the steady state of the subject, (b) lack of an accurate estimate of bronchial flow, (c) the assumption that blood vessel length and blood viscosity are constant throughout the study, and (d) frequently the absence of measurements of the intrathoracic pressure.

In early studies, assessment of the effects of pharmacologic agents on the pulmonary blood volume has depended largely upon changes in the relatively ill-defined intrathoracic or central blood volume (CBV) as determined by the mean transit time or precordial counting methods. Since the introduction of transseptal left heart catheterization, more precise study of alterations in pulmonary blood volume (PBV) by the mean transit time technique has been possible. Admittedly, the volume so estimated probably includes an undetermined portion of the left atrial volume, and accurate measurement of the PBV alone is still not possible.

In order to assure the steady state during the study period and to determine that apparent pharmacologic effects on the pulmonary circulation were not due to the administration of intravenous fluids, 9 patients were studied during sham infusion in our laboratory (Table 12-1). The mean heart rate (HR), cardiac index (CI) and stroke index (SI) did not change. Pulmonary arterial mean pressure (PAm) declined slightly in 7 patients, but the changes were not significant. No change in the left atrial mean (LAm) and pulmonary distending (P_d) pressures was observed. The average PBV was 286 ml/M² during the control period and 287 ml/M² during the sham

TABLE 12-1 Hemodynamic Effects of "Sham" Infusion

Patients	Age	Sex	BSA	Diagnosis	Periods of Study	Blood Flow			Pressures (mm Hg)				Tm (seconds)			Blood Volume (ml/M²)	
						CI	HR	SI	PAm	LAm	Pd	BAm	PA-BA	LA-BA	PA-LA	CBV	PBV
W.W.	50	M	2.02	AS	C	2.33	68	34	16	9	12.5	75	17.4	10.1	7.3	676	284
					S	2.44	71	34	17	13	15	75	16.4	9.8	6.6	668	269
J.S.	56	M	1.72	MS	C	1.84	90	20	23	15	14	90	20.8	11.6	9.2	638	282
					S	1.71	85	20	22	14	13	90	21.0	10.0	11.0	598	314
W.S.	53	M	1.65	AR	C	1.99	60	33	31	22	26.5	81	24.6	15.9	8.7	810	288
				MR	S	2.00	60	33	29	19	24	76	24.8	17.0	7.8	830	272
J.M.	43	F	1.79	MS	C	2.52	68	37	33	20	26.5	95	17.2	9.1	8.1	722	340
				AS	S	2.38	72	33	29	17	23	100	17.9	9.0	8.9	710	352
O.F.	36	M	1.82	AR	C	2.56	81	32	33	24	28.5	83	20.3	12.3	8.0	865	342
				AS	S	2.36	77	31	30	24	27	83	21.1	11.8	9.3	831	366
F.S.	40	M	1.84	AS	C	1.72	73	24	35	23	29	80	24.7	17.2	7.5	708	212
					S	1.65	74	22	32	23	27.5	80	25.3	17.6	7.7	696	212
C.B.	52	F	1.73	MS	C	1.52	81	19	38	15	26.5	90	23.7	12.8	10.9	600	276
					S	1.61	80	20	38	14	26.0	85	23.6	12.4	11.2	643	300
A.C.	34	M	2.00	MS	C	2.37	76	31	40	23	31.5	95	17.2	9.5	7.7	679	304
					S	2.21	80	28	43	24	33.5	97	17.8	10.5	7.3	655	269
I.W.	50	F	1.44	MS	C	1.55	117	13	48	27	37.5	105	23.3	13.8	9.5	603	245
					S	1.55	112	14	45	22	33.5	90	22.8	13.8	9.0	590	233
Control mean						2.04	79.3	27	33.0	19.8	25.8	88.2	21.0	12.5	8.5	700	286
± S.E.						±0.14	±5.6	±3.1	±3.1	±1.88	±2.65	±3.12	±1.06	±0.93	±0.39	±29.8	±13.8
"Sham" mean						1.99	79.0	31.7	31.7	18.9	24.7	86.2	21.2	12.4	8.8	691	287
± S.E.						±0.12	±4.8	±3.1	±3.1	±1.51	±2.37	±2.92	±1.08	±1.04	±0.53	±29.4	±17.0
p value						N.S.	N.S.	N.S.	N.S.	N.S.	N.S.	N.S.	N.S.	N.S.	N.S.	N.S.	N.S.

BSA = Body surface area (M²)
CI = Cardiac index (L/min/M²)
HR = Heart rate (beats/min)
SI = Stroke index (ml/min/beat)
PAm = Pulmonary arterial mean
LAm = Left atrial mean
Pd = Pulmonary distending
BAm = Systemic arterial mean
Tm = Mean transit time
PA-BA = Pulmonary artery to systemic artery

LA-BA = Left atrium to systemic artery
PA-LA = Pulmonary artery to left atrium
CBV = "Central" blood volume
PBV = Pulmonary blood volume
AS = Aortic stenosis
MS = Mitral stenosis
AR = Aortic regurgitation
MR = Mitral regurgitation
C = Control period
S = During "sham" infusion

infusion. Similarly, values for the CBV were the same during the two periods. Data are presented only for the control and sham infusion periods. Four patients were also studied during a 15 to 20 minute recovery period following the infusion; again, no significant differences were observed in any parameter. Thus, a steady state was maintained with reasonable assurance in most patients for periods of 30 to 40 minutes or longer.

The classification of pharmacologic agents used in the studies reported in this chapter is adapted from that proposed by Aviado.[2] We have included only those agents which have been studied extensively for their effects on the pulmonary circulation, those which are frequently used in medical practice, or those which may show promise in ameliorating pulmonary hypertension.

Cardiovascular Drugs

Digitalis Glycosides

Studies in animals and in man have recently demonstrated that the digitalis glycosides (hereafter referred to as digitalis) act pharmacologically at two major sites, myocardial and peripheral.[3-8] In the myocardium, their effects are (a) positive inotropic, with increased strength of myocardial contraction; (b) negative chronotropic, with depression of sinoatrial impulse formation; and (c) negative dromotropic, with slowing of atrioventricular conduction. Peripherally, digitalis causes arterial constriction resulting in augmented peripheral vascular resistance and venous constriction tending to diminish venous return.

Almost uniformly, normal subjects and patients with cardiopulmonary disease show evidence of a positive inotropic effect on the myocardium following the administration of digitalis.[9-14] This effect is manifested by (a) an increase in the rate of rise of systolic pressure in the ventricular pressure pulse (dp/dt), (b) augmented myocardial contractility measured by strain gauge arch or by the changes in force-velocity relationship, (c) shortening of the left ventricular pre-ejection period, and (d) a significant increase in left ventricular stroke work (LVsw) in the presence of a lower left ventricular end-diastolic pressure (LVd) at rest and during exercise.

In normal subjects some workers observed a slight decrease in cardiac output (CO) after acute digitalization,[15] while others indicated no change in either CO or pulmonary vascular pressure.[16,17] Maseri and associates recently reported in more detail the effects of intravenous lanatoside-C in 7 normal subjects.[18] The following changes were observed: (a) an early reduction in HR; (b) a transient decline in CO; (c) a rise in stroke volume (SV) initially, associated with an increased end-diastolic volume and no change in the systolic rate of emptying, followed later by an increased systolic emptying rate and decreased ventricular volume; and (d) an increase in PBV.

In patients with enlarged hearts but no evidence of congestive failure, digitalis usually caused an increase in CO, SV and LVsw with the LVd unchanged or lower.[9,10,19-22]

In patients with mitral stenosis, digitalis frequently, but not always, increased the CO.[23-25] PAm and pulmonary wedge pressure (Pw) declined slightly.

In patients with chronic pulmonary disease and cor pulmonale, three types of response have been reported, depending upon the change in CO. The first was an immediate increase in CO accompanied by little change or an elevation of the right ventricular systolic pressure and PAm.[26-29] The increase in CO was not as great as that observed in patients with left ventricular failure. The second type of response was an immediate decrease in CO frequently accompained by a rise in PAm.[26,28,29] The third was a delayed decrease in CO associated with a fall in PAm.[28] Berglund and associates reported little or no beneficial effects of digitalis in 8 patients with chronic pulmonary disease with or without failure.[30]

In patients with left ventricular failure, CO increased consistently, regardless of the digitalis preparation given.[10,19,26,27,31-33] PAm declined as left ventricular emptying improved and LVd and LAm declined. No change in right atrial or central venous pressures was observed, however.

Kim and Aviado reported that in anesthetized dogs intravenous injection of acetyl strophanthidin caused a slight decrease in PAm, a marked reduction in pulmonary venous flow and an increase in pulmonary vascular resistance (PVR).[34] The increased PVR was interpreted as a result of two combined factors: (a) decreased blood flow and (b) local vasoconstriction of perfused lung.

We studied the effects of acetyl strophanthidin in 23 patients with various types of cardiac disease with particular reference to the PBV. After control studies, acetyl strophanthidin, 0.05 mg/ml in physiological saline, was infused through the pulmonary arterial catheter. The total dose was approximately 0.017 mg/kg, given over a 9 to 12 minute period on the average. The electrocardiogram, systemic arterial pressure (BAm) and LAm were monitored continuously and PAm intermittently. The CO, CBV and PBV were measured 12 to 15 minutes after termination of the infusion. The results are summarized in Table 12-2. The patients were classified arbitrarily into two groups according to their pulmonary pressure-volume responses to acetyl strophanthidin.

In the first group (Group A) of 11 patients, the LVd, LAm and/or PAm declined significantly. Concurrently, the CBV and PBV fell in 9 patients and was unchanged in 2. The CI and SI either increased or remained the same. The LVd was at least

Table 12-2 Effects of Acetyl Strophanthidin on Pulmonary Hemodynamics and Pulmonary Blood Volume

Group	No. of Cases	Periods of Study		Blood Flow			Pressures (mm Hg)					Blood Volume (ml/M²)	
				CI	HR	SI	PAm	LAm	P_d	LVd	BAm	CBV	PBV
I	11	C	mean	2.39	106	24	28.1	24.6	27.8	23.6	98.0	708	371
			±SE	±0.19	±8.9	±3.2	±2.3	±1.7	±2.2	±3.2	±3.7	±33	±27.6
		D	mean	2.60	95	29	18.5	13.1	16.8	12.1	95.0	652	262
			±SE	±0.19	±9.2	±3.4	±2.3	±2.1	±2.3	±2.7	±4.6	±47	±23.0
			Diff in mean (D-C)	0.21	−11	−5.0	−9.6	−11.5	−11.0	−11.0	−3.0	−56	−55
			p value	NS	<0.01	<0.05	<.01	<.01	<0.01	<0.01	NS	<0.025	<0.01
II	12	C	mean	2.83	84	35	20.0	13.0	16.5	12.0	97.0	701	304
			±SE	±0.18	±3.5	±2.9	±1.8	±2.4	±2.2	±2.2	+5.9	±48	±22
		D	mean	2.98	80	39	19.0	12.0	15.5	12.0	101.0	713	313
			±SE	±0.19	±4.1	±3.4	±2.0	±2.3	±2.1	±2.6	±4.2	±46	±23.4
			Diff in mean (D-C)	0.15	−4	4.0	−1.0	−1.0	−1.0	0	4.2	12	9
			p value	<0.02	<0.01	<0.01	NS	NS	NS	NS	NS	NS	NS

C = control period; D = after administration of acetyl strophanthidin.
Other symbols and abbreviations are identical to those used in Table 12-1

moderately elevated in 8 of the 10 patients in whom it was measured. Improved left ventricular function after acetyl strophanthidin was manifested by a decline in LVd and an increase in effective LVsw.

In the second group (Group B) of 12 patients, the LVd, LAm and PAm were not affected. The CI and SI also remained the same or increased only slightly. Effective LVsw increased in more than half the patients. In general, CBV and PBV were unchanged or slightly augmented. The LVd was elevated in only 3 of the 12 patients. Little change in the normal LVd in 9 patients would be expected after acute digitalization. Among the 3 patients with high LVd, 1 had a restrictive cardiomyopathy and 2 had aortic stenosis with normal CI. As noted previously, patients with restrictive cardiomyopathy usually failed to respond to acute digitalization, probably because of a thickened and noncompliant myocardium. The absence of a pressure response in the other 2 patients has not been adequately explained.

These data clearly indicate that LVd, LAm and PAm must fall before the CBV and PBV change. Thus, patients in Group A may be those with more advanced disease or at least disease in which left ventricular function may be appreciably improved by digitalis. The reduction in PBV is an effect of improved left ventricular emptying. The concordant changes in the pressure-volume relationship in the pulmonary vascular bed after acute digitalization are predominantly passive.

Antiarrhythmic Drugs

The commonly used antiarrhythmic drugs include quinidine, procainamide, lidocaine, diphenylhydantoin and propranolol.

Quinidine is considered to be myocardial depressant and a systemic vasodilating agent, causing a decrease in CO and BAm.[35-38]

Quinidine administered directly into the sinus node artery of the dog caused sinus acceleration in small doses and depression in larger doses.[39] Acceleration of the heart rate by quinidine *in vivo* depends on an intact sympathetic nervous system.[40] If sympathetic nervous activity is suppressed by pharmacologic or surgical means, quinidine depresses the pacemaker.

When atrial fibrillation is converted to sinus rhythm with quinidine, hemodynamic improvement is usually observed.[41,42] The effects include an increase in CO, a decrease in BAm, right atrial mean pressure (RAm) and PAm and a reduction in CBV. Multiple factors may be responsible for these changes, including slowing of the HR with improved ventricular filling, restoration of "atrial kick" effect, and more efficient ventricular emptying. Whether the drug itself has important direct effects is undetermined, although an earlier report indicated that the increase in CO and the fall in PAm after quinidine resulted from reduced systemic vascular resistance due to the vasodilating action of the drug.[48] In the absence of evidence favoring active pulmonary vasodilatation, however, the decline in PAm was probably passive.

Decreased myocardial contractility was also observed after administration of procainamide.[36,38,44-46] Intravenous procainamide caused a reduction in PAm in some patients but not in others.[47,48]

Hemodynamic effects of lidocaine have been reported by several workers.[45,46] Depressed myocardial contractile force and BAm were observed in animals,[46] but no appreciable effect on the myocardium was detected in man.[45]

Mixter and collaborators demonstrated myocardial depressant as well as peripheral vasodilating actions of diphenylhydantoin in dogs.[49] Similarly, depressed left ventricular function after the drug was observed by other workers.[37] Conn and associates reported hemodynamic effects of diphenylhydantoin in 12 patients with cardiac disease.[50] CO, PAm and BAm did not change. Lieberson and co-workers found an increase in LVd and a decrease in LV dp/dt and LVsw.[51] These changes, however, lasted less than 25 minutes. CO and HR were not affected. These workers felt that diphenylhydantoin exerted a transient depressant action on the myocardium.

We have not studied the effects of these four antiarrhythmic drugs on the pulmonary circulation. We know of no specific reports concerning their effects on PBV.

The action of propranolol is discussed in a subsequent section of this chapter.

Autonomic Drugs

Adrenergic Activators

In 1948 Ahlquist proposed that adrenergic receptor sites may be classified into two general types: alpha and beta adrenergic activators.[52] The alpha activators act as pressor or excitatory agents on the smooth muscles in the blood vessels (skin, kidneys), causing vasoconstriction. They do not affect the myocardium. The classical example of this type of drug is methoxamine. Beta adrenergic activators act on smooth muscle in the blood vessels (coronaries, skeletal muscles), and they affect the myocardium as well. They depress or inhibit peripheral vessels and cause vasodilatation. They exert a positive inotropic action on

the myocardium, however. An excellent example of this type of drug is isoproterenol. Other adrenergic activators may affect both alpha and beta adrenergic receptor sites. For instance, norepinephrine activates the alpha receptors of peripheral vessels causing vasoconstriction, and at the same time stimulates the beta receptors of the myocardium producing a positive inotropic action.

Epinephrine. Epinephrine affects both alpha and beta adrenergic receptors. The drug acts predominantly as a vasoconstrictor and as a powerful stimulant on the myocardium as well.[53] In many species of animals, intravenous epinephrine has usually caused PAm and BAm to rise and CO to increase.[54-56] In some instances, LAm also rose. The increase in PAm in animal studies after epinephrine has been explained on the basis of (a) rise in LVd and LAm, (b) increased pulmonary blood flow, (c) redistribution of blood volume from the peripheral to the pulmonary circulation, and (d) a direct pulmonary vasoconstricting effect.

Employing a special canine preparation, Borst and co-workers injected epinephrine into one lung, using the other as a control.[57] Redistribution of flow served as the indicator of vasomotor activity instead of changes in PAm and PVR. The ipsilateral pulmonary blood flow decreased consistently. PAm rose in more than half the dogs, and LAm declined in more than 80%. Thus, the authors concluded that epinephrine caused pulmonary vasoconstriction.

Feeley and associates reported an average 24% increase in PBV in dogs after epinephrine,[58] in spite of the stiffening and vasoconstricting effect previously demonstrated in the isolated lung.[59,60] The differences in response of the pulmonary vascular bed in isolated lungs and in intact animals are readily explained if the changes are regarded as the resultants of two opposing factors: (a) increased pulmonary vasomotor tone as a direct action of epinephrine, and (b) increased transmural distending pressure, resulting from action of the drug on the heart and the systemic circulation. In the isolated preparation only the first of these forces operates; in the intact animal, on the other hand, the net effect depends on the relative magnitude of both.

Epinephrine caused a rise in PAm in normal subjects and in patients with various types of cardiopulmonary disease.[61-65] CO, HR and SV all rose. Pw was usually unaffected or rose only slightly. Witham and Fleming reported a fall in the CBV in 5 of 13 patients, and in 4 of the 5 the CO remained constant.[63] Whether PBV decreases or increases after epinephrine remains to be determined.

Norepinephrine. Norepinephrine also has both alpha and beta stimulating effects. In animals, intravenous norepinephrine has been shown to cause a consistent rise in PAm and an increase in CO if the HR was accelerated.[55,56,66-70] Borst and associates found that pulmonary blood flow and LAm both declined in the majority of dogs studied.[57] The PAm response was variable. They felt that norepinephrine caused pulmonary vasoconstriction. In perfused lung the PBV usually decreased as a consequence of pulmonary vasoconstriction. In the intact animal changes in the PBV were variable. Feeley and associates reported an average 25% increase of PBV in dogs after administration of norepinephrine.[58]

In anesthetized dogs, Aramendia and associates found that norepinephrine and isoproterenol infused together increased CO and PBV and reduced

BAm with almost no change in PAm.[71] The expected isoproterenol induced fall in PAm was probably counteracted by the pulmonary vasoconstricting effect of norepinephrine. Pulmonary blood flow usually decreased or failed to change.

In man, PAm has been observed to increase consistently after norepinephrine, an effect most workers have explained as secondary to a rise in LVd and LAm.[72-75] Patel and associates, however, found a significant elevation in PVR, indicated by an increase in the PAm-Pw gradient which was disproportionate to the pulmonary blood flow.[73] They interpreted these observations as strong evidence in favor of active pulmonary vasoconstriction. The change in CO was usually minimal, although some workers reported a slight increase after norepinephrine.

Bousvaros studied the effects of intravenous norepinephrine in 21 patients and in one normal subject.[76] In the majority of patients the increase in PAm preceded the rise in LAm by 20 to 40 seconds. This early widening of the PAm to LAm pressure gradient was interpreted as evidence of active vasoconstriction. The available information indicates that PBV should decrease after norepinephrine.

Metaraminol. The hemodynamic effects of metaraminol, available commercially as Aramine, have been generally considered similar to those of norepinephrine.[53,55] Sarnoff and co-workers reported an increase in CO after metaraminol administration.[77] The effects of metaraminol depend upon the presence of catecholamines in the tissue. Harrison and associates demonstrated depressed arterial and myocardial responses to metaraminol in the dog when the catecholamine content of the heart had been depleted by the prior administration of reserpine.[78] When metaraminol was given to dogs not receiving reserpine, norepinephrine was released, causing a rise in PAm.

Livesay and co-workers studied the effects of metaraminol in normal man.[79] PAm usually rose without a corresponding change in pulmonary blood flow. The LAm and Pw were not measured. Malmcrona and associates reported that metaraminol administered to normal subjects caused a consistent rise in BAm, Pw and PAm associated with variable change in CO.[80] Eliasch and collaborators observed an increase in Pw, PAm and PVR in patients with mitral valve disease after metaraminol. There was an augmentation of CO in half of the patients.

Metaraminol would be expected to cause a decrease in PBV similar to that expected after norepinephrine.

Phenylephrine. The hemodynamic actions of phenylephrine (Neo–synephrine) have not been extensively reported. This agent is primarily an alpha adrenergic activator.

In both dogs and man phenylephrine has consistently reduced CO.[55,82] Beck and associates reported the effects of phenylephrine in 8 patients with mitral stenosis and in 2 with pulmonary hypertension.[83] CO declined as a result of reflex bradycardia. In the initial period PAm rose and Pw declined. Subsequently, both PAm and Pw rose. The initial response was attributed to pulmonary vasoconstriction and the subsequent effect was explained as a result of systemic vasoconstriction, causing an increase in LVd. Phenylephrine might be expected to cause an early decrease in PBV followed by a later increase.

Isoproterenol. Since the original studies of Konzett in 1940,[84] the hemodynamic effects of isoproterenol, commercially available as Isuprel, have

been investigated in animals, in normal subjects and in patients with cardiopulmonary disease.[85-94] This drug is a beta adrenergic activator. After isoproterenol, heart rate and CO increased in association with reduction in the PAm and in the PAm-Pw gradient. The PVR declined in most cases. In anesthetized dogs an increase of 31% in PBV was reported.[58] In dogs subjected to acute pulmonary embolization, there was an increase in PBV after isoproterenol compared with that prior to the administration of the drug.[95] Using implanted pulmonary artery electromagnetic flowmeters, however, Rudolph and Scarpelli found no evidence of a direct pulmonary vasomotor effects of isoproterenol.[96] On the other hand, employing a new method for measuring the pressure and resistance to flow in the pulmonary vascular bed of dogs, Brody and Stemmler found active dilatation of both pulmonary arteries and veins after intravascular infusion of isoproterenol.[97]

McGaff and co-workers reported an increase in PBV and a reduction in PAm and LAm in 7 patients with rheumatic heart disease 20 to 30 minutes after sublingual isoproterenol.[98] The results were interpreted as evidence of active pulmonary vasodilatation.

Harrison and co-workers demonstrated a decline in end-systolic dimension of both ventricles after isoproterenol infusion.[99] This change was interpreted as supporting evidence for the positive inotropic action of the drug on the myocardium.

The effects of intravenous isoproterenol on the pulmonary circulation were studied in 35 patients in our laboratory. The results have recently been published elsewhere,[94] and a summary is presented in Table 12-3.

In 5 patients with primary myocardial disease, the average CI, HR and

Table 12-3   Effects of Isoproterenol on Pulmonary Hemodynamics and Pulmonary Blood Volume

Group and Diagnosis	No. of Cases	Periods of Study		Blood Flow			Pressures (mm Hg)				Blood Volume (ml/M²)	
				CI	HR	SI	PAm	LAm	P_d	BAm	CBV	PBV
I		C	mean	2.28	80	29	20	11	15.3	99	672	261
			±SE	±0.20	±3.8	±4.2	±4.6	±1.4	±3.8	±6.7	±57.2	±12.5
		I	mean	3.42	90	38	14	6	10.0	89	757	300
	5		±SE	±0.27	±2.7	±1.8	±0.9	±1.8	±1.3	±10.9	±76.6	±12.0
PMD			Diff in mean (I-C)	1.14	10.0	9.0	−6.0	−5.0	−5.3	−10.0	85	39
			p value	<0.01	<0.02	<0.02	NS	<0.05	NS	<0.02	<0.02	<0.02
II		C	mean	2.20	76	29	30	19	24.5	91	668	315
			±SE	±0.14	±3.4	±2.4	±2.9	±1.2	±1.9	±3.2	±24.0	±16.4
	18	I	mean	2.90	98	31	36	23	29.6	87	730	377
			±SE	±0.20	±5.2	±2.9	±3.8	±1.9	±3.0	±2.5	±29.1	±21.2
MS			Diff in mean (I-C)	0.70	22	2.0	6.0	4.0	5.1	−4.0	62	62
			p value	<0.01	<0.01	NS	<0.01	<0.01	<0.01	<0.05	<0.01	<0.01
III		C	mean	2.40	73	33	20	13	16.5	93	709	267
			+SE	±0.14	±2.9	±1.6	±1.7	±1.8	±1.7	±3.7	±25.2	±7.3
	11	I	mean	3.38	92	37	18	9	13.7	89	734	283
			+SE	±0.16	±4.6	±1.9	±2.6	±2.2	±2.4	±4.2	±22.0	±8.1
AVD			Diff in mean (I-C)	0.98	19	4.0	−2.0	−4.0	−2.8	−4.0	25	15
			p value	<0.01	<0.01	<0.01	NS	<0.01	<0.02	<0.02	NS	< 0.05

PMD = primary myocardial disease;   MS = mitral stenosis;   AVD = aortic valve disease;
C = control period;   I = during isoproterenol infusion.
Other symbols and abbreviations are identical to those used in Table 12-1

SI increased significantly, accompanied by a consistent decline in PAm and LAm. The BAm was also reduced in 4 of the 5. In each of 2 patients in whom the measurement was made, the LVd also declined. In the group as a whole, CBV and PBV both increased significantly. Similar changes were observed during isoproterenol infusion in a subject with no cardiovascular disease.

In 18 patients with predominant mitral stenosis CI and HR both increased, and SI remained unchanged. PAm and LAm rose significantly. CBV and PBV both increased considerably.

In 11 patients with predominant aortic valvular disease, isoproterenol caused CI, HR and SI to increase and LAm and BAm to decline. With one exception, the PAm was also reduced. Despite the fall in the pulmonary vascular pressures, the CBV and PBV were unaffected.

These effects may be explained by the multiple actions of the drug. First, isoproterenol exerts an active vasodilating effect on the pulmonary vascular bed, resulting in an increase in volume accompanied by a decline in pressure. These changes were most pronounced in 5 patients with primary myocardial disease and in 1 normal subject. They were less conspicuous in 11 patients with aortic valvular disease. Second, the positive inotropic action of isoproterenol was responsible for the increase in CO and SV accompanied by a decline in the LVd. Ordinarily, positive inotropic action on the ventricle would passively reduce the PBV. The augmented volume in some of our patients suggests that the active pulmonary vasodilating action of isoproterenol overcame its inotropic effect in this regard. Third, the sympathomimetic increase in HR and the augmented cardiac output were probably responsible for the elevation of LAm and PAm in patients with predominant mitral stenosis. In such patients slight increase in a mitral flow is accompanied by a disproportionate rise in the diastolic pressure gradient from left atrium to left ventricle. Thus, an increase in LAm and, in turn, PAm would be expected. The elevated pressure would cause passive dilatation of the pulmonary vessels resulting in augmented PBV. Under this circumstance, any concomitant active pulmonary vasodilatation would be masked by superimposed passive vasodilatation. Thus, pulmonary vascular pressure and volume would both increase.

The effects of isoproterenol upon bronchomotor tone and intra-alveolar pressure may also influence the pulmonary vascular pressure considerably.[100] Isoproterenol is a powerful bronchodilator, and decreased intra-alveolar pressure might be expected to induce a secondary fall in PAm. Our study, however, was not designed to demonstrate objectively the circulatory consequences of the bronchodilator action of isoproterenol.

Mephentermine. Mephentermine, available commercially as Wyamine, possesses both alpha and beta adrenergic effects. The mechanism is probably the release of catecholamines, inasmuch as these actions are prevented by the prior administration of reserpine.[101-103] A consistent rise in CO and a decrease in PVR were observed in animals, in normal subjects, in patients with mitral stenosis and in those with chronic pulmonary disease.[104-108]

The individual actions of this agent are similar to those of isoproterenol: namely, cardiac stimulation, pulmonary vasodilatation and probable bronchodilatation. Mephentermine differs from isoproterenol in its systemic pressor effect, since as isoproterenol usually lowers the BAm.

We have studied the effects of mephentermine on pulmonary circulatory dynamics in 2 patients with mitral stenosis who developed vasodepressor reactions during cardiac catheterization (Table 12-4). Mephentermine given during such reactions caused a significant increase in CI mainly as a result of increased HR. BAm, LAm and PAm were uniformly elevated and CBV and PBV were increased. These effects may be explained by (a) peripheral vasodilatation, decreased venous return and CO, and movement of blood from the thorax to the periphery during a vasodepressor reaction (Chapter 11); and (b) peripheral vasoconstriction, augmented venous return and CO, and displacement of blood from the periphery to the thorax after mephentermine.

Methoxamine. Methoxamine, known commercially as Vasoxyl, is a pure alpha adrenergic activator. Its primary vasoconstricting action on the peripheral blood vessels causes a rise in BAm and peripheral vascular resistance (TSR), because no positive inotropic action on the myocardium has been observed. [53,109, 110] Elevated BAm results in reflex vagal bradycardia via the carotid sinus baroreceptors. A reduction in CO and pulmonary blood flow usually follows. The peripheral action of methoxamine is independent of release of catecholamines because its pressor action was not reduced or abolished by reserpine.

In some animals, reduction in PAm was largely secondary to a fall in the pulmonary blood flow.[55] If the LAm was elevated because of systemic pressor action, usually the PAm rose accordingly.[109,110]

We have reported previously that methoxamine caused a consistent decrease in CO and HR accompanied by a marked increase in the arteriovenous oxygen difference in normal subjects

Table 12-4 Hemodynamic Effects of Mephentermine in Patients with Mitral Valve Disease and Vasodepressor Reaction

Patient	Sex	BSA	Diagnosis	FC	Periods of Study	Blood Flow			Pressures (mm Hg)				Tm (seconds)			Blood Volume (ml/M²)	
						CI	HR	SI	PAm	LAm	P_d	BAm	PA-BA	LA-BA	PA-LA	CBV	PBV
MP.	54	1.58	MS	II	V	1.67	56	30	13	12	12.5	54	16.7	8.9	7.8	465	248
	F				M	2.38	75	32	21	17	19.0	86	16.4	9.2	7.2	655	275
E.F.	55	1.48	MS	III	V	2.36	40	59	18	10	14.0	42	17.6	10.6	7.0	692	275
	F				M	3.45	85	40	47	27	37.0	92	14.5	8.9	5.6	830	323

V = period of vasodepressor reactions; M = after mephentermine administration

FC = functional classification

Other symbols and abbreviations are identical to those used in Table 12-1

Table 12-5 Hemodynamic Effects of Methoxamine in Patients with Mitral Valve Disease

Patient	Sex	BSA	Diagnosis	FC	Periods of Study	Blood Flow			Pressures (mm Hg)				Tm (seconds)			Blood Volume (ml/M²)	
						CI	HR	SI	PAm	LAm	P_d	BAm	PA-BA	LA-BA	PA-LA	CBV	PBV
J.B.	30	1.44	MS	I	C	2.56	68	37	15	9	12.0	70	14.3	9.4	4.9	612	210
	F		MR		M	2.44	65	37	22	18	20.0	94	16.7	11.1	5.6	680	227
G.B.	33	1.64	MS	II	C	2.90	100	29	16	10	13.0	104	10.8	6.4	4.6	524	222
	F				M	2.60	80	33	16	10	13.0	130	15.5	8.3	7.2	670	314
A.M.	34	1.36	MR	III	C	2.50	81	31	31	25	28.0	68	15.5	9.5	6.0	644	250
	F				M	2.30	74	31	47	31	39.0	82	17.1	8.9	8.2	657	315
J.P.	41	1.62	MR	III	C	1.80	67	27	38	24	33.0	86	27.0	18.9	8.1	625	242
	F		MS		M	1.40	60	23	40	31	35.5	108	28.4	15.8	13.6	683	317

C = control period; M = period after methoxamine administration

Other symbols and abbreviations are identical to those used in Table 12-1

and in patients with mitral disease.[111] Characteristically, patients with predominant mitral regurgitation responded with significant increments in Pw and PAm. Patients with predominant mitral stenosis showed no change in either Pw or PAm, because any potential increase in Pw secondary to elevated LVd was counteracted by reduced mitral valve flow.

Subsequent studies in our laboratory by combined right and transseptal left heart catheterization confirmed the previous results and demonstrated that the direction of change in LAm is similar to that for Pw.[112] Furthermore, PBV usually increased, associated with a rise or no change in LAm and PAm (Table 12-5). These effects were consistent with passive dilatation of the pulmonary vascular bed as a result of peripheral vascular constriction and displacement of blood into the thorax.

Adrenergic Inhibitors

The adrenergic inhibitors are divided into alpha and beta adrenergic blocking agents and anti-adrenergic or sympatholytic agents.

Adrenergic Blocking Agents. The pharmacologic agents which are capable of interfering with the action of neurotransmitter or of administered sympathomimetic amines on the effector cells are known as adrenergic blocking agents.

Alpha blocking agents. Blockade by members of this group of drugs is limited to the alpha sympathetic receptors which cause vasoconstriction. The beta type of receptors which stimulate the myocardium and cause smooth muscle relaxation are not affected. The vasoconstrictor effect of administered catecholamines is more easily blocked than that of sympathetic nerve stimulation.

This category of drugs includes two subgroups, the first of which consists of those agents which act largely by competitive inhibition. An example is tolazoline (Priscoline). Perfusion of dog lung with tolazoline failed to produce local vasodilatation.[113] In patients with primary pulmonary hypertension, mitral stenosis, congenital heart disease, or chronic pulmonary disease, however, tolazoline has been reported to cause a fall in PAm, usually accompanied by an increase in CO or pulmonary blood flow.[114-121] Changes in PVR were variable. Reduction in PVR cannot be interpreted as active pulmonary vasodilatation because the accompanying increase in pulmonary blood flow may account for the decrease in calculated resistance. No information is available concerning the possible effects of tolazoline on the PBV.

The second subgroup of alpha receptor blocking drugs consists of those agents with predominant adrenolytic and minimal sympatholytic effects. One notable example is phentolamine (Regitine), the major use of which in the past has been in the diagnosis of pheochromocytoma. We have observed no appreciable effects of phentolamine on PAm and PVR in dogs.[122] Intravenous phentolamine caused a reduction in PAm in a patient with pheochromocytoma which was unrelated to CO.[123] A similar fall in the PAm has been reported in patients with mitral stenosis.[124]

Taylor and associates recently reported the effects of 5 mg of intravenous phentolamine on the CBV in 6 normal subjects and in 6 hypertensive patients.[125] They observed a transient but definite immediate increase in CBV, invariably followed by a rapid fall which was greatest between the third and fifth minute after injection. At the same time, BAm, PAm and Pw all declined, and pulmonary blood flow increased. These findings were interpreted as evidence of an increase in the volume distensibility of the pulmonary vascular bed, although the mechanism was obscure. A direct effect of phentolamine on the pulmonary vessels was suspected in view of the rapidity of the pulmonary vascular responses. The possible effects of phentolamine on PBV remain uncertain.

Beta-blocking agents. The recently discovered beta-blocking agents interfere with receptors which are concerned with the relaxation of smooth muscles in the coronary and systemic arterial blood vessels and which exert a positive inotropic effect on the heart.

In 1958 Powell and Slater discovered dichloroisoproterenol (DCI) which blocked selectively the vaso-inhibitory but not the cardioexcitatory effects of the sympathomimetic amines.[126] The effects of the drug were complicated, however, by its intrinsic sympathomimetic action on the heart, resulting in prolonged tachycardia.

Subsequently, Black and Stephenson in 1962 reported the beta-blocking effects of nethalide (also known as pronethalol or Alderlin), with minimal intrinsic sympathomimetic-like action.[127] Dornhorst and Robinson reported the following observations after nethalide was given to normal human volunteers:[128] (a) significant slowing of HR without electrocardiographic changes, (b) attenuation of the increase in HR after exercise, (c) no apparent effect on BAm or the peripheral circulation, (d) no effect on respiratory changes during and after exercise, and (e) total blockade of the action of infused catecholamines on the heart.

Harrison and associates found that nethalide did not alter the CO at rest in 5 normal subjects.[129] Tachycardia

induced by exercise was reduced by premedication with nethalide, and the cardiac response to isoproterenol was blocked. Similar observations were reported by Schröder and Werkö in 10 patients with essential hypertension.[130]

The most recent beta-blocking agent is propranolol, available commercially as Inderal. This drug has been studied clinically in normal subjects and cardiac patients by many workers. In general, HR was reduced at rest as well as during exercise, with or without associated prolonged atrioventricular conduction. The drug lowered CI in most cases.

McKenna and colleagues observed that in intact anesthetized dogs beta adrenergic blockade caused a decrease in CO and cardiac work at rest associated with an increase in arteriovenous oxygen difference and reduced cardiovascular response to simulated exercise.[131] Both PAm and BAm remained unchanged, but the calculated total pulmonary and systemic resistances were increased.

Sowton and Hamer reported a reduction of 20% in CO and LVsw at rest as well as during exercise in a group of cardiac patients after beta adrenergic blockade.[132] Both the absolute and per cent increase in PAm were higher during exercise compared with that before the administration of the beta adrenergic blocking agent.

Braunwald and co-workers infused propranolol into 6 patients during submaximal exercise.[133] Depression of the circulatory response began 1 to 2 minutes after the injection and a new steady state was achieved within 5 minutes at lower level of CO. The average decrease in HR was 21% and in CO, 18%.

Epstein and associates reported that propranolol reduced the endurance time for maximum exercise by an average of 40% of control.[134] In 7 normal subjects the CO and BAm were measured during two periods of exercise, control and immediately after propranolol. The drug caused a significant reduction in CO (−22%), BAm (−15%), LVsw (−34%) and increased arteriovenous oxygen difference (+12%) and central venous pressure (+2.8% mm Hg). The results of exercise studies were similar in 4 patients with heart disease although the minute oxygen uptake and CO during both exercise periods were usually lower.

Cumming and Carr also reported a decrease in CO and an increase in LVd during exercise after propranolol in patients with mitral valve disease.[135] Despite slowing of HR, the cardiac performance was impaired.

Vogel and Blount reported the effects of propranolol on the pulmonary circulation in 5 human subjects.[136] The dose of the drug varied from 0.074 to 0.092 mg/Kg. PAm and total pulmonary resistance (TPR) both increased as CO and HR declined. The BAm responded to the Valsalva maneuver with a "square wave" response. The authors suggested that propranolol causes pulmonary arterial vasoconstriction and that beta receptors play an active role in the regulation of the pulmonary circulation.

Recently, the actions of two new beta blocking agents, MJ 1998 and MJ 1999, were reported.[137-139] These two phenethanolamine compounds appear to block the adrenotropic action of isoproterenol on the cardiac muscle of the tested animals. MJ 1999 was found to block beta adrenergic receptors without cardiac depressant effects.

We have studied the effects of intravenous propranolol (0.15 mg/kg) on pulmonary blood pressure and volume in 11 patients with various types of cardiac disease (Table 12-6). There was a consistent decrease in CI and HR in all patients, A reduction in SI and BAm was observed in most of the patients. In more than half the patients, LAm and PAm increased, accompanied by inconsistent changes in the PBV. The increase in LAm and PAm probably resulted from elevation of the LVd and depressed cardiac performance. No definite evidence of pulmonary vasoconstriction was demonstrated.

Antiadrenergic Agents. This group of new drugs consists of agents with properties described as antiadrenergic, sympatholytic, or sympathetic nerve blocking. Their major action is blockade of sympathetic nerve stimulation. Their interference with the effects of injected catecholamines is much less conspicuous. The three drugs included here are bretylium, guanethidine and reserpine.

Bretylium. Bretylium blockade most likely results from interference with release of norepinephrine at sympathetic nerve endings. This effect is usually preceded by an initial release of stored catecholamines, which may explain the occurrence of transient early cardiac stimulation and systemic hypertension.

Bretylium has been reported to cause a rise in PAm and PVR in man, in the sheep, and in the dog.[140-142] Whether the increased PVR was related to the blockade or to the initial release of stored catecholamines was not clear. In man, CO was reduced 40 to 60 minutes after intravenous bretylium,[143-144] whereas in animals the drug produced an early increase in CO.[141,145] The persistent reduction in CO was explained on the basis of blockade of sympathetic nerves to the heart and the peripheral blood vessels. McGaff and Leight reported a slight augmentation of PBV in dogs after bretylium.[142]

Guanethidine. Guanethidine de-

Table 12-6 Effects of Propranolol on Pulmonary Hemodynamics and Pulmonary Blood Volume

Patient	Age	Sex	BSA	Diagnosis	Condition	Blood Flow			Pressures (mm Hg)				Blood Volume (ml/M²)	
						CI	HR	SI	PAm	LAm	P_d	BAm	CBV	PBV
E.W.	33	M	1.84	PMD	C	2.94	68	44	13	7	10.0	105	482	218
					P	2.36	60	39	16	7	11.5	105	526	290
L.B.	53	M	1.92	PMD	C	1.68	70	24	14	8	11.0	100	400	205
					P	1.36	60	23	16	9	12.5	95	367	143
N.R.	46	M	2.15	PMD	C	2.82	90	32	16	8	12.0	110	720	365
					P	2.30	78	30	19	12	15.5	105	640	297
M.B.	45	F	1.62	MS	C	2.06	90	23	14	9	11.5	85	485	212
					P	1.84	72	26	13	7	10.0	83	438	232
H.M.	55	M	1.90	MR	C	2.78	60	45	15	8	11.5	103	623	284
					P	2.11	52	41	20	13	16.5	97	577	277
A.A.	60	F	1.65	MS	C	1.62	162	10	17	10	13.5	103	623	284
					P	1.22	140	9	20	15	17.5	97	577	277
M.P.	54	F	1.58	MS	C	2.10	110	19	22	13	17.5	82	475	152
				MR	P	1.64	84	14	19	11	15.0	75	408	144
F.M.	44	M	1.54	MS	C	1.85	65	28	32	20	26.0	108	605	272
					P	1.28	45	29	26	17	21.5	92	555	273
F.S.	45	M	1.61	AS	C	3.25	94	34	14	11	12.5	82	530	265
				AR	P	3.00	86	35	18	13	15.5	90	333	245
F.G.	40	M	2.10	AS	C	2.35	70	34	15	5	10.0	93	454	191
					P	1.95	60	32	16	7	11.5	92	462	220
J.F.	52	M	1.93	AS	C	2.76	60	46	19	15	17.0	95	666	278
				AR	P	1.97	48	41	21	17	19.0	90	611	291

PMD = primary myocardial disease; C = control period; P = after administration of propranolol
Other symbols and abbreviations are identical to those used in Table 12-1

pletes catecholamines in the sympathetic nerve endings by causing excessive release or by blocking their synthesis. Initial release of stored catecholamines precedes the blockade, an effect similar to that of bretylium. The early release of catecholamines is manifested by transient elevation in BAm.

The reported hemodynamic effects of guanethidine have been variable. The most consistent effects were those related to blockade of sympathetic nerves, manifested by a significant decline in BAm and TSR.[140,146-148] The decline in blood pressure was associated with either a reduction in CO[146,147] or no appreciable change in CO.[148] Harris and associates, however, reported that PVR was not reduced after guanethidine in normotensive patients breathing low oxygen.[149] On the other hand, Taylor and co-workers noted a significant fall in BAm, PAm and PVR

and no change in CO in hypertensive patients.[150]

Reserpine. Recent studies have shown that reserpine acts by continuously depleting catecholamines. Intravenous reserpine reduced PAm and PVR without associated changes in Pw in patients with mitral stenosis and in others with chronic pulmonary disease, presumably an effect of blockade of vasoconstriction.[151-154]

CO usually decreased in normal subjects, but the CO did not change consistently in hypertensive patients.[155-157] The reduction in CO was probably caused by a decrease in venous return resulting from interference with venomotor reflexes and by blockade of the sympathetic nerves to the heart.

Recently, Brutsaert demonstrated reduction in pulmonary vascular responses to hypoxia and tyramine after pretreatment with reserpine in cats.[158]

He concluded that pulmonary stores of catecholamines may be important in inducing pulmonary vasoconstriction during hypoxia. No information is available concerning the possible effects of bretylium, guanethidine or reserpine on PBV in man.

Cholinergic Activators

Acetylcholine, one of the most commonly used cholinergic activators, has its major action on the neuro-effector junctions of the vagus nerve. In 1933 Gaddum and Holtz and in 1935 Alcock and associates showed a fall in PAm after a small dose of acetylcholine was injected into isolated lung.[159,160] In 1955 Harris demonstrated that acetylcholine decreased PAm in patients with pulmonary hypertension when a carefully regulated dose was injected into the right heart or pulmonary artery.[161-163] The effects were more pronounced in patients with pulmonary hypertension than in those with mild or severe pulmonary hypertension. CO, BAm and indirect LAm were usually not affected, because the drug was quickly destroyed or metabolized in the lung.

In 1956 Cournand and associates reported the pulmonary circulatory dynamics in man during continuous infusion of acetylcholine to one branch of the pulmonary artery.[164] In 1958 Fritts and co-workers reported that acetylcholine caused a slight reduction in PAm and no change in pulmonary blood flow in normal subjects.[165] The reduction in pressure was greater if the drug was administered during inhalation of low oxygen. The authors suggested that acetylcholine caused active dilatation of the pulmonary vessels because of the following observations: (a) a consistent fall in PAm, (b) constant or increased pulmonary blood flow, (c) constant indirect LAm, (d)

unchanged extravascular pressure within the lungs and thorax as indicated by steady minute ventilation and respiratory frequency and the absence of respiratory symptoms, and (e) constant HR, BAm and CBV.

Studies by other workers in patients with pulmonary hypertension associated with various types of cardiac or pulmonary disease confirmed that acetylcholine reduced PAm in association with a slight increase or no change in pulmonary blood flow and no change in the indirect or direct LAm.[166-181] In the majority of cases, PVR declined. The evidence indicated that acetylcholine acted primarily on pulmonary arteries with little or no effect on pulmonary capillaries and veins.

During the past 8 years we have studied the effects of acetylcholine in a number of patients with pulmonary hypertension. The primary diagnosis in most of them was mitral stenosis or idiopathic pulmonary hypertension. Several patients with pulmonary hypertension associated with congenital heart disease were also studied. Acetylcholine chloride was freshly prepared with 5% dextrose in water and infused into the right heart or main pulmonary artery at the rate of 2 to 5 mg per minute. In several patients the dose was 8 to 12 mg per minute.

Our initial studies of acetylcholine in 18 patients with mitral stenosis demonstrated (a) a decrease in PAm and PVR with no change in Pw, (b) an increase in CI, and SI, (c) an increase in CBV.[173]

Our subsequent studies in another 14 patients with predominant mitral stenosis confirmed these findings. In addition we showed that acetylcholine increased PBV without affecting LAm. The decline in PAm accompanied by an increase in PBV strongly suggested active pulmonary vasodilatation (Figure

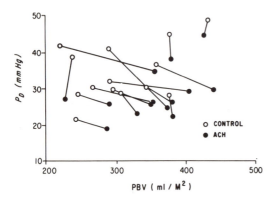

EFFECTS OF ACETYLCHOLINE IN MITRAL STENOSIS

Figure 12-1. In 14 patients with predominant mitral stenosis and pulmonary hypertension there was a reduction in pulmonary distending pressure (P_d) associated with an increase or no change in the pulmonary blood volume (PBV) following intravenous infusion of acetylcholine (ACH). The discordant pressure-volume changes suggest active vasodilatation of the pulmonary vascular bed.

12-1). Table 12-7 summarizes the effects of acetylcholine in patients with predominant mitral stenosis and pulmonary hypertension. There was a decrease in PAm associated with an increase in both CBV and PBV. The changes were statistically significant.

Furthermore, as mentioned in Chapter 16, our results also supported the observation of Fritts and associates that acetylcholine infused into the pulmonary circulation counteracted hypoxic vasoconstriction and caused active vasodilatation, despite continuing hypoxia. The vasodilating effects were manifested by a decrease in the PAm and P_d and an increase in the PBV.

Our experience with acetylcholine in idiopathic or primary pulmonary hypertension, however, differed from that reported by others. Acetylcholine failed to alter the PAm or PBV in 5 patients with this disease (Table 12-8),

in sharp contrast to the marked reduction observed in patients with predominant mitral stenosis and almost the same degree of pulmonary hypertension. The results in these two groups of patients are shown in Figure 12-2. The divergent responses to acetylcholine led us to conclude that the marked increase in PVR in patients with idiopathic or primary pulmonary hypertension was primarily a result of structural changes in the vessels with little or no functional vasoconstriction. On the other hand, functional vasoconstriction was a major factor in augmenting PVR in patients with mitral stenosis and marked pulmonary hypertension.

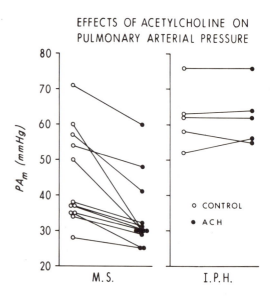

EFFECTS OF ACETYLCHOLINE ON PULMONARY ARTERIAL PRESSURE

Figure 12-2. Effects of intravenous infusion of acetylcholine on the pulmonary arterial pressure in patients with mitral stenosis (left panel) and in those with idiopathic pulmonary hypertension (right panel). A reduction in the pulmonary arterial pressure was observed in all patients with mitral stenosis but not in those with idiopathic pulmonary hypertension. The lack of response in the latter group may indicate significant degree of structural change of the pulmonary vascular bed.

Table 12-7 Hemodynamic Effects of Acetylcholine Infusion in Mitral Stenosis

Patient	Age	Sex	BSA	Periods of Study	Blood Flow			Pressures (mm Hg)				Tm (seconds)			Blood Volume (ml./M²)	
					CI	HR	SI	PAm	LAm	P_d	BAm	PA-BA	LA-BA	PA-LA	CBV	PBV
J.M.	54	M	1.65	C	1.81	49	37	28	15	21.5	60	20.4	12.3	8.1	611	243
				A	1.80	47	39	25	13	19	60	19.6	10.0	9.6	590	288
G.W.	38	M	1.90	C	2.32	93	25	34	27	30.5	92	14.8	5.9	8.9	575	342
				A	2.57	89	29	29	24	26.5	92	12.8	4.0	8.8	550	378
H.F.	50	F	1.74	C	1.91	87	22	35	23	29	85	20.2	10.6	9.6	642	306
				A	2.14	89	24	25	22	23.5	75	19.4	10.2	9.2	691	328
J.W.	21	F	1.59	C	2.30	70	33	35	25	30	70	15.4	6.7	7.7	583	296
				A	2.81	80	35	30	22	26	70	12.8	5.5	7.3	596	350
S.R.	30	F	1.54	C	2.18	75	29	36	21	28.5	75	18.5	8.2	10.3	670	376
				A	2.21	81	27	27	18	22.5	75	18.5	8.2	10.3	685	380
S.K.	21	F	1.49	C	2.13	81	26	37	20	28.5	77	14.1	7.3	6.8	501	244
				A	2.49	75	34	30	22	26	76	13.3	6.2	7.1	532	291
E.F.	55	F	1.48	C	3.07	74	41	37	22	30.5	77	14.3	9.1	5.3	730	266
				A	3.30	74	44	31	22	26.5	77	14.5	8.1	6.4	800	352
E.We.	24	F	1.67	C	3.07	83	37	38	27	32.5	80	10.5	4.8	5.7	537	292
				A	2.95	96	31	32	27	29.5	83	12.2	4.0	8.2	600	403
A.L.	31	F	1.48	C	1.89	111	17	50	28	39	108	13.0	5.5	7.5	410	238
				A	1.65	103	16	30	24	27	96	14.3	6.1	8.2	395	226
A.A.	43	M	1.81	C	2.01	110	18	54	32	37	100	23.3	12.6	10.7	778	356
				A	2.21	81	21	48	26	30	84	24.5	12.3	12.3	816	440
E.W.	34	F	1.46	C	1.60	62	26	57	27	42	72	18.1	10.1	8.0	485	229
				A	1.90	48	40	41	29	35	60	19.5	8.7	11.2	617	354
H.C.	39	M	1.86	C	3.40	127	29	60	24	42	100	10.8	5.7	5.1	615	289
				A	3.10	77	34	30	20	25	84	12.5	5.3	7.2	647	372
F.L.	57	F	1.72	C	2.05	74	27	60	30	45	102	21.9	11.0	10.9	745	374
				A	2.43	72	33	49	28	38.5	97	20.2	10.8	9.3	812	377
J.M.	26	F	1.45	C	1.61	75	22	71	28	49.5	75	31.3	15.2	16.1	845	432
				A	2.07	75	27	60	30	45	70	25.7	13.5	12.2	885	424
Control mean ± S.E.					2.24 ±0.15	63.6 ±5.6	27.8 ±1.9	45.1 ±3.5	24.9 ±1.2	34.7 ±2.1	83.4 ±3.8	17.6 ±1.50	8.9 ±0.84	8.6 ±0.77	623 ±32.6	306 ±16.5
Acetylcholine mean ± S.E.					2.40 ±0.13	77.6 ±4.2	31.0 ±2.1	34.8 ±2.8	23.4 ±1.2	28.6 ±1.8	78.5 ±3.1	17.1 ±1.22	8.1 ±0.81	9.1 ±0.50	658 ±35.7	355 ±15.2
p value					<0.05	N.S.	<0.025	<0.01	<0.05	<0.01	<0.01	N.S.	<0.05	N.S.	<0.05	<0.01

C = control period; A = during acetylcholine infusion; N.S. = not significant
Other symbols and abbreviations are identical to those used in Table 12-1

Table 12-8 Effects of Acetylcholine in Idiopathic Pulmonary Hypertension

Patient	Age Sex	BSA	Periods of Study	CI	HR	SI	Sa_{O_2}	PA (S/D)	(m)	(LAm)	BA (S/D)	(m)	CBV	PBV	TBV	TPR	PVR
J.H.	35	1.88	C	2.10	108	19	92.3	116/56	74	10*	106/66	76	525	—	—	1550	1350
	M		A	2.11	100	21	92.8	116/60	76	—	108/66	76	520	—	—	1550	—
V.S.	27	1.37	C	1.86	66	28	95.0	94/39	58	8	120/75	90	510	249	—	1800	1580
	F		A	1.71	88	20	—	85/31	55	7	110/70	85	510	274	—	1880	1640
R.S.	39	1.55	C	2.06	84	26	92.2	92/32	52	9*	147/97	111	525	—	2860	1440	1190
	F		A	2.27	80	28	—	92/34	56	—	126/84	105	545	—	2910	1320	—
L.T.	24	1.51	C	2.31	64	36	93.7	92/50	62	—	92/50	65	480	—	—	1420	—
	F		A	2.45	70	35	—	92/50	62	—	94/51	66	490	—	—	1340	—
M.R.	30	1.62	C	1.76	66	27	97.7	111/72	85	7*	113/72	85	413	—	3790	1800	1480
	F		A	1.53	63	25	95.1	112/75	90	—	112/75	90	410	—	—	1920	—

Sao_2 = arterial blood oxygen saturation(%); S/D m = systolic, diastolic and mean; TBV = total blood volume; TPR = total pulmonary resistance; PVR = pulmonary vascular resistance; * = pulmonary wedge mean pressure
Other symbols and abbreviations are identical to those used in Table 12-1

Cholinergic Inhibitors

Ganglionic Blocking Agents. The three most commonly used ganglionic blocking agents are tetraethylammonium chloride(TEAC), hexamethonium, and trimethaphan(Arfonad). Although TEAC was the first compound demonstrated by Acheson and Moe to cause ganglionic blockade,[182] it is no longer used because of side effects which tend to counteract the expected result. Earlier studies of Fowler and associates on the actions of TEAC in patients with pulmonary hypertension suggested that increased PVR in man may be partly mediated through the autonomic nervous system.[183] Hexamethonium has been studied more extensively than the other agents, and most of the information in this section is derived from reports concerning this drug. Hexamethonium has the disadvantage that its hypotensive action is relatively prolonged. Trimethaphan is a newer compound and is unique as a hypotensive agent because it may be given by continuous intravenous infusion and its action can be quickly controlled or terminated by adjusting the rate of infusion. At present, it is the drug of choice for ganglionic blockade.

Intravenous hexamethonium caused a simultaneous decline in BAm and PAm in normal subjects and in patients with various diseases.[184-199] The response of pulmonary blood flow was inconstant, but in most cases PVR declined. Studies by Sancetta and associates suggested that reduction in PAm could be attributed in part to pulmonary vasodilatation.[196] Hexamethonium has been used successfully to relieve pulmonary edema in man,[200-202] apparently because of shifting of blood from the lungs to the dilated peripheral vessels and possibly because of improved left ventricular function.

McGaff and co-workers studied the effects of acute ganglionic blockade on pulmonary circulation in closed chest dogs.[203] CO, PAm and LAm decreased, but no significant change in PBV was observed. These workers interpreted the findings as suggestive evidence of relaxation of walls of the pulmonary vessels.

Our initial study of the effects of hexamethonium on the pulmonary circulation in 27 patients with mitral stenosis demonstrated (a) a decline in BAm, PAm and Pw in most cases; (b) an insignificant change in CO, HR and SI; and (c) a decrease in PAm-Pw gradient and in calculated PVR in a

Table 12-9   Hemodynamic Effects of Hexamethonium
in Patients with Valvular Heart Disease

Pat-ient	Age	Sex	BSA	Diag-nosis	Periods of Study	Blood Flow			Pressures (mm Hg)				Tm (seconds)			Blood Volume (ml/M²)	
						CI	HR	SI	PAm	LAm	P_d	BAm	PA-BA	LA-BA	PA-LA	CBV	PBV
M.C.	50	F	1.67	MS	C	3.56	78	45	28	21	24.5	75	20.0	10.8	9.2	1116	550
				MR	Hex	3.24	70	45	20	17	18.5	64	20.2	10.6	9.6	1080	530
J.B.	46	M	2.00	MS	C	1.50	79	19	36	24	30	90	25.4	15.4	10.0	632	331
				MR	Hex	1.00	62	16	16	11	13.5	56	27.0	15.0	12.0	452	200
D.L.	33	M	1.89	MS	C	2.60	123	21	48	31	39.5	88	20.3	9.9	10.4	876	450
				MR	Hex	1.60	123	13	36	22	29	64	20.9	12.9	8.0	556	213
W.M.	56	M	1.82	MS	C	1.72	100	16	76	36	56	116	22.6	12.9	9.7	650	278
				MR	Hex	1.58	80	19	36	14	25	52	25.0	15.3	9.7	656	255
Control mean						2.35	95	25	47	28	37.5	92	22.1	12.3	9.8	818	402
±S.E.						±0.47	±10.6	±6.7	±10.5	±3.4	±6.9	±8.6	±1.3	±1.2	±0.3	±114	±61
Hexamethonium mean						1.86	84	23	27	16	21.5	59	23.3	13.5	9.8	686	299
±S.E.						±0.48	±13.6	±7.4	±5.3	±2.4	±3.4	±3.0	±1.6	±1.1	0.9	±138	±78
p value						<0.10	<0.10	N.S.	<0.05	<0.05	<0.05	<0.05	<0.10	N.S.	N.S.	N.S.	N.S.

C = control period; Hex = after hexamethonium administration
Other symbols and abbreviations are identical to those used in Table 12-1

small number of cases.[198] Subsequent studies in 4 patients with mitral valve disease yielded similar results (Table 12-9).[112] The direction and magnitude of the change in LAm were the same as those of the Pw. In all 4 cases PBV declined. The decline in PAm together with reduced PBV strongly suggests passive movement of blood from the lungs to the peripheral vessels. The reduction in PBV excludes pulmonary vasodilatation. It is clear that reduction in the calculated PVR following hexamethonium as observed by many workers can not be interpreted as evidence of pulmonary vasodilatation.

Intravenous trimethaphan in normal subjects and in patients with mitral stenosis also caused a decrease in PAm and calculated PVR and a slight increase in CO.[204-206] Thus, the PBV might be excepted to fall, as it does following hexamethonium.

Atropine. Atropine has been reported to counteract or prevent almost all the effects of acetylcholine or vagal stimulation on the pulmonary circulation. Atropine has been reported to cause an increase in HR and CO in man.[207-213] Although RAm declined, no consistent change in PAm has been observed.[214-217] Daly and associates reported reduction in PAm, PBV and Vc in normal subjects following atropine.[218]

Musculotropic Drugs

Aminophylline

The actions of aminophylline have been studied frequently in patients with bronchial asthma, pulmonary emphysema or cardiovascular disease.[219-231] In general, CO increased or was unaffected, and the PAm and PAm-Pw gradient declined. The calculated PVR was reduced in the majority of cases. Most workers interpreted these effects as evidence of pulmonary vasodilatation.

We have studied the effects of intravenous aminophylline on the pulmonary circulation in 32 patients with valvular heart disease. Eighteen patients had predominant mitral and 14 had predominant aortic valvular disease. Details have been published elsewhere,[231] and Table 12-10 summarizes the results.

In patients with mitral valve disease, no significant change was observed in CI, HR, SI, or BAm, but

Table 12-10   Effects of Aminophylline on Pulmonary Hemodynamics and Pulmonary Blood Volume

Group and Diagnosis	No. of Cases	Periods of Study		Blood Flow			Pressures (mm Hg)				PBV (ml/M²)
				CI	HR	SI	PAm	LAm	P_d	BAm	
I		C	mean	2.19	79.2	27.7	37.3	22.9	30.6	95.0	284
	17		± SE	±0.14	±3.7	±2.1	±3.0	±1.6	±2.0	±3.4	±12.5
MVD		Am	mean	2.21	82.8	27.0	31.4	18.8	25.6	92.0	311
			± SE	±0.15	±5.1	±2.5	±4.1	±1.7	±2.8	±3.8	±14.0
			Diff in mean (Am-C)	0.02	3.6	—0.7	—5.9	—4.1	—5.0	—3.0	27
			p value	NS	NS	NS	<0.01	<0.01	<0.01	NS	<0.025
II		C	mean	2.44	71.2	34.3	21.9	12.1	17.0	89.0	285
	14		± SE	±0.10	±2.8	±2.4	±2.5	±1.4	±1.8	±3.5	±10.3
AVD		Am	mean	2.42	76.9	31.5	17.3	9.9	13.8	85.5	316
			± SE	±0.10	±4.3	±2.1	±2.2	±1.8	±2.0	±3.8	±18.8
			Diff in mean (Am-C)	—0.02	5.7	—2.8	—4.6	—2.2	—3.2	—3.5	31
			p value	NS	<0.01	<0.02	<0.01	<0.01	<0.01	<.05	<0.01

C = control period;   Am = after administration of aminophylline.
Other symbols and abbreviations are identical to those used in Table 12-1.

PAm, LAm and calculated PVR declined significantly. Considering the group as a whole, aminophylline caused a statistically significant increase in the PBV.

In patients with aortic valve disease, again CI was not affected, but HR increased, accompanied by a slight increase in SI. As in the mitral group, a significant decline in PAm and LAm was accompanied by an increase in PBV. The calculated PVR decreased moderately.

Thus, these data provide new evidence favoring a direct active vasodilating effect of aminophylline on the pulmonary vasculature. The data presently available, however, do not establish the mechanism or the site of this action. Rodbard has observed that similar effects could result from drug-induced bronchodilatation, an uncertain factor in our patients.[100] None, however, had clinically apparent bronchospasm. Recent studies by Parker and associates demonstrated a significant decrease in PAm in patients with cor pulmonale following aminophylline.[229] These authors suggested that the changes were too large to be explained by an isolated effect on transmural pressure secondary to bronchodilatation.

Glyceryl Trinitrate (Nitroglycerin)

In 1940 Hochrein first reported that PAm fell in patients with pulmonary hypertension following glyceryl trinitrate.[232] Eldridge and colleagues described the beneficial effects of glyceryl trinitrate in patients with cardiac asthma.[233] Johnson and associates demonstrated a decrease in Pw, PAm and calculated PVR in patients with left ventricular failure.[234,235] Gorlin and co-workers also found a fall in calculated PVR in normal man and in patients with coronary artery disease.[236,237] An increase in the SV of normal subjects was reported by Wégria and associates.[228] Müller and Rorvik found that glyceryl trinitrate could prevent the elevation of Pw which occurred after exercise as well as during a spontaneous attack of angina pectoris.[239]

Rowe and co-workers studied the effects of erythrol tetranitrate in 5 subjects with normal cardiovascular systems, 4 patients with systemic hypertension and 6 patients with a history of angina.[240] They found a reduction in CO, BAm, PAm, and coronary vascular resistance. They supported the hypothesis that the effectiveness of nitrites is due to reduction of cardiac work into a range compatible with attainable coronary blood flow.

Recent reports by many workers demonstrated that in normal subjects and cardiac patients nitroglycerin or amyl nitrite not only reduced CO, PAm and LAm (or Pw) at rest but also increased the exercise tolerance.[241-244] Frick and associates studied hemodynamic effects of nitroglycerin in patients with angina pectoris by atrial pacing.[245] At all heart rates studied, nitroglycerin allowed the heart to be driven at a higher rate without production of anginal pain. The results reflected a decreased oxygen requirement of the heart after nitroglycerin.

We have studied the effects of glyceryl trinitrate in 1 patient with mitral stenosis (Table 12-11). The drug caused a significant decrease in PAm and had little effect on LAm. The CI and PBV declined slightly. The results reported by Johnson and associates suggest that glyceryl trinitrate exerted its primary action on the myocardium and the peripheral circulation.[234,235] Reduction in the PAm and presumably in the PBV was secondary to improved ventricular emptying.

Angiotensin

The mode of action of angiotensin has been reviewed recently in two articles.[246,247] The vasconstrictor action of angiotensin is a direct stimulation of vascular smooth muscle. The precapillary vessels are most affected, and the postcapillary venules and veins are only minimally involved. Angiotensin usually caused a significant rise in BAm, LAm or Pw, and PAm in patients with normal cardiovascular systems.[248-252] The PAm-Pw gradient was unaffected. In general, CO decreased or remained the same. The nature of positive inotropic action of angiotensin on ventricular myocardium was recently reported by Koch-Weser.[253]

We have studied the effects of angiotensin on the pulmonary circulation in 11 patients with mitral valve disease (Table 12-12), data from 5 of whom (A.G., M.K., C.C., J.R., and C.C.) have been reported previously.[112] CI decreased significantly, accompanied by inconsistent changes in HR and SV. BAm, LAm, and PAm were elevated significantly (Figure 12-3). The most unexpected effect was a decrease in the CBV and PBV in most cases. If the pulmonary vascular bed reacted passively to angiotensin, one would have expected an increase in PBV secondary to the increase in P_d. The rise in pressure and fall in volume

Table 12-11   Hemodynamic Effects of Nitroglycerin in a Patient with Predominant Mitral Stenosis

Periods of Study	Blood Flow			Pressures (mm/Hg)				Tm (seconds)			Blood Volume (ml/M²)	
	CI	HR	SI	PAm	LAm	P_d	BAm	PA-BA	LA-BA	PA-LA	CBV	PBV
Control	1.73	100	17	53	21	37.0	87	23.4	10.4	13.0	673	374
After Nitroglycerin												
2 min.	—	100	—	50	21	35.5	—	—	—	—	—	—
6 min.	1.73	104	17	53	21	37.0	87	22.8	—	—	655	—
11 min.	1.50	103	15	40	18	29.0	82	26.7	12.5	14.2	668	355
21 min.	1.50	102	15	42	20	31.0	88	26.1	12.5	13.5	652	338

The symbols and abbreviations are identical to those used in Table 12-1

strongly suggested that angiotensin caused pulmonary vasoconstriction, a view shared by other workers.[70,250]

Chemical Constituents of the Blood

Histamine

Perfusion of the lungs of several species of animals has demonstrated a local constricting action of histamine.[57,254-256] In intact animals, however, histamine has been reported to induce either a rise or a fall in the PAm.[257-262] The effects of pulmonary blood flow have also been inconsistent. Some workers have observed an increase in pulmonary blood flow which they explained by one or more of the following effects: (a) sympathetic stimulation and release of catecholamines, (b) positive inotropic action on the myocardium, (c) hypoxia secondary to bronchoconstriction, (d) release of potassium and (e) release of bradykinin. Other investigators found pulmonary blood flow decreased, an effect which might have several explanations: (a) systemic shock, (b) reduction in venous return secondary to peripheral vasodilatation, and (c) cardiac decompensation with elevation of the LAm.

Feeley and associates found that in dogs histamine produced active pulmonary venoconstriction and passive distention in proximal vessels.[58] When venoconstriction was marked, PBV declined. When venoconstriction was only moderate, the increase in Vc was predominant and PBV was sometimes increased. Thus, the change in PBV after histamine was variable, depending upon the degree of pulmonary venoconstriction.

In man, the response of the PAm to histamine has also been inconsistent.[263-269] Some authors reported no change, others observed a fall, and still others a rise in PAm. Pulmonary blood flow increased, associated with decrease in PVR. Some of the explanations listed under animal studies may also apply to the divergent results observed in man.

Storstein and co-workers studied pulmonary hemodynamic responses to subcutaneous histamine in 21 patients with various chronic lung diseases.[270] PAm declined with no accompanying change in Pw or pulmonary blood flow. Thus, the calculated PVR was usually reduced. The increase in bronchomotor tone produced by histamine in some patients did not influence the pressure or resistance in the pulmonary vascular bed.

5-Hydroxytryptamine

Administration of 5-hydroxytryptamine (5-HT) during experimental perfusion of the lungs of guinea pigs, sheep, cats and dogs usually caused local pulmonary vasoconstriction.[57,270-275] In intact, anesthetized animals there was usually a rise in PAm after administration of 5-HT.[276-286] Various segments of the pulmonary vessels constricted, as manifested by selective pressure elevation in the pulmonary arteries and pulmonary veins proximal to the junction between pulmonary veins and left atrium.[281,282,285] Despite an increase in the PVR, pulmonary blood flow usually increased as well. In other words, the rise in the PAm-Pw gradient in most cases was disproportionate to the rise in pulmonary blood flow.[281,282,286] The increase in pulmonary blood flow may be related to two factors: (a) peripheral vascular activity increasing venous return, and (b) pulmonary venoconstriction reflexly augmenting right ventricular output.

In the dog, McGaff and Milnor found that PBV decreased approximately 26% after 5-HT, probably

Table 12-12 Hemodynamic Effects of Angiotensin Infusion in Patients with Valvular Heart Disease

Patients	Age	Sex	BSA	Diagnosis	Periods of Study	Blood Flow CI	HR	SI	Pressures (mm Hg) PAm	LAm	P_d	BAm	Tm (seconds) PA-BA	LA-BA	PA-LA	Blood Volume (mL/M²) CBV	PBV
D.T.	29	M	1.56	MR	C	2.98	110	27	14	10	12	84	11.6	7.3	4.3	580	213
				MS	AN	2.58	90	29	30	22	26	116	13.1	10.0	3.1	568	128
D.Ov.	56	F	1.58	MR	C	1.68	76	22	15	11	13	75	23.0	12.2	10.8	645	302
				MS	AN	1.51	80	19	20	17	18.5	118	25.6	14.7	10.3	645	261
A.G.	15	F	1.37	MR	C	4.25	117	36	17	12	14.5	96	7.4	3.3	4.1	520	293
				MS	AN	2.80	70	40	23	19	21	132	9.1	3.4	5.7	472	264
D.O.	57	M	1.62	MR	C	2.52	90	28	18	7	12.5	104	24.2	13.6	10.6	1020	444
					AN	1.89	84	23	37	23	30	123	28.9	16.8	12.1	925	380
M.K.	52	F	1.63	MS	C	1.58	64	25	18	10	14	100	15.5	7.8	7.7	412	204
					AN	1.29	106	12	22	12	17	120	18.3	11.0	7.3	393	158
E.W.	35	F	1.45	MR	C	1.54	71	21	19	10	14.5	100	23.8	14.5	9.3	615	240
					AN	1.16	75	15	35	32	33.5	135	30.1	23.5	6.6	580	128
E.S.	52	F	1.54	MR	C	2.00	97	20	19	12	15.5	90	16.6	8.3	8.3	555	276
					AN	1.75	122	14	33	25	29	120	20.6	10.7	9.9	598	288
J.R.	46	M	1.88	MR	C	3.50	112	31	20	16	18	100	10.9	5.3	5.6	642	327
				MS	AN	2.70	80	34	52	40	46	128	11.7	6.1	5.6	527	252
C.C.	38	M	2.12	MR	C	2.20	60	37	21	15	18	94	24.6	15.6	9.0	896	330
				MS	AN	1.30	48	27	26	23	24.5	116	25.4	14.8	10.6	554	230
S.S.	37	F	1.67	MR	C	2.26	53	43	21	16	18.5	80	21.1	13.0	8.1	800	305
				AR	AN	1.58	55	29	27	24	25.5	95	28.2	17.8	10.4	743	274
M.G.	50	F	1.35	MS	C	2.15	80	27	22	18	20	88	21.8	13.4	8.4	780	300
				AR	AN	1.56	86	18	29	20	24.5	125	18.5	9.6	8.9	480	232
Control	mean					2.42	84.6	28.8	18.6	12.5	15.5	91.9	18.2	10.4	7.8	678	294
	± S.E.					±0.26	±6.7	±2.0	±0.76	±1.01	±0.82	±2.82	±1.85	±1.24	±0.69	±53.6	±19.8
Angiotension	mean					1.83	81.5	23.6	30.4	23.4	26.9	120.7	20.9	12.6	8.2	590	236
	± S.E.					±0.18	±6.3	±2.7	±2.70	±2.25	±2.41	±3.19	±2.22	±1.71	±0.83	±43.6	±22.6
	p value					<0.01	N.S.	<0.02	<0.01	<0.01	<0.01	<0.01	<0.02	<0.05	N.S.	<0.05	<0.01

C = control period; AN = during angiotensin infusion
Other symbols and abbreviations are identical to those used in Table 12-1

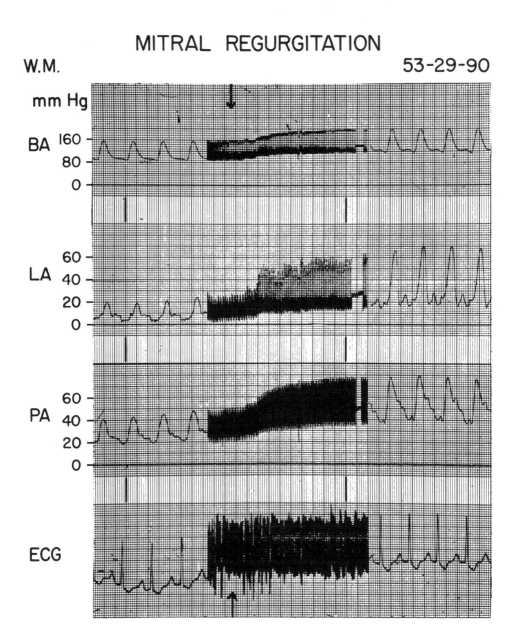

Figure 12-3. In a patient with predominant mitral regurgitation, a significant rise in brachial arterial (BA), left atrial (LA) and pulmonary arterial (PA) pressures was recorded after intravenous injection of angiotensin. The arrow indicates the time at which the injection was made. Note the prominent regurgitant wave in the left atrial pressure tracing. The paper speed in the beginning and at the end was 25 mm per second, and in the middle it was 2.5 mm per second.

directly reflecting the decreased diameter of the constricted pulmonary venous bed.[287] Recent studies by Rudolph and Scarpelli have also provided evidence of a direct pulmonary vasoconstricting response after 5-HT in both conscious and anesthetized dogs. [288]

Infusion of 5-HT into man has had various effects on the PAm.[279-291] Harris and associates gave a continuous infusion of 1.85 to 6.5 μg/kg/min to 7 patients and found that the most consistent effect was an increase in HR.[291] An unequivocal rise in PAm occurred in only 1 patient. CO did not change. The same workers studied the effects of 5-HT given by a single rapid injection in 3 patients. One patient received a dose of 4 μg/kg into the right artium and developed transient ventricular arrest and systemic hypotension followed by a sustained rise in both PAm and BAm. This response was interpreted as a Bezold-like reflex, and the investigation was therefore discontinued.

No reports of effects on the PBV following 5-HT in man have appeared, but the drug would probably decrease PBV by pulmonary vasoconstriction.

Bradykinin

Bradykinin, an endogenous polypeptide, is a powerful vasodilator in the systemic circulation.[292,293] It was first described in 1949 and the pure product was isolated in 1960.

Some investigators reported an increase in CO and HR associated with a decrease in BAm, PAm and TPR in animals.[294,295] Similar results in man were observed by other workers.[296,297] Carlier found an increase in CO without associated reduction in PAm.[298]

Recently, Freitas and associates published two studies of the effects of bradykinin in man.[299,300] The first included 10 patients, 6 of whom had

essential hypertension, and 4 of whom had no detectable cardiovascular disease. The dose of synthetic bradykinin infused intravenously was usually less than 1 μg/kg/min. CI, HR, and SI increased as BAm and TSR declined. PAm and LAm were unaffected, but the calculated PVR decreased consistently. No information was included concerning changes in PBV. The authors suggested that the decreased PVR was probably a manifestation of active pulmonary vasodilatation, independent of changes in the systemic circulation.

These authors' second study reported the effects of synthetic bradykinin in 21 patients with pulmonary hypertension secondary to mitral valve disease. Bradykinin was infused intravenously at 0.75 to 1.42 μg/kg/min (average dose 0.98 μg/kg/min) until the reduction in BAm or the increase in HR or both were stable. Bradykinin reduced calculated TSR manifested by a fall in BAm and an increase in CO. Despite an increase in both LAm and PAm, calculated PVR decreased noticeably. No significant change in PBV was evident. The authors interpreted the changes in the pulmonary circulation as mechanical or reflex effects, secondary to the action of bradykinin on the systemic arteries and heart and not as direct effects of the drug on the pulmonary vessels.

Inhalation Anesthetics, Barbiturates and Morphine

Inhalation Anesthetics

Ether. Divergent observations have shown that inhalation of ether increased or decreased CO.[301-303] Increase in CO was considered a result of catecholamine release; decrease in CO was explained as resulting from depressant activity of the agent on myocardium.[304-308] In some patients a rise in PAm was observed, probably as a consequence of increased pulmonary blood flow. An increase in calculated PVR during ether inhalation was reported by Johnson.[309] Sjöstrand demonstrated a reduction in CBV in animals, with corresponding increase in the volume of the peripheral circulation.[310] In human subjects the response of the CBV was variable.[301,309]

Cycloproprane. During cyclopropane anesthesia, Etsten and associates observed a decrease in CO, a rise in PAm, and an increase in the calculated PVR.[311] Other workers have also found a decrease in CO in man during cyclopropane anethesia,[312,313] but Jones reported an increase in some patients.[314] No information concerning the effect of this agent on PBV is available.

Halothane. Information concerning the effects of halothane on the pulmonary circulation in man is scanty. Depression of myocardial contractility has been demonstrated in the dog and in man,[315,316] but CO has not been shown to change consistently during halothane anesthesia.[317-319] An increase in PAm and TPR has been reported by other workers.[320]

Barbiturates

In most patients barbiturates have caused a reduction in CO and inconsistent variations in the PAm.[321-324] Johnson observed a decrease in CBV which was not affected by the supplementary use of curare or by oxygen inhalation.[309] Etsten and Li also reported reduction in the intrathoracic blood volume.[323] The reduction in CBV was attributed to redistribution and pooling of blood in the periphery.

Morphine

Pur-Shahriari and associates studied the effects of morphine injected into the right atrium of the dog.[325] CO, HR, and BAm all decreased. They speculated that the beneficial effects of morphine in the treatment of acute pulmonary edema might be explained on the basis of (a) peripheral venous pooling of blood resulting in pulmonary decongestion, an apparently short-lasting action, and (b) a sustained decrease in left ventricular minute work with no apparent change in myocardial contractility.

Other workers also reported pooling of blood in the peripheral vessels of dogs after morphine, associated with a decrease in venous return.[326]

In supine patients morphine exerted little effect on CO, HR, BAm, or pulmonary circulation.[327,328] Glassman and associates, however, reported a slight increase in CO, little change or some increase in PBV and a decrease in PVR. They interpreted the results as evidence of direct action of morphine to increase the distensibility of pulmonary vessels.[329]

Roy and co-workers reported the effects of morphine sulfate on the hemodynamics and PBV in 4 men who had previously experienced high altitude pulmonary edema (Table 12-13).[330] Studies were performed 20 to 67 days after recovery from pulmonary edema. Morphine in a 10 mg dose was injected through a cardiac catheter into the pulmonary artery of each patient. The immediate response was reduction in the CO, SV, BAm, PAm, and left and right ventricular work. CBV and PBV both decreased. The authors suggested that the reduction in PBV was probably an effect of redistribution of blood toward the peripheral circulation. We have studied the effects of morphine sulfate on the pulmonary

Table 12-13 Effects of Morphine on Pulmonary Hemodynamics and Pulmonary Blood Volume

Case No.	Sex	BSA	Periods of Study	Blood Flow			Pressures (mm/Hg)				Blood Volume (ml/M²)		Remark
				CI	HR	SI	PAm	LAm	P_d	BAm	CBV	PBV	
1	M	1.67	A	5.8	100	58	17	4.0	10.5	115	1102	397	(a)
			B	4.1	84	49	13	1.5	7.2	105	786	335	
2	M	1.66	A	4.1	90	46	14	6.0	10.0	102	956	198	(a)
			B	3.9	90	43	12	4.0	8.0	90	902	156	
3	M	1.65	A	7.8	90	87	13	4.0	8.5	88	1573	468	(a)
			B	6.6	80	83	12	4.0	8.0	85	1202	278	
4	M	1.66	A	3.1	54	57	22	10.0	16.0	84	775	285	(a)
			B	2.8	50	56	20	9.0	14.5	93	765	233	
5	M	1.80	A	3.5	84	44	28	23.0	26.5	90	824	355	(b)
			B	3.4	84	43	25	17.0	22.0	90	777	307	

(a) = data after Roy and co-workers; (b) = data obtained from a patient with aortic regurgitation studied in our laboratory.

Other symbols and abbreviations are identical to those used in Table 12-1

hemodynamics and blood volume in 1 patient with mitral valve disease. As shown in Table 12-13, the results were similar to those reported by Roy and co-workers. P_d and PBV both diminished, suggesting that the effect on the pulmonary vascular bed is passive as Roy and co-workers proposed.

REFERENCES

1. Fowler, N.O.: Effects of pharmacologic agents on the pulmonary circulation. Am. J. Med., 28, 927, 1960.

2. Aviado, D. M.: The Lung Circulation, vols. 1 and 2, New York, Pergamon Press, Inc., 1965.

3. Cotten, M., deV., and Stopp, P.E.: Action of digitalis on the non-failing heart of the dog. Am. J. Physiol., 192, 114, 1958.

4. Ross, J., Waldhausen, J. A., and Braunwald, E.: Studies on digitalis. I. Direct effects on peripheral vascular resistence. J. Clin. Invest., 39, 930, 1960.

5. Rodman, T., and Pastor, B.H.: The hemodynamic effects of digitalis in the normal and diseased heart. Am. Heart J., 65, 564, 1963.

6. Braunwald, E., Bloodwell, R.D., Goldberg, L.I., and Morrow, A.G.: Studies on digitalis. IV. Observations in man on the effects of digitalis preparations on the contractility of the non-failing heart and on total vascular resistance. J. Clin. Invest., 40, 52, 1961.

7. Mendez, C., Aceves, J., and Mendez, R.: Inhibition of adrenergic cardiac acceleration by cardiac glycosides. J. Pharmacol. & Exp. Ther., 131, 191, 1961.

8. James, T.N., and Nadeau, R.A.: The chronotropic effects of digitalis studied by direct perfusion of the sinus node. J. Pharmacol. & Exp. Ther., 139, 42, 1963.

9. Mason, D.T., and Braunwald, E.: Studies on digitalis. IX. Effects of Ouabain on the non-failing human heart. J. Clin. Invest., 42, 1105, 1963.

10. Murphy, G.W., Schreiner, B.F., Bleakley, P.L., and Yu, P.N.: Left ventricular performance following digitalization in patients with and without heart failure. Circulation, 30, 358, 1964.

11. Weissler, A.M., Gamel, W.G., Grode, H.E., Cohen, S., and Schoenfeld, C.D.: The effect of digitalis on ventricular ejection in normal human subjects. Circulation, 29, 721, 1964.

12. Weissler, A.M., Kamen, A.R., Bornstein, R.S., Schoenfeld, C.D., and Cohen, S.: Effect of deslanoside on the duration of the phases of ventricular systole in man. Am. J. Cardiol., 15, 153, 1965.

13. Braunwald, E., Mason, D.T., and Ross, J.: Studies of cardiocirculatory actions of digitalis. Medicine, 44, 233, 1965.

14. Sonnenblick, E.H., Williams, J.F., Glick, G., Mason, D.T., and Braunwald, E.: Studies on digitalis. XV. Effects of cardiac glycosides on myocardial force-velocity relations in non-failing human heart. Circulation, 34, 532, 1966.

15. Williams, M.H., Zohman, L.R., and Ratner, A.C.: Hemodynamic effects of cardiac glycosides on normal human subjects during rest and exercise. J. Appl. Physiol., 13, 417, 1958.

16. Selzer, A., Hultgren, H.N., Ebnother, C.L., Bradley, H.W., and Stone, A.O.: Effect of digoxin on the circulation in normal man. Brit. Heart J., *21*, 335, 1959.

17. Dresdale, D.T., Yuceoglu, Y.Z., Michtom, R.J., Schultz, M., and Lunger, M.: Effects of lanatoside C on cardiovascular hemodynamics. Acute digitalizing doses in subjects with normal hearts and with heart disease without failure. Am. J. Cardiol., *4*, 88, 1959.

18. Maseri, A., Bianchi, R., Giusti, C., Toni, P., and Donato, L.: Early effects of digitalis on central hemodynamics in normal subjects. Am. J. Cardiol., *15*, 162, 1965.

19. Lagerlöf, H., and Werkö, L.: Studies on circulation in man; the effect of Cedilanid (lanatoside C) on cardiac output and blood pressure in the pulmonary circulation in patients with compensated and decompensated heart disease. Acta Cardiol., *4*, 1, 1949.

20. Bayliss, R.I.S., Etheridge, M.J., Hyman, A.L., Kelly, H.G., McMichael, J., and Reid, E.A.S.: The effect of digoxin on the right ventricular pressure in hypertensive and ischaemic heart failure. Brit. Heart J., *12*, 317, 1950.

21. Harvey, R.M., Ferrer, M.I., Cathcart, R.T., and Alexander, J.K.: Some effects of digoxin on the heart and circulation in man. Digoxin in enlarged hearts not in clinical congestive failure. Circulation, *4*, 366, 1951.

22. Selzer, A., and Malmborg, R.O.: Hemodynamic effects of digoxin in latent cardiac failure. Circulation, *25*, 695, 1962.

23. Ferrer, M.I., Harvey, R.M., Cathcart, R.T., Cournand, A., and Richards, D.W.: Hemodynamic studies in rheumatic heart disease. Circulation, *6*, 688, 1952.

24. Yu, P.N., Nye, R.E., Lovejoy, F.W., Macias, J. de J., Schreiner, B.F., and Lux, J.J.: Effects of acetyl strophanthidin on pulmonary circulation in patients with cardiac failure and mitral stenosis. Am. Heart J., *54*, 235, 1957.

25. Greene, M.A., Gordon, A., and Boltax, A.J.: Effects of intravenous lanatoside-C upon cardiodynamics in patients with mitral stenosis and regular sinus rhythm. Am. Heart J., *61*, 622, 1961.

26. McMichael, J.: Pharmacology of the failing human heart. Brit. Med. J., *2*, 927, 1948.

27. Bloomfield, R.A., Rapoport, B., Milnor, J.P., Long, W.K., Mebane, J.G., and Ellis, L.B.: The effects of the cardiac glycosides upon the dynamics of the circulation in congestive heart failure. I. Ouabain. J. Clin. Invest., *27*, 588, 1948.

28. Ferrer, M.I., Harvey, R.M., Cathcart, R.T., Webster, C.A., Richards, D.W., and Cournand, A.: Some effects of digoxin upon the heart and circulation in man. Digoxin in chronic cor pulmonale. Circulation, *1*, 161, 1950.

29. Mounsey, J.P.D., Ritzmann, L.W., Selverstone, N.J., Briscoe, W.A., and McLemore, G.A.: Circulatory changes in severe pulmonary emphysema. Brit. Heart J., *14*, 153, 1952.

30. Berglund, E., Widimsky, J., and Malmberg, R.: Lack of effect of digitalis in patients with pulmonary disease with and without failure. Am. J. Cardiol., *11*, 477, 1963.

31. Stead, E.A., Warren, J.V., and Brannon, E.S.: Effect of lanatoside C on the circulation of patients with congestive heart failure. Arch. Int. Med., *81*, 282, 1948.

32. Harvey, R.M., Ferrer, M.I., Cathcart, R.T., Richards, D.W., and Cournand, A.: Some effects of digoxin upon the heart and circulation in man. Digoxin in left ventricular failure. Am. J. Med., *7*, 439, 1949.

33. Ferrer, M.I., Conroy, R.J., and Harvey, R.M.: Some effects of digoxin upon the heart and circulation in man. Digoxin in combined (left and right) ventricular failure. Circulation, *21*, 372, 1960.

34. Kim, Y.S., and Aviado, D.M.: Digitalis and pulmonary circulation. Am. Heart J., *62*, 680, 1961.

35. Carney, E.K., Ross, J., and Cooper, T.: The effect of large doses of quinidine on myocardial function in the normothermic and hypothermic dog. J. Thorac. Cardiov. Surg., *43*, 372, 1962.

36. Angelakos, E.T., and Hastings, E.P.: The influence of quinidine and procaine amide on myocardial contractility in vivo. Am. J. Cardiol., *5*, 791, 1960.

37. Mierzwiak, D.S., Mitchell, J.H., and Shapiro, W.: The effect of diphenylhydantoin (Dilantin) and quinidine on left ventricular function in dogs. Am. Heart J., *74*, 780, 1967.

38. Folle, L.E., and Aviado, D.M.: Cardiopulmonary effects of quinidine and procaine amide. J. Pharmacol. & Exp. Ther., *154*, 92, 1966.

39. James, T.N., and Nadeau, R.A.,: The mechanism of action of quinidine on the sinus node studied by direct perfusion through its artery. Am. Heart J., *67*, 804, 1964.

40. Roberts, J., Stadter, R.P., Cairoli, V., and Modell, W.: Relationship between adrenergic activity and cardiac action of quinidine. Circ. Res., *11*, 758, 1962.

41. Hansen, W.R., McClendon, R.L., and Kinsman, J.M.: Auricular fibrillation: Hemodynamic studies before and after conversion with quinidine. Am. Heart J., *44*, 499, 1952.

42. Storstein, O., and Tveten, H.: The hemo-dynamic effects of restoring normal sinus rhythm in patients with auricular fibrillation. Scand. J. Clin. Lab. Invest., 7, 167, 1955.

43. Ferrer, M.I., Harvey, R.M., Werkö, L., Dresdale, D.T., Cournand A., and Richards, D.W.: Some effects of quinidine sulfate on the heart and circulation in man. Am. Heart J., 36, 816, 1948.

44. Allard, J.R., Ware, W.H., and Bennett, L.L.: Negative chronotropism and inotropism of procaine amide in the heart. J. Lab. & Clin. Med., 55, 129, 1960.

45. Harrison, D.C., Sprouse, J.H., and Morrow, A.G.: The antiarrhythmic properties of lidocaine and procaine amide. Clinical and physiologic studies of their cardiovascular effects in man. Circulation, 28, 486, 1963.

46. Austen, W.G., and Moran, J.M.: Cardiac and peripheral vascular effects of lidocaine and procaine amide. Am. J. Cardiol., 16, 701, 1965.

47. McClenden, R.L., Hansen, W.R, and Kinsman, J.M.: Hemodynamic changes following procaine amide administered intravenously. Am. J.Med. Sci., 222, 375, 1951.

48. Lucas, B. G. B., and Short, D.S.: Procaine amide in the control of cardiac arrhythmias. Brit. Heart J., 14, 470, 1952.

49. Mixter, C.G., Moran, J.M., and Austen, W.G.: Cardiac and peripheral vascular effects of diphenylhydantoin sodium. Am. J. Cardiol., 17, 332, 1966.

50. Conn, R.D., Kennedy, J.W., and Blackmon, J.R.: Hemodynamic effects of diphenylhydantoin. Am. Heart J., 73, 500, 1967.

51. Lieberson, A.D., Schumacher, R.R., Childress, R.H., Boyd, D.L., and Williams, J.F.: Effect of diphenylhydantoin on left ventricular function in patients with heart disease. Circulation, 36, 692, 1967.

52. Ahlquist, R.P.: A study of the adrenotropic receptors. Am. J. Physiol., 153, 586, 1948.

53. Goldberg, L.I., Bloodwell, R.D., Braunwald, E., and Morrow, A.G.: The direct effects of norepinephrine, epinephrine and methoxamine on myocardial contractile force in man. Circulation, 22, 1125, 1960.

54. Rose, J.C., Fries, E.D., Hufnagel, C.A., and Massullo, E.A.: Effects of epinephrine and nor-epinephrine in dogs studied with a mechanical left ventricle. Demonstration of active vasoconstriction in the lesser circulation. Am. J. Physiol, 182, 197, 1955.

55. Aviado, D.M., and Schmidt, C.F.: Effects of sympathomimetic drugs on pulmonary circulation with special reference to a new pulmonary vasodilator. J. Pharmacol. & Exp. Ther., 120, 512, 1957.

56. Duke, H.N., and Stedeford, R.D.: Pulmonary vasomotor responses to epinephrine and norepinephrine in the cat. Circ. Res., 8, 640, 1960.

57. Borst, H.G., Berglund, E., and McGregor, M.: The effects of pharmacologic agents on the pulmonary circulation in the dog. Studies on epinephrine, nor-epinephrine, 5-hydroxytryptamine, acetylcholine, histamine and aminophylline. J. Clin. Invest., 36, 669, 1957.

58. Feeley, J.W., Lee, T.D., and Milnor, W.R.: Active and passive components of pulmonary vascular response to vasoactive drugs in the dog. Am. J. Physiol., 205, 1193, 1963.

59. Gaddum, J.H., and Holtz, P.: The localization of the action of drugs on the pulmonary vessels of dogs and cats. J. Physiol., 77, 139, 1933.

60. Suetuna, M.: Pharmacological studies of the pulmonary blood vessels. Igaku Kenkyu Acta Medica, 24, 1158, 1954.

61. Goldenberg, M., Pines, K.L., Baldwin, E., deF., Greene, D.G., and Roh, C.E.: The hemodynamic responses of man to norepinephrine and epinephrine and its relation to the problem of hypertension. Am. J. Med., 5, 792, 1948.

62. Condorelli, L.: Physiopathologie de la circulation artérielle pulmonarie. Schweiz med. Wschr., 80, 986, 1950.

63. Witham, A.C., and Fleming, J.W.: The effects of epinephrine on the pulmonary circulation in man. J. Clin. Invest., 30, 707, 1951.

64. Forman, S., May, L.G., Bennett, A., Kobayashi, M., and Gregory, R.: Effects of pressor and depressor agents on pulmonary and systemic pressures of normotensives and hypertensives. Proc. Soc. Exp. Biol. & Med., 83, 847, 1953.

65. Nelson, R.A., May, L.G., Bennett, A., Kobayashi, M., and Gregory, R.: Comparison of the effects of pressor and depressor agents and influences on pulmonary and systemic pressures of normotensive and hypertensive subjects. Am. Heart J., 50, 172, 1955.

66. Konzett, H., and Hebb, C.O.: Vaso- and bronchomotor actions of noradrenaline (Arterenol) and of adrenaline in the isolated perfused lungs of the dogs. Arch. Int. de Pharmacodyn. et de Ther., 78, 210, 1949.

67. Shadle, O.W., Moore, J.C., and Billig, D.M.: Effects of 1-arternol on "central blood volume" in the dog. Circ. Res., 3, 385, 1955.

68. Levy, M.N., and Brind, S.H.: Influence of 1-norepinephrine upon cardiac output in anesthetized dogs. Circ. Res., 5, 85, 1957.

69. Patel, D.J., Mallos, A.J., and Freitas, F.M., de: Importance of transmural pressure and lung volume in evaluating drug effect on pulmonary vascular tone. Circ. Res., *9*, 1217, 1961.

70. Fowler, N.O., and Holmes, J.C.: Pulmonary pressor action of 1-norepinephrine and angiotensin. Am. Heart J., *70*, 66, 1965.

71. Aramendia, P., Fermoso, J.D., Barrios, A., and Taquini, A.C.: Response of the pulmonary circulation to infusion of norepinephrine and isoproterenol. Acta physiol. Lat. Amer., *13*, 20, 1963.

72. Fowler, N.O., Westcott, R.N., Scott, R.C., and McQuire, J.: The effect of nor-epinephrine upon pulmonary arteriolar resistance in man. J. Clin. Invest., *30*, 517, 1951.

73. Patel, D.J., Lange, R.L., and Hecht, H.H.: Some evidence for active constriction in the human pulmonary vascular bed. Circulation, *18*, 19, 1958.

74. Regan, T.J., Defazio, V., Binak, K., and Hellems, H.K.: Norepinephrine induced pulmonary congestion in patients with aortic valve regurgitation. J. Clin. Invest., *38*, 1564, 1959.

75. Tuckman, J., and Finnerty, F.A.: Cardiac index during intravenous levarterenol infusion in man. Circ. Res., *7*, 988, 1959.

76. Bousvaros, G.A.: Effects of norepinephrine on human pulmonary circulation. Brit. Heart J., *24*, 738, 1962.

77. Sarnoff, S.J., Case, R.B., Berglund, E., and Sarnoff, L.C.: Ventricular function. V. The circulatory effects of Aramine: mechanism of action of "vasopressor" drugs in cardiogenic shock. Circulation, *10*, 84, 1954.

78. Harrison, D.C., Chidsey, C.A., and Braunwald E.: Studies on the mechanism of action of metaraminol (Aramine). Ann. Int. Med., *59*, 297, 1963.

79. Livesay, W.R., Moyer, J.H., and Chapman, D.W.: The cardiosvscular and renal hemodynamic effects of Aramine. Am. Heart J., *47*, 745, 1954.

80. Malmcrona, R., Schröder, G., and Werkö, L.: Hemodynamic effects of meteraminol. I. Normal subjects. Am. J. Cardiol., *13*, 10, 1964.

81. Eliasch, H., Malmborg, R.O., Pernow, B., and Zetterquist, S.: The effects of Aramine (metaraminol) on the sphanchnic, the cardiopulmonary and the systemic circulation in patients with mitral valvular disease. Acta med. Scand., *175*, 167, 1964.

82. Horvath, S.M., and Knapp, D.W.: Hemodynamic effects of neosynephrine. Am. J. Physiol., *178*, 387, 1954.

83. Beck, W., Shrire, V., and Vogelpoel, L.: The hemodynamic effects of amyl nitrite and phenylephrine in patients with mitral stenosis and severe pulmonary hypertension. Am. Heart J., *64*, 631, 1962.

84. Konzett, H.: Neue broncholytisch hockwinksame Körper der Adrenalinreihe. Arch. Exp. Path. Pharmak, *197*, 27, 1940.

85. Kaufman, J., Iglauer, A., and Herwitz, G.K.: Effect of Isuprel (isopropylepinephrine) on circulation of normal man. Am. J. Med., *11*, 442, 1951.

86. Lands, A.M., and Howard, J.W.: A comparative study of the effects of 1-arterenol, epi- and iso-propylarterenol on the heart. J. Pharmacol. & Exp. Ther., *106*, 65, 1952.

87. Weissler A.M., Leonard, J.J., and Warren, J.V.: The hemodynamic effects of isoproterenol in man; with observations on the role of the central blood volume. J. Lab. & Clin. Med., *53*, 921, 1959.

88. Dodge, H.T., Lord, J.D., and Sandler, II: Cardiovascular effects of isoproterenol in normal subjects and subjects with congestive heart failure. Am. Heart J., *60*, 94, 1960.

89. Gorton, R., Gunnells, J.C., Weissler, A.M., and Stead, E.A.: Effects of atropine and isoproterenol on cardiac output, central venous pressure, and mean transit time of indicators placed at three different sites in the venous system. Circ. Res., *9*, 979, 1961.

90. Whalen, R.E., Cohen, A.I., Sumner, R.G., and McIntosh, H.D.: Hemodynamic effects of isoproterenol infusion in patients with normal and diseased mitral valves. Circulation, *27*, 512, 1963.

91. Williams, J.F., White, D.H., and Behnke, R.H.: Changes in pulmonary hemodynamics produced by isoproterenol infusion in emphysematous patients. Circulation, *28*, 396, 1963.

92. Lee, T.D., Roveti, G.C., and Ross, R.S.: The hemodynamic effects of isoproterenol on pulmonary hypertension in man. Am. Heart J., *65*, 361, 1963.

93. Cox, A.R., Cobb, L.A., and Bruce, R.A.: Differential hemodynamic effects of isoproterenol on mitral stenosis and left ventricular diseases. Am. Heart J., *65*, 802, 1963.

94. Schreiner, B.F., Murphy, G.W., James, D.H., and Yu, P.N.: Effects of isoproterenol on the pulmonary blood volume in patients with valvular heart disease and primary myocardial disease. Circulation, *37*, 220, 1968.

95. Hyman, A.L., Myers, W.D., and Meyer, D.: The effect of acute pulmonary embolus upon

cardiopulmonary hemodynamics. Am. Heart J., *67*, 313, 1964.

96. Rudolph, A.M., and Scarpelli, E.M.: Drug action on pulmonary circulation of unanesthetized dogs. Am. J. Physiol., *206*, 1201, 1964.

97. Brody, J.S, and Stemmler, E.J.: Differential reactivity in the pulmonary circulation. J. Clin. Invest., *47*, 80, 1968.

98. McGaff, C.J., Roveti, G.C., Glassman, E., and Milnor, W.R.: The pulmonary blood volume in rheumatic heart disease and its alteration by isoproterenol. Circulation, *27*, 77, 1963.

99. Harrison, D.C., Glick, G., Goldblatt, A., and Braunwald, E.: Studies on cardiac dimensions in intact, unanesthetized man. IV. Effects of isoproterenol and methoxamine. Circulation, *29*, 186, 1964.

100. Rodbard, S.: Bronchomotor tone. Am. J. Med., *15*, 356, 1953.

101. Egar, E.I., and Hamilton, W.K.: The effect of reserpine on the action of various vasopressors. Anesthesiology, *20*, 641, 1959.

102. Swaine, C.R., Perlmutter, J., and Sydney, E.: Mechanism of action of mephentermine. Fed. Proc., *19*, 122, 1960.

103. Fawaz, G.: The effect of mephentermine on isolated dog hearts, normal and pretreated with reserpine. Brit. J. Pharmacol., *16*, 309, 1961.

104. Brofman, B.L., Hellerstein, H.K., and Caskey, W.H.: Mephentermine — an effective pressor amine. Clinical and laboratory observations. Am. Heart. J., *44*, 396, 1952.

105. Welch, G.H., Braunwald, E., Case, R.B., and Sarnoff, S.J.: The effect of mephentermine sulfate on myocardial oxygen consumption, myocardial efficiency and peripheral vascular resistance. Am. J. Med., *24*, 871, 1958.

106. Barrera, F., Regalado, G.G., Changsut, R.L., and Dominguez, J.C.: Cardiovascular-respiratory actions of mephentermine in mitral stenosis and its effects on pulmonary function in chronic pulmonary emphysema. Circ. Res., *9*, 1185, 1961.

107. Li, T.H., Shimosato, S., and Etsten, B.: Hemodynamics of mephentermine in man. New Engl. J. Med., *267*, 180, 1962.

108. Li, T.H., Shimosato, S., Gamble, C.A., and Etsten, B.E.: Hemodynamics of mephentermine during spinal anesthesia in man. Anesthesiology, *24*, 817, 1963.

109. Brewster, W.R., Osgood, P.F., Isaacs, J.P., and Goldberg, L.I.: Hemodynamic effects of a pressor amine (methoxamine) with prominent vasoconstrictor activity. Circ. Res., *8*, 980, 1960.

110. West, J.W., Faulk, A.T., and Guzman, S.V.: Comparative study of effects of levarterenol and methoxamine in shock associated with acute myocardial ischemia in dogs. Circ. Res., *10*, 712, 1962.

111. Stanfield, C.A., and Yu, P.N.: Hemodynamic effects of methoxamine in mitral valve disease. Circ. Res., *8*, 859, 1960.

112. Oakley, C., Glick, G., Luria, M.N., Schreiner, B.F., and Yu, P.N.: Some regulatory mechanisms of the human pulmonary vascular bed. Circulation, *26*, 917, 1962.

113. Rose, J.C.: Studies on properties of pulmonary blood vessels. Bull. Georgetown Univ. Med. Ctr., *10*, 147, 1957.

114. Dresdale, D.T., Schultz, M., and Michtom, R.J.: Primary pulmonary hypertension. I. Clinical and hemodynamic study. Am. J. Med., *11*, 686, 1951.

115. Dresdale, D.T., Michtom, R.J., and Schultz, M.: Recent studies in primary pulmonary hypertension including pharmacodynamic observations on pulmonary vascular resistance. Bull. N.Y. Acad. Med., *30*, 195, 1954.

116. Mackinnon, J., Vickers, C.F.H., and Wade, E.G.: The effects of adrenergic-blocking agents on the pulmonary circulation in man. Brit. Heart J., *18*, 442, 1956.

117. Gardiner, J. M.: The effect of "priscol" in pulmonary hypertension. Australasian Ann. Med., *3*, 59, 1954.

118. Braun, K., Izak, G., and Rosenberg, S.Z.: Pulmonary arterial pressure after Priscoline in mitral stenosis. Brit. Heart J., *19*, 217, 1957.

119. Wood, P.: The Eisenmenger syndrome or pulmonary hypertension with reversed central shunt. Brit. Med. J., *2*, 755, 1958.

120. Grover, R.F., Reeves, J.T., and Blount, S.G.: Tolazoline hydrochloride (Priscoline): An effective pulmonary vasodilator. Am. Heart J., *61*, 5, 1961.

121. Rudolph, A.M., Paul, M.H., Sommer, L.S., and Nadas, A.S.: Effects of tolazoline hydrochloride (Priscoline) on circulatory dynamics of patients with pulmonary hypertension. Am. Heart J., *55*, 424, 1958.

122. Finlayson, J.K., Luria, M.N., and Yu, P.N.: Some circulatory effects of thoracotomy and intermittent positive pressure respiration in dogs. Circ. Res., *9*, 862, 1961.

123. Paley, H.W., Tsai, S.Y., Johnson, J.E., Kennoyer, W.C., May, L.G., and Gregory, R.: The effects of histamine and regitine on the pulmonary artery pressure in a case of pheochromocytoma. J. Lab. & Clin. Med., *44*, 905, 1954.

124. Storstein, O., Elgvin, T., Helle, I., and Sebelien, J.: The effect of phentolamine (Regitine) on the pulmonary circulation. Scand. J. Clin. & Lab. Invest., *9*, 150, 1957.

125. Taylor, S.H., Sutherland, G.R., MacKenzie, G.J., Staunton, H.P., and Donald, K.W.: The circulatory effects of intravenous phentolamine in man. Circulation, *31*, 741, 1965.

126. Powell, C.E., and Slater, I.H.: Blocking of inhibitory adrenergic receptors by a dichloroanalogue of isoproterenol. J. Pharmacol. & Exp. Ther., *122*, 480, 1958.

127. Black, J.W., and Stevenson, J.S.: Pharmacology of a new adrenergic beta-receptor-blocking compound (Nethalide). Lancet, *2*, 311, 1962.

128. Dornhorst, A.C., and Robinson, B.F.: Clinical pharmacology of a beta-adrenergic-blocking agent. Lancet, *2*, 314, 1962.

129. Harrison, D.C., Braunwald, E., Glick, G., Mason, D.T., Chidsey, C.A., and Ross, J.: Effects of beta adrenergic blockade on the circulation, with particular reference to observations in patients with hypertrophic subaortic stenosis. Circulation, *29*, 84, 1964.

130. Schröder, G., and Werkö, L.: Nethalide, a beta adrenergic blocking agent. Clin. Pharmacol. Ther., *5*, 159, 1964.

131. McKenna, D.H., Corliss, R.J., Sialer, S., Zarnstorff, W.C., Crumpton, C.W., and Rowe, G.G.: Effect of propranolol on systemic and coronary hemodynamics at rest and during simulated exercise. Circ. Res., *19*, 520, 1966.

132. Sowton, E., and Hamer, J.: Hemodynamic changes after beta adrenergic blockade. Am. J. Cardiol., *18*, 317, 1966.

133. Braunwald, E., Sonnenblick, E.H., Ross, J., Glick, G., and Epstein, S.E.: An analysis of the cardiac response to exercise. Circ. Res., *20*, Suppl. *1*, 44, 1967.

134. Epstein, S.E. Robinson, B.F., Kahler, R.L., and Braunwald, E.: Effects of beta-adrenergic blockade on the cardiac response to maximal and submaximal exercise in man. J. Clin. Invest., *44*, 1745, 1965.

135. Cumming, G.R., and Carr, W.: Hemodynamic response to exercise after beta-adrenergic blockade with propranolol in patients with mitral valve obstruction. Canad. Med. Ass. J., *95*, 527, 1966.

136. Vogel, J.H.K., and Blount, S.G.: Role of beta adrenergic receptors in the regulation of the pulmonary circulation. Circulation, *32*, Suppl. 2, 212, 1965.

137. Lish, P.M., Weikel, J.H., and Dungan, K.W.: Pharmacological and toxicological properties of two new beta-adrenergic receptor antagonists. J. Pharmacol. & Exp. Ther., *149*, 161, 1965.

138. Stanton, H.C., Kirchgessner, T., and Parmenter, K.: Cardiovascular pharmacology of two new beta-adrenergic receptor antagonists. J. Pharmacol. & Exp. Ther., *149*, 174, 1965.

139. Levy, J.V., and Richards, V.: Inotropic and metabolic effects of three beta-adrenergic receptor blocking drugs on isolated rabbit left atria. J. Pharmacol. & Exp. Ther., *150*, 361, 1965.

140. Taylor, S.H., and Donald, K.W.: The circulatory effects of bretylium tosylate and guanethidine. Lancet, *2*, 389, 1960

141. Halmágyi, D.F.J., and Colebatch, H.J.H.: Effect of bretylium tosylate (Darenthin) on pulmonary circulation. Circ. Res., *9*, 136, 1961.

142. McGaff, C.J., and Leight, L.: Pulmonary hypertensive effects of bretylium tosylate in the dog. Am. Heart J., *65*, 240, 1963.

143. Conway, J.: Clinical pharmacology of bretylium tosylate: Preliminary observations. Ann. N.Y. Acad. Sci., *88*, 956, 1960.

144. Doyle, A.E., Fraser, J.R.E., and Smith, P.K.: Effects of bretylium tosylate on blood pressure, cardiac output and renal function in hypertension. Brit. Med. J., *2*, 422, 1960.

145. Aviado, D.M., and Dil, A.H.: The effects of a new sympathetic blocking drug (bretylium) on cardiovascular control. J. Pharmacol. & Exp. Ther., *129*, 328, 1960.

146. Richardson, D.W., Wyso, E.M., Magee, J.H., and Cavell, G.C.: Circulatory effects of guanethidine. Clinical, renal and cardiac responses to treatment with a novel antihypertensive drug. Circulation, *22*, 184, 1960.

147. Rokseth, R., Storstein, O., Voll, A., Abrahamsen, A.M., and Ofstad, J.: Circulatory and respiratory effects of guanethidine. Brit. Heart J., *24*, 195, 1962.

148. Chamberlain, D.A., and Howard, J.: Guanethidine and methyldopa: A hemodynamic study. Brit. Heart J., *26*, 528, 1964.

149. Harris, P., Bishop, J.M., and Segel, N.: The influence of guanethidine on hypoxic pulmonary hypertension in normal man. Clin. Sci., *21*, 295, 1961.

150. Taylor, S.H., Sutherland, G.R., Hutchison, D.C.S., Kidd, B.S.L., Robertson, P.C., Kennelly, B.M., and Donald, K.W.: The effects of intravenous guanethidine on the systemic and pulmonary circulations in man. Am. Heart J., *63*, 239, 1962.

151. Halmágyi, D., Felkai, B., Czipott, Z., and Kovacs, G.: The effect of Serpasil in pulmonary hypertension. Brit. Heart J., *19*, 375, 1957.

152. Angelino, P.F., Garbabni, R., and Tartara, D.: Hypotensive effect of reserpine on pulmo-

nary hypertension in mitral patients. Proc. 3rd European Congr. Cardiol., *2*, 441, 1960.

153. Reusch, C.S.: The cardiorenal hemodynamic effects of antihypertensive therapy with reserpine. Am. Heart J., *64*, 643, 1962.

154. Widimský, J., Kasalicky, J., Dejdar, R., Vysloužil, Z., and Lukeš, M.: Effect of reserpine on the lesser circulation in chronic pulmonary diseases. Brit. Heart J., *24*, 274, 1962.

155. Gaffney, T.E., Bryant, W.M., and Braunwald, E.: Effects of reserpine and guanethidine on venous reflexes. Circ. Res., *11*, 889, 1962.

156. Mahon, W.A., and Mashford, M.L.: The pressor effect of tyramine in man and its modification by reserpine pretreatment. J. Clin. Invest., *42*, 338, 1963.

157. Faraco, E.Z., Nedel, N., Azevedo, D.F., and Freitas, F.M., de.: The acute effect of reserpine on the pulmonary circulation. Acta Cardiol. (Brux), *18*, 105, 1963.

158. Brutsaert, D.: Influence of reserpine and of adrenolytic agents on the pulmonary arterial pressure response to hypoxia. Arch. int. Pharmacodyn., *147*, 587, 1964.

159. Gaddum, J.H., and Holtz, P.: The localization of the action of drugs on the pulmonary vessels of dogs and cats. J. Physiol., *77*, 139, 1933.

160. Alcock, P., Berry, J.L., and Daly, I., de B.: The action of drugs on the pulmonary circulation. Quart. J. Exp. Physiol., *25*, 369, 1935.

161. Harris, P.: A study of the effects of disease on the pressures in the pulmonary artery and right ventricle in man. Thesis, University of London, 1955.

162. Harris, P., Fritts, H.W., Clauss, R.H., Odell, J.E., and Cournand, A.: Influence of acetylcholine on human pulmonary circulation under normal and hypoxic conditions. Proc. Soc. Exp. Biol. & Med., *93*, 77, 1956.

163. Harris, P.: Influence of acetylcholine on the pulmonary arterial pressure. Brit. Heart J., *19*, 272, 1957.

164. Cournand, A., Fritts, H.W., Harris, P., and Himmelstein, A.: Preliminary observations on the effects in man of continuous perfusion with acetylcholine of one branch of the pulmonary artery upon the homolateral pulmonary blood flow. Trans. Ass. Am. Phys., *69*, 163, 1956.

165. Fritts, H.W., Harris, P., Clauss, R.H., Odell, J.E., and Cournand, A.: The effect of acetylcholine on the human circulation under normal and hypoxic conditions. J. Clin. Invest., *37*, 99, 1958.

166. Wood, P., Besterman, E.M., Towers, M.K., and McIlroy, M.B.: The effect of acetylcholine on pulmonary vascular resistance and left atrial pressure in mitral stenosis. Brit. Heart J., *19*, 279, 1957.

167. Shepherd, J.T., Semler, H.J., Helmholz, H.F., and Wood, E.H.: Effects of infusion of acetylcholine on pulmonary vascular resistance in patients with pulmonary hypertension and congenital heart disease. Circulation, *20*, 381, 1959.

168. Marshall, R.J., Helmholz, H.F., and Shepherd, J.T.: Effect of acetylcholine on pulmonary vascular resistance in a patient with idiopathic pulmonary hypertension. Circulation, *20*, 391, 1959.

169. Söderholm, B., and Werkö, L.: Acetylcholine and the pulmonary circulation in mitral valvular disease. Brit. Heart J., *21*, 1, 1959.

170. Crittenden, I.H., Adams, F.H., and Latta, H.: Preoperative evaluation of the pulmonary vascular bed in patients with pulmonary hypertension associated with left to right shunts. I. Effects of acetylcholine: Preliminary report. Pediatrics, *24*, 448, 1959.

171. Chidsey, C.A., Fritts, H.W., Zocche, G.P., Himmelstein, A., and Cournand, A.: Effect of acetylcholine on the distribution of pulmonary blood flow in chronic pulmonary emphysema. Mal. Cardiovas., *1*, 15, 1960.

172. Samet, P., Bernstein, W.H., and Widrich, J.: Intracardiac infusion of acetylcholine in primary pulmonary hypertension. Am. Heart J., *60*, 433, 1960.

173. Stanfield, C.A., Finlayson, J.K., Luria, M.N., Constantine, H., Flatley, F.J., and Yu, P.N.: Effects of acetylcholine on hemodynamics and blood oxygen saturation in mitral stenosis. Circulation, *24*, 1164, 1961.

174. Charms, B.L.: Primary pulmonary hypertension. Effect of unilateral pulmonary artery occlusion and infusion of acetylcholine. Am. J. Cardiol., *8*, 94, 1961.

175. Charms, B.L., Givertz, B., and Toshihiko, I.: Effect of acetylcholine on the pulmonary circulation in patients with chronic pulmonary disease. Circulation, *25*, 814, 1962.

176. Bateman, M., Davidson, L.A.G., Donald, K.W., and Harris, P.: A comparison of the effect of acetylcholine and 100% oxygen on the pulmonary circulation of patients with mitral stenosis. Clin. Sci., *22*, 223, 1962.

177. Söderholm, B., Werkö, L., and Widimský, J.: The effect of acetylcholine and gas exchange in cases of mitral stenosis. Acta Med. Scand., *172*, 95, 1962.

178. Bernstein, W.H., Samet., P., and Littwak, R.S.: The effect of intracardiac acetylcholine infusion upon right heart dynamics in patients with rheumatic heart disease studied during exercise. Am. Heart J., *63*, 86, 1962.

179. Schlant, R.C., Tsagaris, T.J., Robertson, R.J., Winter, T.S., and Edwards, F.K.: The effect of acetylcholine upon arterial saturation. Am. Heart J., *64*, 512, 1962.

180. Behnke, R.H., Williams, J.F., and White, D.H.: The effect of acetylcholine infusion upon cardiac dynamics in patients with pulmonary emphysema. Am. Rev. Resp. Dis., *87*, 57, 1963.

181. Irnell, L., and Nordgren, L.: Effects of acetylcholine infusion on the pulmonary circulation in patients with bronchial asthma. Acta Med. Scand., *179*, 385, 1966.

182. Acheson, G.H., and Moe, G.K.: The action of tetraethyl-ammonium on the mammalian circulation. J. Pharmacol. & Exp. Ther., *87*, 220, 1946.

183. Fowler, N.O., Westcott, R.N., Hauenstein, V.D., Scott, R.C., and McQuire, J.: Observation on autonomic participation in pulmonary arteriolar resistance in man. J. Clin. Invest., *29*, 1387, 1950.

184. Gilmore, H.R., Kopelman, H., McMichael, J., and Milne, I.G.: The effect of hexamethonium bromide on the cardiac output and pulmonary circulation. Lancet, *2*, 898, 1952.

185. Halmágyi, D., Felkai, B., Ivanyi, J., Zsoter, T., Tenyi, M., and Szücs, Z.: The role of the nervous system in the maintenance of pulmonary arterial hypertension in heart failure. Brit. Heart J., *15*, 15, 1953.

186. Rakita, L., and Sancetta, L.M.: Acute hemodynamic effects of hexamethonium in normotensive man. Circ. Res., *1*, 499, 1953.

187. Wilson, V.H., and Keeley, K.J.: The hemodynamic effects of hexamethonium bromide in patients with pulmonary hypertension and heart failure. S. Afr. J. Med. Sci., *18*, 125, 1953.

188. Freis, E.D., Rose, J.C., Partenope, E.A., Higgins, T.F., Kelley, R.T., Schnaper, H.W., and Johnson, R.L.: The hemodynamic effects of hypotensive drugs in man. III. Hexamethonium. J. Clin. Invest., *32*, 1285, 1953.

189. Davies, L.G., Goodwin, J.F., and Van Leuven, B.D.: The nature of pulmonary hypertension in mitral stenosis. Brit. Heart J., *16*, 440, 1954.

190. Storstein, O., and Tveten, H.: The effect of hexamethonium bromide on the pulmonary circulation. Scand. J. Clin. & Lab. Invest., *6*, 169, 1954.

191. Judson, W.E., Hollander, W., and Arrowwood, J.G.: Studies on the pulmonary circulation: Effects of anoxia, exercise and hexamethonium in patients with and without thoracic sympathetic denervation. J. Clin. Invest., *33*, 946, 1954.

192. Burch, R.R.: The effects of intravenous hexamethonium on venous pressure of normotensive and hypertensive patients with and without congestive heart failure. Circulation, *11*, 271, 1955.

193. Sancetta, S.M.: Acute hemodynamic effects of hexamethonium (C6) in patients with emphysematous pulmonary hypertension. Am. Heart J., *49*, 501, 1955.

194. Wade, E.G., MacKinnon, J., and Vickers, C.F.H.: The nature of the increased pulmonary vascular resistance in mitral stenosis. Brit. Heart J., *18*, 458, 1956.

195. Balchum, O.J., Gensini, G., and Blount, S.G.: The effect of hexamethonium upon the pulmonary vascular resistance in mitral stenosis. J. Lab. & Clin. Med., *50*, 186, 1957.

196. Sancetta, S.M.: Acute hemodynamic effects of total head-down body tilt and hexamethonium in normal and pulmonary emphysematous subjects. J. Lab. & Clin. Med., *49*, 684, 1957.

197. Goodwin, J.F., Hollman, A., and O'Donnell, T.V.: Ganglion-blocking agents in mitral valve disease. Lancet, *2*, 1251, 1958.

198. Yu, P.N., Nye, R.E., Lovejoy, F.W., Schreiner, B.F., and Yim, B.J.B.: Studies of pulmonary hypertension. IX. The effects of intravenous hexamethonium on pulmonary circulation in patients with mitral stenosis. J. Clin. Invest., *37*, 194, 1958.

199. Aviado, D.M.: Hemodynamic effects of ganglion blocking drugs. Circ. Res., *8*, 304, 1960.

200. Finlayson, J.K., Luria, M.N., Stanfield, C.A., and Yu, P.N.: Hemodynamic studies in acute pulmonary edema. Ann. Int. Med., *54*, 244, 1961.

201. Ellstad, M.H., and Olson, W.H.: Use of intravenously given ganglionic blocking agents for acute pulmonary edema. Preliminary report. J.A.M.A., *161*, 49, 1956.

202. Perry, A.W.: Hexamethonium in the treatment of acute pulmonary edema. Canad. Med. Ass. J., *85*, 202, 1961.

203. McGaff, C.J., and Leight, L.: Effects of acute ganglionic blockade on the pulmonary circulation of the dog. Am. J. Med. Sci., *246*, 319, 1963.

204. Sarnoff, S.J., Goodale, W.T., and Sarnoff, L.C.: Graded reduction of arterial pressure

in man by means of a Thiophanium derivative (Ro 2-2222). Preliminary observations on its effect in acute pulmonary edema. Circulation, *6*, 63, 1952.

205. Lepine, C.: Etude de la petite circulation dans l'hypertension arterielle pulmonaire. II. Effect d'un ganglioplégique (Arfonad) sur les pressions, les résistances vasculaires et le débit sanguin. Un Med. Canada, *87*, 528, 1958.

206. Sobol, B.J., Kessler, R.H., Rader, B., and Eichna, L.W.: Cardiac, hemodynamic and renal functions in congestive heart failure during induced peripheral vasodilatation; relationship to Starling's law of the heart in man. J. Clin. Invest., *38*, 557, 1959.

207. Nalefski, L.A., and Brown, C.F.G.: Action of atropine on the cardiovascular system in normal persons. Arch. Int. Med., *86*, 898, 1950.

208. Hamilton, W.F.: The physiology of pulmonary circulation. J. Allergy, *22*, 397, 1951.

209. Gorlin, R., McMillan, I.K.R., Medd, W.E., Matthews, M.B., and Daley, R.: Dynamics of the circulation in aortic valvular disease. Am. J. Med., *18*, 855, 1955.

210. Weissler, A.M., Leonard, J.J., and Warren, J.V.: Effects of posture and atropine on the cardiac output. J. Clin. Invest., *36*, 1656, 1957.

211. Gorlin, R.: Studies on the regulation of the coronary circulation in man. I. Atropine-induced changes in cardiac rate. Am. J. Med., *25*, 37, 1958.

212. Berry, J.N., Thompson, H.K., Miller, D.E., and McIntosh, H.D.: Changes in cardiac output, stroke volume, and central venous pressure induced by atropine in man. Am. Heart J., *58*, 204, 1959.

213. Kahler, R.L., Gaffney, T.E., and Braunwald, E.: The effects of autonomic nervous system inhibition on the circulatory response to muscular exercise. J. Clin. Invest., *41*, 1981, 1962.

214. Condorelli, L.: Physiopathologie de la circulation artérielle pulmonaire. Schweiz med. Wcshr, *80*, 986, 1950.

215. Wade, E.G., MacKinnon, J., and Vickers, C.F.G.: The nature of the increased pulmonary vascular resistance in mitral stenosis. Brit. Heart J., *19*, 458, 1956.

216. Williams, M.H., Zohman, L.R., and Bertrand, C.A.: Effect of atropine on the pulmonary circulation during rest and exercise in patients with chronic airway obstruction. Dis. Chest, *37*, 597, 1960.

217. Greene, M.A., Boltax, A.J. and Ulberg, R.J.: Cardiovascular dynamics of vasovagal reaction in man. Circ. Res., *9*, 12, 1961.

218. Daly, W.J., Ross, J.C., and Behnke, R.H.: The effect of changes in the pulmonary vascular bed produced by atropine, pulmonary engorgement, and positive pressure breathing on diffusing and mechanical properties of the lung. J. Clin. Invest., *42*, 1083, 1963.

219. Howarth, S., McMichael, J., and Sharpey-Schafer, E.P.: Circulatory action of theophylline ethylene diamine. Clin. Sci., *6*, 125, 1947.

220. James, D.F., Turner, H., and Merrill, A.J.: Circulatory and renal effects of aminophylline in congestive heart failure. Am. J. Med., *5*, 619, 1948.

221. Werkö, L., and Lagerlöf, H.: Studies on the circulation of blood in man. VII. The effect of a single intravenous dose of theophylline diethanolamine on cardiac output, pulmonary blood volume and systemic and pulmonary blood pressures in hypertensive cardiovascular disease. Scand. J. Clin. & Lab. Invest., *2*, 181, 1950.

222. Mendelsohn, H.J., Zimmerman, H.A., and Adelman, A.: A study of pulmonary hemodynamics during pulmonary resection. J. Thorac. Surg., *20*, 366, 1950.

223. Zimmerman, H.A.: A study of the pulmonary circulation in man. Dis. Chest, *20*, 46, 1951.

224. Schuman, C., and Simmons, H.G.: Cardiac asthma: Its pathogenesis and response to aminophylline. Ann. Int. Med., *36*, 864, 1952.

225. Dulfano, M.J., Yahni, J., Toor, M., Rosen, N., and Langer, L.: The prognostic value of aminophylline in the selection of patients for mitral valvotomy. J. Lab. & Clin. Med., *48*, 329, 1956.

226. Sweet, H.C., Peden, B.W., Kistner, W.F., and Mudd, J.G.: The effect of aminophylline on the emphysematous patient. Missouri Med., *55*, 1079, 1958.

227. Storstein, O., Helle, I., and Rokseth, R.: The effect of theophylline ethylene-diamine on the pulmonary circulation. Am. Heart J., *55*, 781, 1958.

228. Maxwell, G.M., Crumpton, C.W., Rowe, G.G., White, D.H., and Castillo, C.A.: The effects of theophylline ethylene-diamine (aminophylline) on the coronary hemodynamics of normal and diseased hearts. J. Lab. & Clin. Med., *54*, 88, 1959.

229. Parker, J.O., Kekar, K., and West, R.O.: Hemodynamic effects of aminophylline in cor pulmonale. Circulation, *33*, 17, 1966.

230. Parker, J.O., Kelly, G., and West, R.O.: Hemodynamic effects of aminophylline in heart failure. Am. J. Cardiol., *17*, 232, 1966.

231. Murphy, G.W., Schreiner, B.F., and Yu, P.N.: Effects of aminophylline on the pulmonary circulation and left ventricular performance in patients with valvular heart disease. Circulation, *37*, 361, 1968.

232. Hochrein, M.: O klinickim problemima plucnog krvotoka. Lijeen Vjesn, *62*, 471, 1940.

233. Eldridge, F.L., Hultgren, H.N., Stewart, P., and Proctor, D.: The effect of nitroglycerin upon the cardiovascular system. Stanford Med. Bull., *13*, 273, 1955.

234. Johnson, J.B., Cross, J.F., and Hale, E.: Effects of sublingual administration of nitroglycerin on pulmonary-artery pressure in patients with failure of the left ventricle. New Engl. J. Med., *257*, 1114, 1957.

235. Johnson, J.B., Fairley, A., and Carter, C.: Effects of sublingual nitroglycerin on pulmonary arterial pressure in patients with left ventricular failure. Ann. Int. Med., *50*, 34, 1959.

236. Brachfeld, N., Bozer, J., and Gorlin, R.: Action of nitroglycerin on the coronary circulation in normal and in mild cardiac subjects. Circulation, *19*, 697, 1959.

237. Gorlin, R., Brachfeld, N., MacLeod, C., and Bopp, P.: Effect of nitroglycerin on the coronary circulation in patients with coronary artery disease or increased left ventricular work. Circulation, *19*, 705, 1959.

238. Wégria, R., Nickerson, J.L., Case, R.B., and Holland, J.F.: Effect of nitroglycerin on the cardiovascular system of normal persons. Am. J. Med., *10*, 414, 1951.

239. Müller, O., and Rorvik, K.: Hemodynamic consequences of coronary heart disease. With observations during anginal pain and on the effect of nitroglycerin. Brit. Heart J., *20*, 302, 1958.

240. Rowe, G.G., Chelins, C.J., Afonso, S., Gurtner, H.P., and Crumpton, C.W.: Systemic and coronary hemodynamic effects of erythrol tetranitrate. J. Clin. Invest., *40*, 1217, 1961.

241. Christensson, R., Karlefors, T., and Westling, H.: Hemodynamic effects of nitroglycerin in patients with coronary artery disease. Brit. Heart J., *27*, 511, 1965.

242. Parker, J.O., Giorgi, S., Di, and West, R.O.: Hemodynamic study of acute coronary insufficiency precipitated by exercise with observations on the effects of nitroglycerin. Am. J. Cardiol., *17*, 470, 1966.

243. Leon, A.C., de, and Perloff, J.K.: The pulmonary hemodynamic effects of amyl nitrite in normal man. Am. Heart J., *72*, 337, 1966.

244. Najmi, M., Griggs, D., Kasparian, H., and Novack, P.: Effects of nitroglycerin on hemodynamics during rest and exercise in patients with coronary insufficiency. Circulation, *35*, 46, 1967.

245. Frick, M.H., Balcon, R., Cross, D., and Sowton, E.: Hemodynamic effects of nitroglycerin in patients with angina pectoris, studied by an atrial pacing method. Circulation, *37*, 160, 1968.

246. Taquini, A.C., and Taquini, A.C.: The renin-angiotensin system in hypertension. Am. Heart J., *62*, 558, 1961.

247. Page, I.H., and Bumpus, F.M.: A new hormone, angiotensin. Clin. Pharmacol. Ther., *3*, 758, 1962.

248. Lichlen, P.V., Bühlmann, A., and Schaub, F.: Untersuchungen uber die blutdrucksteigernde Wirkung von synthetischem Hypertensin. II. am normotenen Menschen. Cardiologia, *35*, 139, 1959.

249. Sancetta, S.M.: General and pulmonary hemodynamic effects of pure decapeptide angiotensin in normotensive man. Circ. Res., *8*, 616, 1960.

250. Segel, N., Harris, P., and Bishop, J.M.: The effects of synthetic hypertension on the systemic and pulmonary circulations in man. Clin. Sci., *20*, 49, 1960.

251. Yu, P.N., Luria, M.N., Finlayson, J.K., Stanfield, C.A., Constantine, H., and Flatley, F.J.: The effects of angiotensin on pulmonary circulation and ventricular function. Circulation, *24*, 1326, 1961.

252. Johnson, W.P., and Bruce, R.A.: Hemodynamic and metabolic effects of angiotensin. II. During rest and exercise in normal healthy subjects. Am. Heart J., *63*, 212, 1962.

253. Koch-Weser, J.: Nature of the inotropic action of angiotensin on ventricular myocardium. Circ. Res., *16*, 230, 1965.

254. Dixon, W.E., and Premankur, De: The action of certain quinine derivatives with special reference to local anesthesia and pulmonary edema. J. Pharmacol. & Exp. Ther., *31*, 407, 1927.

255. Alcock, P., Berry, J.L., Daly, I., de B., and Narayana, B.: The action on perfused lungs of drugs injected into the bronchial vascular system. Quart. J. Exp. Physiol., *26*, 13, 1935.

256. Daly, I., de B., Foggie, P., and Hebb, C.O.: An experimental analysis of the action of adrenaline and histamine on different parts of the pulmonary vascular bed. Quart. J. Exp. Physiol., *30*, 21, 1940.

257. Abe, K.: Effects of the restriction of the pulmonary artery on the blood pressure and

on the volume of some organs, and the cause of the arterial blood pressure, due to the so-called "paradoxical vasodilatory substances." Tohoku J. Exp. Med., *1*, 398, 1920.

258. Woodbury, R.A., and Hamilton, W.F.: The effect of histamine on the pulmonary blood pressure of various animals with and without anesthesia. J. Pharmacol. & Exp. Ther., *71*, 293, 1941.

259. Ellis, C.H., Van Harreveld, A., and Wolfgram, F.J.: A study of the hemodynamic actions of histamine and 1, 10-diaminodecane in cats. Arch. Int. Pharmacodyn., *97*, 287, 1954.

260. Delaunois A.L,, Kordecki, R., Polet, H., and Ryzeuski, J.: Cardiac output, arterial blood pressure and pulmonary arterial pressure in histamime shock. Arch. Int. Pharmacodyn., *120*, 114, 1959.

261. Storstein, O., Cudkowicz, L., and Attwood, H.D.: Effect of histamine on the pulmonary circulation in dogs. Circ. Res., *7*, 360, 1959.

262. Chien, S., and Krakoff, L.: Hemodynamics of dogs in histamine shock, with special reference to splanchnic blood volume and flow. Circ. Res., *12*, 29, 1963.

263. Weiss, S., Robb, G.P., and Ellis, L.B.: The systemic effects of histamine in man with special reference to the responses of the cardiovascular system. Arch. Int. Med., *49*, 360, 1932.

264. Memir, P., Stone, H.H., Mackrell, T.N., and Hawthorne, H.R.: Studies on pulmonary embolism utilizing the method of controlled unilateral pulmonary artery occlusion. Surg. Forum, *5*, 210, 1954.

265. Spitzbarth, H., Gersmeyer, E.F., Weyland, H., and Gasteyer, K.H.: Der Pulmonalarterendruck des Menschen bei Kreislaufveränderungen im Phenothiazin-schlaf. Klin Wschr., *35*, 87, 1957.

266. Lambertini, A., Lanari, A., and Lanari Zubiaur, F.: La presión arterial pulmonar en ataque de asma espontineos e inducidos por histamina. Medicina (B. Aires), *20*, 93, 1960.

267. Lindell, S.E., Svanborg, A., Söderholm, B., and Westling, H.: Hemodynamic changes in chronic constrictive pericarditis during exercise and histamine infusion. Brit. Heart J., *25*, 35, 1963.

268. Westling, H.: Effects of histamine on the pulmonary circulation in man. Proc. First Internat'l. Pharmacol. Meet., Pergamon Press, *9*, 117, 1963.

269. Lindell, S.E., Söderholm, B., and Westling, H.: Hemodynamic effects of histamine in mitral stenosis. Brit. Heart J., *26*, 180, 1964.

270. Storstein, O., Calabresi, M., Nims, R.G., and Gray, F.D.: The effect of histamine on the pulmonary circulation in man. Yale J. Biol. Med., *32*, 197, 1959.

271. Gaddum, J.H., Hebb, C.O., Silver, A., and Swan, A.A.B.: 5-Hydroxytryptamine. Pharmacological action and destruction in perfused lungs. Quart J. Exp. Physiol., *38*, 255, 1953.

272. Bhattacharya, B.K.: A pharmacological study on the effect of 5-hydroxytryptamine and its antagonists on the bronchial musculature. Arch. Int. Pharmacodyn., *103*, 357, 1955.

273. Rose, J.C., and Lazaro, E.J.: Pulmonary vascular responses to serotonin and effects of certain serotonin antagonists. Circ. Res., *6*, 283, 1958.

274. Rudolph, A.M., and Auld, P.A.M.: Physical factors affecting normal and serotonin-constricted pulmonary vessels. Am. J. Physiol., *198*, 864, 1960.

275. Halmágyi, D.F.J., and Colebatch, H.J.H.: Serotonin-like cardiorespiratory effects of a serotonin antagonist. J. Pharmacol. & Exp. Ther., *134*, 47, 1961.

276. Comroe, J.H., Van Linden, B., Stroud, R.C., and Roncoroni, A.: Reflex and direct cardiopulmonary effects of 5-OH-tryptamine (serotonin). Their possible role in pulmonary embolism and coronary thrombosis. Am. J. Physiol., *173*, 379, 1953.

277. MacCanon, D.M., and Horvath, S.M.: Some effects of serotonin in pentobarbital anesthetized dogs. Am. J. Physiol., *179*, 131, 1954.

278. Rudolph, A.M., and Paul, M.H.: Pulmonary and systemic vascular response to continuous infusion of 5-hydroxytryptamine (serotonin) in the dog. Am. J. Physiol., *189*, 263, 1957.

279. Rudolph, A.M., Kurland, M.D., Auld, P.A.M., and Paul, M.H.: Effects of vasodilator drugs on normal and serotonin-constricted pulmonary vessels of the dog. Am. J. Physiol., *197*, 617, 1959.

280. Maxwell, G.M., Castillo, C.A., Clifford, J.E., Crumpton, C.W., and Rowe, G.G.: Effect of serotonin (5-hydroxytryptamine) on the systemic and coronary vascular bed of the dog. Am. J. Physiol., *197*, 736, 1959.

281. Kabins, S.A., Molina, C., and Katz, L.N.: Pulmonary vascular effects of serotonin (5-OH-tryptamine) in dogs: Its role in causing pulmonary edema. Am. J. Physiol., *197*, 955, 1959.

282. Shepherd, J.T, Donald, D.E., Linder, E., and Swan, H.J.C.: Effect of small doses of 5-hydroxytryptamine (serotonin) on pulmonary circulation in the closed-chest dog. Am. J. Physiol., *197*, 963, 1959.

283. Crumpton, C.W., Castillo, C.A., Rowe, G.G., and Maxwell, G.M.: Serotonin and the dynamics of the heart. Ann. N.Y. Acad. Sci., *80*, 960, 1959.

284. Aviado, D.M.: Pulmonary venular responses to anoxia, 5-hydroxytryptamine and histamine. Am. J. Physiol., *198*, 1032, 1960.

285. Rudolph, A.M.: Pulmonary venomotor activity. Med. Thorac., *19*, 376, 1962.

286. Duteil, J.J., and Aviado, D.M.: Factors influencing pulmonary hypertensive response to 5-hydroxytryptamine. Circ. Res., *11*, 466, 1962.

287. McGaff, C.J., and Milnor, W.R.: Effects of serotonin on pulmonary blood volume in the dog. Am. J. Physiol., *202*, 957, 1962.

288. Rudolph, A.M., and Scarpelli, E.M.: Drug action on pulmonary circulation of anesthetized dogs. Am. J. Physiol., *206*, 1201, 1964.

289. Nemir, P., Stone, H.H., Mackrell, T.N., and Hawthorne, H.R.: Studies on pulmonary embolism utilizing the method of controlled unilateral pulmonary artery occlusion. Surg. Forum, *5*, 210, 1954.

290. Stone, H.H., and Nemir, P.: Study of the role of 5-hydroxytryptamine (serotonin) and histamine in the pathogenesis of pulmonary embolism in man. Ann. Surg., *152*, 890, 1960.

291. Harris, P., Fritts, H.W., and Cournand, A.: Some circulatory effects of 5-hydroxytryptamine in man. Circulation, *21*, 1134, 1960.

292. Rocha e Silva, M., Beraldo, W.T., and Rosenfeld, G.: Bradykinin, a hypotensive and smooth muscle stimulating factor released from plasma globulin by snake venoms and by trypsin. Am. J. Physiol., *156*, 261, 1949.

293. Elliott, D.F., Lewis, G.P., and Horton, E.W.: Isolation of bradykinin. Plasma kinin from ox blood. Biochem. J., *74*, 15, 1960.

294. Maxwell, G.M., Elliott, R.B., and Kneebone, G.M.: Effects of bradykinin on the systemic and coronary vascular bed of the intact dog. Circ. Res., *10*, 359, 1962.

295. Rowe, G.G., Afonso, S., Castillo, C.A., Lioy, F., Lugo, J.E.,, and Crumpton, C.W.: The systemic and coronary hemodynamic effects of synthetic bradykinin. Am. Heart J., *65*, 656, 1963.

296. Kontos, H.A., Magee, J.H., Shapiro, W., and Patterson, J.L.: General and regional circulatory effects of synthetic bradykinin in man. Circ. Res., *14*, 351, 1964.

297. Bishop, J.M., Harris, P., and Segal, N.: The effect of synthetic bradykinin on the pulmonary and systemic circulation in man. J. Physiol., *165*, 37P, 1963.

298. Carlier, J.: Effets hémodynamiques de la bradykinine synthétique chez le chien. Arch. Int. Physiol., *71*, 253, 1963.

299. Freitas, F.M., de, Faraco, F.Z., and Azevedo, D.F., de: General circulatory alterations induced by intravenous infusion of synthetic bradykinin in man. Circulation, *29*, 66, 1964.

300. Freitas, F.M., de, Faraco, E.Z., Azevedo, D.F., de, and Lewin, I.: Action of bradykinin on human pulmonary circulation. Circulation, *34*, 385, 1966.

301. Boniface, K.J., Brown, J.M., and Kronen, P.S.: The influence of some inhalation anesthetic agents on the contractile force of the heart. J. Pharmacol. & Exp. Ther., *113*, 64, 1955.

302. Fletcher, G., Pender, J.W., and Wood, E.H.: Hemodynamic effects of ether anesthesia and surgery in 11 cases. Current Res. in Anesth. & Analg., *35*, 18, 1956.

303. Greisheimer, E.M.: The circulatory effects of anesthetics. *In* W.F. Hamilton and P. Dow (eds), *Handbook of Physiology*, Section 2, Vol. 3, p. 2477, Washington, D.C., American Physiological Society, 1965.

304. McAllister, F.F., and Root, W.S.: The circulatory responses of normal and sympathectomized dogs to ether anesthesia. Am. J. Physiol., *133*, 70, 1941.

305. Brewster, W.R., Isaacs, J.P., and Wain-Andersén, T.: Depressant effect of ether on myocardium of the dog and its modification by reflex release of epinephrine and norepinephrine. Am. J. Physiol., *175*, 399, 1953.

306. Watts, D.T.: Epinephrine in the circulating blood during ether anesthesia. J. Pharmacol. & Exp. Ther., *114*, 203, 1955.

307. Richardson, J.A., Woods, E.F., and Richardson, A.K.: Plasma concentrations of epinephrine and norepinephrine during anesthesia. J. Pharmacol. & Exp. Ther., *119*, 378, 1957.

308. Price, H.L., Linde, H.W., Jones, R.E., Black, G.W., and Price, M.L.: Sympatho-adrenal responses to general anesthesia in man and their relation to hemodynamics. Anesthesiology, *20*, 563, 1959.

309. Johnson, S.R.: The effects of some anesthetic agents on the circulation in man, with special reference to the significance of pulmonary blood volume for the circulatory regulation. Acta chir. Scand., *102*, Suppl. 158, 1951.

310. Sjörstrand, T.: Determination of changes in the intrathoracic blood volume in man. Acta Physiol. Scand., *22*, 114, 1951.

311. Etsten, B., Reynolds, R.N., and Li, T.H.: The effects of controlled respiration on circulation during cyclopropane anesthesia. Anesthesiology, *16*, 365, 1955.

312. Li, T.H., and Etsten, B.: Effect of cyclopropane anesthesia on cardiac output and related hemodynamics in man. Anesthesiology, *18*, 15, 1957.

313. Thompson, M.C., Patrick, R.T., and Wood, E.H.: Effects of cyclopropane anesthesia on the circulation of human beings. J.A.M.A., *164*, 389, 1957.

314. Jones, R.E., Guldmann, N., Linde, H.W., Dripps, R.D., and Price, H.L.: Cyclopropane anesthesia. III. Effects of cyclopropane on respiration and circulation in normal man. Anesthesiology, *21*, 380, 1960.

315. Mahaffey, J.E., Aldinger, E.E., Sprouse, J.H., Darby, T.D., and Throner, W.B.: The cardiovascular effects of halothane. Anesthesiology, *22*, 982, 1961.

316. Shimosato, S., Li, T.H., and Etsten, B.: Ventricular function during halothane anesthesia in closed chest dog. Circ. Res., *12*, 63, 1963.

317. Payne, J., P., Gardiner, D., and Verner, I.R.: Cardiac output during halothane anesthesia. Brit. J. Anaesth., *31*, 87, 1959.

318. Kubota, Y., and Vandam, L.D.: Circulatory effects of halothane in patients with heart disease. Clin. Pharmacol. Ther., *3*, 153, 1962.

319. Deutsch, S., Linde, H.W., Dripps, R.D., and Price, H.L.: Circulatory and respiratory actions of halothane in man. Anesthesiology, *23*, 631, 1962.

320. Wyant, G.M., Merriman,, J.E., Kilduff, C.J., and Thomas, E.T.: The cardiovascular effects of halothane. Canad. Anaesth. Soc. J., *5*, 384, 1958.

321. Elder, J.D., Nagano, S.M., Eastwood, D.W., and Harnagel, D.: Circulatory changes associated with thiopental anesthesia in man. Anesthesiology, *16*, 394, 1955.

322. Fieldman, E.J., Ridley, R.W., and Wood, E.H.: Hemodynamic studies during thiopental sodium and nitrous oxide anesthesia in humans. Anesthesiology, *16*, 473, 1955.

323. Etsten, B., and Li, T.H.: Hemodynamic changes during thiopental anesthesia in humans; cardiac output, stroke volume, total peripheral resistance and intrathoracic blood volume. J. Clin. Invest., *34*, 500, 1955.

324. Dobkin, A.B., and Wyant, G.M.: The physiological effects of intravenous anesthesia on man. Canad. Anaesth. Soc., J., *4*, 295, 1957.

325 Pur-Shahriari, A.A., Mills R.A., Hoppin, F.G., and Dexter, L.: Comparison of chronic and acute effects of morphine sulfate on cardiovascular function. Am. J. Cardiol., *20*, 654, 1967.

326. Henney, R.P., Vasko, J.S., Brawley, R.K., Oldham, H.N., and Morrow, AG.: The effects of morphine on the resistance and capacitance vessels of the peripheral circulation. Am. Heart J., *72, 2*, 1966.

327. Drew, J.H., Dripps, R.D., and Comroe, J.H.: Clinical studies on morphine; effects of morphine upon the circulation of man and upon the circulatory and respiratory responses to tilting. Anesthesiology, *7*, 44, 1946.

328. Fejfar, Z., Bergmann, K., Fejfarová, M., and Valach, A.: The effect of morphine on pulmonary hemodynamics in mitral stenosis. Cardiologia, *31*, 461, 1957.

329. Glassman, E., Baliff, R.J., Weinstein, C., and Castro, E., de: Hemodynamic actions of morphine on the human pulmonary circulation. Circulation, *28*, 726, 1963.

330. Roy, S.B., Singh, I., Bhatia, M.L., and Khanna, P.K.: Effect of morphine on pulmonary blood volume in convalescents from high altitude pulmonary oedema. Brit. Heart J., *27*, 876, 1965.

Section III

CHAPTER 13

Technique and Methodology for Measuring Pulmonary Capillary Blood Volume

General Principles

One major function of the lung is to provide for the exchange of gases between alveolar sacs and blood in the pulmonary capillaries. Gases move across the alveolo-capillary membrane by simple diffusion, a process which is subject to several influences.[1-4]

(1) The initial pressure gradient across the alveolo-capillary membrane is the difference between the partial pressure of the gas in the alveoli and that in the mixed venous blood entering the pulmonary capillaries.

(2) The duration of contact between the alveolar gas and blood flowing in the pulmonary capillaries is governed by the rate of blood flow and the size, dimensions and geometry of the pulmonary capillary bed.

(3) The diffusion characteristics of the alveolo-capillary membrane are affected by its intrinsic physical, biochemical and enzymatic characteristics.

(4) The coefficient of diffusion of a gas varies inversely as the square root of its molecular weight. In the gas phase, partial pressure is directly and linearly related to its concentration. When a gas is dissolved in a liquid, its concentration is equal to its partial pressure multiplied by its solubility.

(5) A gas may combine with hemoglobin in the red blood cell.

Diffusion within the alveolar gas itself is not a significant limitation to the passage of a gas into the blood. It should be emphasized that the critical area for diffusion is the surface of the *functional alveoli* in contact with *functional capillaries.*

Utilizing the diffusion characteristics of carbon monoxide (CO) across the alveolo-capillary membrane of the lung, Roughton and Forster described the theoretical basis for the measurement of total pulmonary diffusing capacity for CO (D_{LCO}).[5,6] They further demonstrated that such measurements enabled the total pulmonary diffusing capacity to be subdivided into (*a*) membrane diffusing capacity (D_{MCO}); (*b*) the rate of uptake of CO by the red cells (Θ); and (*c*) the pulmonary capillary blood volume at any instant (Vc). They proposed the equation $\frac{1}{D_L} = \frac{1}{D_L} + \frac{1}{\Theta \cdot Vc}$. McNeill, Rankin and Forster have described these components in terms of resistance.[7] $\frac{1}{D_L}$ may be considered the total resistance to the uptake of CO, which is composed of the sum of $\frac{1}{D_M}$, the membrane resistance, and $\frac{1}{\Theta \cdot Vc}$, the red cell uptake resistance.

The principles and theory of the measurement of diffusing capacity of the lungs have been described and discussed by many workers.[1-12] The D_{LCO} is defined as the number of milliliters of CO (at STPD) which can cross the alveolo-capillary membrane per minute at a pressure gradient of 1 mm Hg of CO. This diffusing capacity depends on the amount and distribution of inspired gas, the surface area and thickness of the alveolar membrane, the volume of blood in the pulmonary capillaries and the amount of circulating hemoglobin.

Various methods of measuring pulmonary diffusing capacity have been summarized by Forster.[2] The most frequently used ones are breath-holding method and steady-state method.

Techniques and Methods

Single-Breath Method

The breath-holding technique, proposed by Krogh,[13,14] as modified by Forster and co-workers,[15-17] has been extensively used in various centers for determination of D_{LCO} because it is a relatively easy technique and requires little cooperation from the patient. A low fraction of CO and He mixture in ambient air is used for this determination, i.e. 0.3% CO, 10% He, 20.9% O_2, and the remainder N_2. The equation for the calculation of D_L is as follows:

$$D_{LCO} = \frac{(V_A)\ (60)}{(t)\ (BP - 47)} \times$$
$$logN \left(\frac{F_{AHe}}{F_{IHe}} \times \frac{F_{ICO}}{F_{ACOt}} \right)$$

Where V_A = volume of alveolar gas in ml at STPD which can be calculated from the inspired volume plus the residual volume

   t = breath-holding time (usually 10 seconds)

   BP = atmospheric barometric pressure in mm Hg

   47 = water vapor pressure in mm Hg at 37° C

   logN = naperian logarithm

   F_{AHe} = concentration of He in the expired alveolar air

F_{IHe} = concentration of He in the inspired air

F_{ICO} = concentration of CO in the inspired air

F_{ACOt} = concentration of CO in the expired alveolar air at the end of breath-holding time (t)

Helium is used to estimate concentration of CO at the beginning of breath holding:

$$F_{ACOo} = \frac{F_{AHe}}{F_{IHe}} \times F_{ICO}$$

Pulmonary capillary blood volume (Vc) can be estimated by determinations of D_{LCO} at various levels of oxygen tension (usually from 100 to 600 mm Hg). D_{LCO} decreases with increase in the alveolar pO_2, because in the presence of a high oxygen tension, CO is not as readily accepted by hemoglobin and the rate (Θ) of movement of CO from the plasma into the red cells is diminished.[5,6]

As shown in Figure 13-1, if D_{LCO}

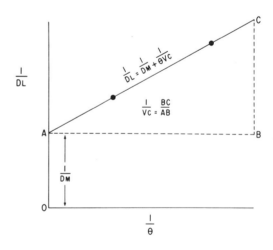

Figure 13-1.   Graphic determination of pulmonary capillary blood volume. The line itself is a plot of red cell resistance against reaction rate resistance per ml of blood (1/Θ); its slope, therefore, is the reciprocal of pulmonary capillary blood volume (1/Vc).

is measured at two or more levels of capillary oxygen tension, corresponding to different values of Θ, and if the reciprocals of D_L measured at various levels are plotted against appropriate values of $1/\Theta$, a straight line, AC, may be shown to connect these points. At the point A the line intersects the ordinate where $1/\Theta$ is virtually zero, and the rate of combination of CO with hemoglobin is infinitely rapid. Hence, at the point of intersection A, the only resistance to the diffusion of CO is that offered by the pulmonary membrane and the value of this intercept is equal to $1/D_M$. If only the triangular area above the intercept is considered, the plotted line is seen to be a graph of red blood cell resistance against reaction rate resistance $(1/\Theta)$. Since the red cell resistance is the product of $1/\Theta$ and $1/Vc$, the slope of the line equals $1/Vc$. The value of Θ, which is the rate of uptake of CO by the red cells, is determined for a specific lambda(λ) which is the ratio of the "permeability" of the red cell interior to that of its membrane. Roughton and Forster have found λ to have a wide range between 1.5 and infinity.[5,6] A λ value of 2.5 is used arbitrarily in nearly all studies, however, because this value is considered to be the most normal value for the ratio of permeability of erythrocyte interior to erythrocyte membrane. For more detailed information, the original papers by Roughton and Forster should be consulted.[5,6]

In cases where the oxygen capacity of the blood is markedly different from the normal value of 20 vol.% which is equivalent to 15 gm of hemoglobin, correction to the normal value is made with the equation:

$$Vc \text{ (corrected)} = Vc \times 15/\text{Hgb Gm. \%}$$

In our laboratory the single breath method is used as modified and standardized by Ogilvie and associates.[17]

This method is also used in many pulmonary function laboratories. With minor modifications, it is described in detail as follows:

Duplicate determinations of D_{LCO} are made at each of the two levels of O_2 tension. The two mixtures consist of 0.3% carbon monoxide (CO) and 10% helium (He), one in room air and the other in O_2.

The patient, either sitting or recumbent, is asked to exhale completely almost to his residual volume. He then takes a rapid maximum inspiration of the CO mixture in room air from the reservoir bag. The inspiration is held for approximately 10 seconds, after which he exhales rapidly. About 750 ml of the first part of the exhaled gas is eliminated, and the remainder is collected in a 3 to 5 liter anesthesia bag for analysis of CO, He and O_2. The inspired volume is recorded by the spirometer. The alveolar volume is the sum of the inspired volume and the residual volume which, in turn, is determined by the closed-circuit helium dilution method of Meneely and Kaltreider.[18]

Prior to the measurement of D_{LCO} at high O_2 tension, the subject breathes 100% O_2 for about 5 minutes. Thereafter, a mixture of CO and He in O_2 is inhaled, and the procedure described in the preceding paragraph is repeated. Between the two successive measurements of D_{LCO} an interval of about 10 minutes is allowed in order to permit the elimination of any He which might have been retained in the subject's lungs.

Before each D_{LCO} determination the gas reservoir bag is thoroughly washed out and refilled with a new supply from the appropriate gas mixture tank.

By means of a pump with a flow rate of 150 ml/min, the mixed expired or end-tidal sample obtained from the subject is pulled through a tube filled with agents which absorb the carbon dioxide and water. The sample is then analyzed for CO, He and O_2. Carbon monoxide is analyzed by using a Beckman L/B Model 15A infra-red analyzer, He by a Collins catherometer, and O_2 by a Beckman Model C_2 paramagnetic analyzer as well as by an Instrumentation Laboratory glass electrode analyzer. For each calculation of D_{LCO} the catherometer reading of He is corrected according to the O_2 concentration of the mixture. Repeated determinations of D_{LCO} inevitably induce a rise in CO hemoglobin and CO back pressure (pCO) in the pulmonary capillary bed. Therefore, in order to approximate the true alveolar to capillary CO gradient for calculation of D_{LCO}, the excessive pCO is subtracted from the measured alveolar pCO according to the formula described by Forster and associates.[19]

Steady-State Method

Some workers have used the steady-state carbon monoxide method as originally described by Filley, McIntosh and Wright for the determination of pulmonary capillary blood volume.[12] The method is briefly summarized as follows. With an indwelling needle or catheter in a systemic artery and with the subject breathing through a mouthpiece connected to a respiratory valve and an open circuit, he inspires 0.1% CO in air for 6 minutes. A 4 minute interval is allowed to attain equilibrium between gas in the lungs and in the inspired gas and to flush the expired air and collecting bag. During the fifth and sixth minutes of CO breathing, expired gas is collected in a Douglas bag at a known respiratory rate, while 15 ml of arterial

blood is withdrawn into a heparinized syringe.

The volume of expired air is determined and samples are analyzed for CO by infra-red analyzer and expressed in absolute CO concentration by reference to standard gases analyzed to one part per million. Concentrations of both O_2 and CO_2 of the expired air samples are determined by micro Scholander method. The arterial blood sample is analyzed for CO_2 and O_2 tension by a glass electrode analyzer. As $D_{LCO} = \dfrac{\dot{V}_{CO}}{P_{ACO}}$, the CO uptake, $\dot{V}_{CO}$, is calculated as follows:

$$\dot{V}_{CO} = \dot{V}_E \times F_{ICO} \times \frac{F_{EN2}}{F_{IN2}} - FECO$$

Where $\dot{V}_{CO}$ = CO volume in ml/min
$\dot{V}_E$ = total gas volume in ml/min (STPD)
F_{ICO} = concentration of CO in inspired volume
F_{EN2} = concentration of N_2 in expired volume
F_{IN2} = concentration of N_2 in inspired volume
F_{ECO} = concentration of CO in expired volume

The P_{ACO} (alveolar air CO tension) is calculated by using the Bohr equation or "alveolar" equation, assuming that the alveolar CO_2 tension, P_{ACO2}, is equal to the arterial CO_2 tension, P_{aCO2}. The equation used is

$$P_{ACO} = (BP - 47)\frac{F_{ECO} - rF_{ICO}}{1 - r}$$

Where $r = \dfrac{V_D}{V_T} = \dfrac{P_{aCO2} - P_{ECO2}}{P_{aCO2}}$
V_D = physiologic dead space
V_T = tidal volume

assuming that the partial pressure of CO in the pulmonary capillary blood is zero.

The steady-state method reported by Bates, Boucot and Dormer is similar, except that the end-tidal pCO is used as the mean alveolar pCO,[10] and this method requires no arterial gas analysis.

The fraction of CO removed from

the respired gas or percentage uptake of CO is calculated as follows.

$$CO_F = \frac{\dot{V}_{CO}}{V_E \cdot F_{ICO} \cdot (F_{EN_2}/F_{IN_2}) - f \cdot d\,(F_{ICO} - F_{ACO})}$$

Where CO_F = amount of CO in ml taken up by blood per ml of CO entering the lungs

f = respiratory rate per minute

d = dead space of apparatus, ml

F_{ACO} = fractional concentration of CO in alveolar air

As in the single breath method, the pulmonary capillary blood volume may be estimated by the determination of D_L at two or three levels of oxygen in the alveolar air.

Rebreathing Method

This method was originally designed by Kruhoffer[20] using $C^{14}O$ and later modified by Lewis and associates utilizing CO and continuous analysis. The technique was fully described by the latter authors.[21]

Comparison between Single-Breath Method and Steady-State Method

In 1955 Forster and co-workers measured D_{LCO} by the single-breath method in 7 normal subjects and compared the results with those obtained by the steady-state D_{LCO} method (Filley).[16] In general, the single-breath D_{LCO} was higher than the steady-state D_{LCO}. The advantages and limitations of each method were discussed. "The steady state D_{LCO} method is subject to theoretical error if inspired gas is not distributed evenly throughout the lung in relation to the pulmonary capillary blood flow, just as the single breath D_{LCO} estimate is subject to error if inspired gas is not distributed evenly with respect to the alveolar volume." Both methods have the disadvantage that CO is a nonphysiologic gas.

In 1958 Shephard demonstrated that higher values of D_{LCO} were obtained by the single-breath method than by the steady-state method (Bates) in a given subject and that higher values of D_{LCO} were obtained with increased alveolar volume.[22]

In 1961 Cadigan and associates also reported that values for the single-breath D_{LCO} were always larger than those by the steady-state D_{LCO} (Filley) in the same subject.[23] Variations of single-breath D_{LCO} between multiple tests were found to be due to variations in the volume of the lungs (V_A) at which the breath was held. A quantitative relationship between D_{LCO} and V_A was demonstrated both at rest and during exercise. In patients with pulmonary disease, greater discrepancy between the results of the single-breath and the steady-state methods was attributed to inequalities of (a) ventilation, (b) perfusion, or (c) ventilation-perfusion ratios.

In 1961 Apthorp and Marshall studied the D_{LCO} by comparing the single-breath method and the steady-state method of Bates and co-workers.[24] In 16 normal subjects at rest the steady state D_{LCO} was about 75% of the single breath D_{LCO}. The steady-state D_{LCO} increased with increasing tidal volume and the steady-state D_{LCO} was approximately the same as single-breath D_{LCO} at maximal tidal volume. In patients with normal pulmonary gas mixing and in those with impaired pulmonary gas mixing but no clinical evidence of emphysema, the steady-state D_{LCO} was about 70% of the single-breath D_{LCO}. On the other hand, in patients with pulmonary emphysema no relationship was observed between the single-breath and the steady-state D_{LCO}. The lack of relationship was attributed to uneven ventilation or inequality of ventilation and perfusion.

Range of Variation and Reproducibility

Ogilvie and his colleagues investigated the reproducibility of D_{LCO} in 24 normal subjects and found that the coefficient of variation for single measurements on a single subject was 8.5%.[17] Variation from day to day was significantly greater than for measurements made within 1 day. Lewis and associates determined Vc in 4 subjects and found it to be reproducible and stable over a period of months.[25] Krumholz showed good reproducibility of D_M and Vc in a study which included 6 subjects who were studied at 1 week intervals.[26] His results showed a mean control D_M and Vc of 81 and 103 ml respectively, and the respective figures after a week were 79 and 95 ml. In our laboratory repeat determinations of D_{LCO} and Vc were made in a series of normal subjects.[27,28] The results are presented in Table 13-1. The daily variations were small.

Limitations and Potential Errors

The sources of error in the determination of diffusing capacity by different methods have been admirably discussed by Forster and associates.[1,4,15-17] It should be recognized that the Vc estimated by carbon monoxide diffusing capacity may not be the true capillary blood volume, inasmuch as a number of assumptions must be made in the final calculation. Determination of Vc by this technique is subject to considerable uncertainty, especially when applied to patients with cardiopulmonary disease. The limiting factors include (a) technical errors in determining the total diffusing capacity for carbon monoxide by either the single-breath or the steady-state method; (b) measurement of the reaction rate of carbon monoxide with hemoglobin only under certain conditions; (c) considerable variation in calculated values for the membrane diffusing capacity and pul-

TABLE 13-1   Multiple Determinations of D_L and Vc in Normal Subjects

Subjects	D_L (ml/mm Hg/min)					Vc (ml/M²)					Interval
	A	B	C	D	E	A	B	C	D	E	
J.P.	25.4	26.7				60.2	50.0				4 weeks
D.S.	38.2	40.6				42.8	44.8				1 week
P.Y.	31.2	28.5				33.2	43.0				2 weeks
C.R.	25.6	29.0				48.2	50.6				1 month
S.H.	24.8	25.1				60.0	62.5				2 weeks
S.N.	29.2	27.2				54.4	53.6				3 weeks
G.C.	29.8	31.0				52.4	47.8				2 weeks
E.M.	33.2	35.0				58.6	53.4				4 months
M.M.	32.4	28.4				44.6	41.0				10 weeks
F.P.	33.2	35.2				48.3	51.2				6 months
P.P.	32.5	32.0	34.6			44.9	39.0				3 weeks
K.G.	34.0	35.8	36.0			53.5	51.2	54.3			22 months
H.C.	21.2	21.0	19.3			32.6	32.3	30.9			2 weeks
J.F.	39.5	32.3	30.5			33.1	31.2	37.6			4 weeks
N.S.	31.2	31.0	30.8	32.1	31.2	55.0	54.3	54.0	54.0	54.3	15 months

D_L = Pulmonary diffusing capacity for carbon monoxide
Vc = Pulmonary capillary blood volume
Interval = Interval between the first and the second determinations or between
      the first and the last determinations
A,B,C,D, and E = Different dates on which the determinations of D_L and Vc
      were made

monary capillary blood volume when slight technical errors are made; (*d*) questionable justifications and reliability of separating the total diffusing capacity (D_L) into D_M and Vc based upon the kinetics of combination of carbon monoxide with hemoglobin; (*e*) the possibility of new error introduced with the various modifications of methods for measuring the diffusing capacity; and (*f*) underestimation of Vc because of uneven distribution of D_L in different parts of the lungs resulting in non-uniform distribution of Vc.[29-32]

In the single-breath method the initial blood carbon monoxide may be assumed to be negligible in non-smokers. In the case of cigarette smokers, however, it is desirable to measure the pulmonary capillary blood CO level before and after the test. Pulmonary capillary CO should be estimated if steady-state D_L method is used or repeat determinations of breath-holding D_L method are employed.

In the steady-state method, appreciable pulmonary capillary tension is assumed to be absent over a short period of breathing inspired gas containing CO, an assumption which may not be valid. Theoretically, an elevation of pulmonary capillary CO may result from slow reaction of CO with the intracellular hemoglobin allowing accumulation of CO in the plasma. Another cause of a significant amount of pulmonary capillary CO may be the presence of sufficient carboxyhemoglobin (CO Hb) to result in a measurable blood CO tension in equilibrium with it.

Staub and associates have extensively studied the small vessel hematocrit in the cat lung and its relation to the measured Vc.[33,34] Using a rapid freezing technique, alveolar capillary hematocrit was determined directly. The average hematocrit in the pulmonary vessels less than 0.5 mm in diameter was 15% less than that in the systemic arteries. The capillary hematocrit was even lower. This implies that Vc measured by diffusing methods actually occupies a larger volume of capillaries *e.g.*, a Vc of 60 ml actually occupies 70 ml or more of capillaries.

Despite the multiplicity of such questions and theoretical pitfalls, many investigators have found the method of measuring D_{LCO} at high and low levels of oxygen is sensitive and reliable enough to register (*a*) a definite and consistent increase in Vc from the sitting to the recumbent position,[25,35,36] (*b*) a substantial increase in Vc during exercise and in association with acute pulmonary vascular congestion,[25,37-41] and (*c*) a significantly increased Vc in patients with large atrial septal defects, returning to normal after successful surgical closure of the defect.[27,42-45]

REFERENCES

1. Forster, R.E.: Exchange of gases between alveolar air and pulmonary capillary blood: Pulmonary diffusing capacity. Physiol. Rev., *37*, 391, 1957.
2. Comroe, J.H., Forster, R.E., DuBois, A.B., Biscoe, W.A., and Carlsen, E.: *The Lung: Clinical Physiology and Pulmonary Function Tests*, 2nd ed., Chicago, Year Book Medical Publishers, Inc., 1962.
3. Staub, N.C.: The interdependence of pulmonary structure and function. Anesthesiology, *24*, 831, 1963.
4. Forster, R.E.: Diffusion of Gases. *In* W.O. Fenn and H. Rahn (eds), *Handbook of Physiology*, Section 3, Respiration, Vol. 1, p. 839, Washington, D.C., American Physiological Society, 1964.
5. Roughton, F.J.W., Forster, R.E., and Cander, L.: Rate at which carbon monoxide replaces oxygen from combination with human hemoglobin in solution and in the red cell. J. Appl. Physiol., *11*, 269, 1957.

6. Roughton, F.J.W., and Forster, R.E.: Relative importance of diffusion and chemical reaction rates in determining rate of exchange of gases in the human lungs, with special reference to true diffusing capacity of the pulmonary membrane and volume of blood in the lung capillaries. J. Appl. Physiol., *11*, 290, 1957.

7. McNeill, R.S., Rankin, J., and Forster, R.E.: The diffusing capacity of the pulmonary membrane and the pulmonary capillary blood in cardiopulmonary disease. Clin. Sci., *17*, 465, 1958.

8. Lilienthal, J.L., Riley, R.L., Proemmel, D.D., and Franke, R.E.: An experimental analysis in man of the oxygen pressure gradient from alveolar air to arterial blood during rest and exercise at sea level and at altitude. Am. J. Physiol., *147*, 199, 1946.

9. Riley, R.L., and Cournand, A.: Analysis of factors affecting partial pressures of oxygen and carbon dioxide in gas and blood of lungs: Theory. J. Appl. Physiol., *4*, 77, 1951.

10. Bates, D.V., Boucot, N.G., and Dormer, A.E.: The pulmonary diffusing capacity in normal subjects. J. Physiol. (London), *129*, 237, 1955.

11. Jones, R.S., and Meade, F.: A theoretical and experimental analysis of anomalies in the estimation of pulmonary diffusing capacity by the single breath method. Quart. J. Exp. Physiol., *46*, 131, 1961.

12. Filley, G.F., McIntosh, D.J., and Wright, G.W.: Carbon monoxide uptake and pulmonary diffusing capacity in normal subjects at rest and during exercise. J. Clin. Invest., *33*, 530, 1954.

13. Krogh, A., and Krogh, M.: On the rate of diffusion of carbonic oxide into the lungs of man. Skand. Arch. f. Physiol., *23*, 236, 1909.

14. Krogh, M.: The diffusion of gases through the lungs of man. J. Physiol., *49*, 271, 1915.

15. Forster, R.E., Fowler, W.S., Bates, D.V., and Van Lingen, B.: The absorption of carbon monoxide by the lungs during breath holding. J. Clin. Invest., *33*, 1135, 1954.

16. Forster, R.E., Cohn, J.E., Briscoe, W.A., Blakemore, W.S., and Riley, R.L.: A modification of the Krogh carbon monoxide breath-holding technique for estimating the diffusing capacity of the lung; a comparison with three other studies. J. Clin. Invest., *34*, 1417, 1955.

17. Ogilvie, C.M., Forster, R.E., Blakemore, W.S. and Morton, J.W.: A standardized breath-holding technique for the clinical measurement of the diffusing capacity of the lung for carbon monoxide. J. Clin. Invest., *36*, 1, 1957.

18. Meneely, G.R., and Kaltreider, N.L.: The volume of the lung determined by helium dilution: Description of the method and comparison with other procedures. J. Clin. Invest., *28*, 129, 1949.

19. Forster, R.E., Roughton, F.J.W., Cander, L., Briscoe, W.A., and Kreuzer, F.: Apparent pulmonary diffusing capacity for CO at varying alveolar O_2 tensions. J. Appl. Physiol., *11*, 277, 1957.

20. Kruhoffer, P.: Studies on the lung diffusion coefficient for carbon monoxide in normal human subjects by means of $C^{14}O$. Acta. Physiol. Scand., *32*, 106, 1954.

21. Lewis, B.M., Lin, T.H., Noe, F.E., and Hayford-Welsing, E.J.: The measurement of pulmonary diffusing capacity for carbon monoxide by a rebreathing method. J. Clin. Invest., *38*, 2073, 1959.

22. Shephard, R.J.: "Breath-holding" measurement of carbon monoxide diffusing capacity. Comparison of field test with steady-state and other measurements. J. Physiol., *141*, 408, 1958.

23. Cadigan, J.B., Marks, A., Ellicott, M., Jones, R.H., and Gaensler, E.A.: An analysis of factors affecting the measurement of pulmonary diffusing capacity by the single breath method. J. Clin. Invest., *40*, 1495, 1961.

24. Apthorp, G.H., and Marshall, R.: Pulmonary diffusing capacity: A comparison of breath holding and steady state methods using carbon monoxide. J. Clin. Invest., *40*, 1775, 1961.

25. Lewis, B.M., Lin, T.H., Roe, F.E., and Komisaruk, R.: The measurement of pulmonary capillary blood volume and pulmonary membrane diffusing capacity in normal subjects; the effects of exercise and position. J. Clin. Invest., *37*, 1061, 1958.

26. Krumholz, R.A.: Pulmonary membrane diffusing capacity and pulmonary capillary blood volume: An appraisal of their clinical usefulness. Am. Rev. Resp. Dis., *94*, 195, 1966.

27. Flatley, F.J., Constantine, H., McCredie, R.M., and Yu, P.N.: Pulmonary diffusing capacity and pulmonary capillary blood volume in normal subjects and in cardiac patients. Am. Heart J., *64*, 159, 1962.

28. Gazioglu, K., and Yu, P.N.: Pulmonary blood volume and pulmonary capillary blood volume in valvular heart disease. Circulation, *35*, 701, 1967.

29. Burrows, B., Niden, A.H., Harper, P.V., and Barclay, W.R.: Non-uniform pulmonary diffusion as demonstrated by the carbon monoxide equilibration technique; mathematical considerations. J. Clin. Invest., *38*, 795, 1960.

30. Dollery, C.T., Dyson, N.A., and Sinclair, J.D.: Regional variations in uptake of radioactive CO in the normal lung. J. Appl. Physiol., *15*, 411, 1960.

31. West, J.B.: Regional differences in gas exchange in the lung of erect man. J. Appl. Physiol., *17*, 893, 1962.

32. Staub, N.C.: The alveolar-arterial oxygen tension gradient due to diffusion. J. Appl. Rhysiol., *18*, 673, 1963.

33. Staub, N.C.: Microcirculation of the lung utilizing very rapid freezing. Angiol., *12*, 469, 1961,

34. Staub, N.C., and Storey, W.F.: Relation between morphological and physiological events in lung studied by rapid freezing. J. Appl. Physiol, *17*, 381, 1962.

35. Lewis, C.M., McElroy, W.T., Hayford-Welsing, E.J., and Samberg, L.C.: The effects of body position, ganglionic blockade and norepinephrine on the pulmonary capillary bed. J. Clin. Invest., *39*, 1345, 1960.

36. Newman, F.: The effect of change in posture on alveolar capillary diffusion and capillary blood volume in the human lung. J. Physiol., *162*, 29, 1962.

37. Jonson, R.L., Spicer, W.S., Bishop, J.M., and Forster, R.E.: Pulmonary capillary blood volume flow and diffusing capacity during exercise. J. Appl. Physiol., *15*, 893. 1960.

38. Krumholz, R.A., King, L.H., and Ross, J.C.: Effect of pulmonary vascular engorgement on D_L during and immediately after exercise. J Appl. Physiol., *18*, 1180, 1963.

39. Ross, J.C., Maddock, G.E., and Ley, G.D.: Effect of pressure suit inflation on pulmonary capillary bood volume. J. Appl. Physiol., *16*, 674, 1961.

40. Daly, W.J., Ross, J.C., and Behnke, R.H.: The effect of change in the pulmonary vascular bed produced by atropine, pulmonary engorgement and positive pressure breathing on diffusing and mechanical properties of the lung. J. Clin. Invest., *42*, 1038, 1963.

41. Daly, W.J., Giammona, S.T., Ross, J.C., and Feigenbaum, H.: Effects of pulmonary vascular congestion on postural changes in the perfusion and filling of the pulmonary vascular bed. J. Clin. Invest., *43*, 68, 1964.

42. Rankin, J., and Collier, Q.C.: The influence of atrial and ventricular septal pefects on the capillary bed of the lung and on the diffusion characteristics of the pulmonary membrane. J. Lab. Clin. Med. *52*, 937, 1958.

43. Bucci, G., Cook, C.D., and Hamann, J.F.: Studies of respiratory physiology in children. VI. Lung diffusing capacity of pulmonary membrane and pulmonary capillary blood volume in congenital heart disease. J. Clin. Invest., *40*, 1431, 1961.

44. McCredie, R.M., Lovejoy, F.W., and Yu, P.N.: Pulmonary diffusing capacity and pulmonary capillary volume in patients with intracardiac shunts. J. Lab. Clin. Med., *63*, 914, 1964.

45. Gazioglu, K., and Yu, P.N.: Pulmonary capillary blood volume in congenital heart disease. Unpublished data.

CHAPTER 14

Pulmonary Capillary Blood Volume in Health

Normal Subjects at Rest

Table 14-1 summarizes the mean and range of pulmonary capillary blood volume (Vc) in more than 200 normal subjects, as reported by a number of workers.[1-17] These values are tabulated according to the methods used, the position of the subjects when the measurements were made and the age range of the subjects studied.

Some workers have reported a decline in overall D_L with increasing age,[18-21] but others found no significant difference in D_L with advancing age in females and only a slight reduction in D_L in the 50 to 59 year old age group of males.[19,22] D_L and Vc are in general less in females than in males. If a correction for body surface area is made, however, no significant sex difference is observed. Hamer found no relation between Vc and age.[23] He attributed decline in D_L with increasing age to a reduction in D_M. Bucci and collaborators found that D_L, D_M, and Vc correlate directly with body surface area, and the association of larger body surface area with greater D_L and Vc is generally recognized.[24]

We have estimated vital capacity, D_L, D_M, and Vc in several groups of normal subjects, ranging in age from 11 to 47 years in both the sitting and recumbent positions (Table 14-2). In the sitting position no significant difference is evident among any of the groups for either D_L or Vc. The Vc is generally higher in the recumbent position than in the sitting position, however, at least for the adult group.

In this and subsequent chapters D_L refers to pulmonary diffusing capacity for carbon monoxide. If reference is made to pulmonary diffusing capacity for oxygen, the expression D_{LO2} is used.

Effects of Physiologic and Mechanical Interventions

Posture

It was generally agreed that D_L increased when subjects assumed a supine from a sitting position.[25,26] D_L also increased from the standing to the sitting position, but the change was usually less significant.

Lewis and co-workers demonstrated that the increase in D_L observed earlier by Ogilvie and associates was due to an increase in Vc.[5] In 4 normal subjects the mean Vc increased from 59.2 ml in the sitting position to 85.9 ml in the supine position. The change was considered a consequence of passive enlargement of the pulmonary capillary bed. Similar findings were reported by Newman.[27]

TABLE 14-1   Pulmonary Capillary Blood Volume (Vc) in Normal Subjects

Year	Authors	No. of Subjects	Age	Position	Vc Mean (Range)	Vc/M² Mean (Range)
1. Single-Breath Method						
1964	McCredie et al.	16	20–45	St	57 (41–91)	31
1965	Johnson et al.	10	8–28	St or S	75 (42–110)	—
1957	Roughton and Forster	7	18–39	S	79 (30–108)	—
1958	McNeill et al.	8	23–48	S	97 (75–116)	49
1958	Lewis et al.	19	21–34	S	65 (39–61)	37
1961	Ross et al.	10	22–47	S	93 (69–125)	—
1963	Daly et al.	7	22–34	S	85 (61–100)	—
1965	Steiner et al.	5	–	S	93 (68–120)	—
1966	Miller and Johnson	5	18–29	S	90 (80–100)	—
1962	Flatley et al.	13	14–70	R	—	43 (27–72)
1963	Daly et al.	8	22–34	R	112 (56–182)	—
1964	Daly et al.	10	22–36	R	99 (74–133)	—
1965	Daly et al.	9	21–29	R	82 (55–114)	—
1967	Gazioglu and Yu	18	16–45	R	—	54 (39–66)
1961	Bucci et al.	59	7–40	—	—	38 (30–48)
1962	Hamer	25	15–59	—	75 (43–187)	—
1966	Krumholz	43	17–35	—	99 (51–171)	—
2. Steady-State Method						
1957	Roughton and Forster	6	18–39	S	59 (32–98)	—
1957	Bates	6	–	—	73 (42–112)	—
1961	Constantine et al.	9	20–49	S	—	45 (29–66)
1964	McCredie	18	8–46	R	—	52 (29–90)
3. Rebreathing Method						
1960	Lewis et al.	8	22–35	R	142 (95–211)	—

St = Standing   R = Recumbent
S = Sitting   Vc = Pulmonary capillary blood volume in ml

TABLE 14-2   DL, DM, and Vc Determined in Normal Subjects of Various Ages

Subjects	No.	Age	BSA	Position	VC Mean (Range)	D_L Mean (Range)	D_M Mean (Range)	Vc Mean (Range)
Preteens	8	11–12	1.51	S	2.1 (1.6–2.4)	17 (13–21)	39 (33–47)	40 (26–60)
Teenagers and Adolescents	23	13–20	1.71	S	2.2 (1.7–2.7)	18 (12–24)	45 (26–118)	42 (24–79)
Adults	8	22–27	1.66	S	2.3 (1.8–2.6)	16 (13–18)	43 (24–77)	37 (27–61)
Preteens and Teenagers	3	11–16	1.69	R	2.0 (1.7–2.3)	15 (14–16)	27 (24–32)	51 (33–63)
Adults	25	20–47	1.85	R	2.4 (1.8–3.2)	18 (12–21)	39 (25–62)	52 (39–66)

S   = Sitting D_L = ml/min/mm Hg/M²
R   = Recumbent D_M = ml/min/mm Hg/M²
VC = Vital capacity (L/M²)   VC = ml/M²

Utilizing the technique of body tilting, Daly and associates demonstrated an increase in D_L and Vc in the position of head-down tilting and a decrease in D_L and Vc in head-up tilting.[11,12] The changes in D_L and Vc were closely parallel to alterations in the central venous and presumably pulmonary vascular pressures. These pressure changes probably resulted in increase or decrease in capillary transmural pressure in the respective positions, a postulation consistent with the notion that the change in the Vc is indeed dependent on the transmural pressure. They further observed that after a small increase in central vascular pressure no further increase in D_L or Vc was observed despite additional large increases in pressure, produced either by head-down tilting or by pressure suit inflation, suggesting that passive enlargement of the pulmonary capillary bed by pressure is limited. Assuming that the increased central vascular pressure did not affect the pulmonary capillary hematocrit, the rate of reaction of carbon monoxide with hemoglobin, or the diffusivity of the membrane per unit area, these observations may be explained by one or both of two alternative mechanisms: (a) increased pulmonary vascular pressure initially recruited previously "empty" capillaries and no further recruitment effect was possible after a relatively small increase in pressure; (b) increased pulmonary vascular pressure produced limited dilatation of already "open" capillaries.

Pressure Suit Inflation

In 1957 Bondurant, Hickam and Isley reported acute central and pulmonary vascular engorgement induced in normal subjects by inflation of pressure suits.[28] Pulmonary compliance decreased concomitantly.

In 1958 Lewis, Forster and Beckman in Philadelphia reported no significant increase in D_L in normal subjects during antigravity pressure suit inflation.[29]

In 1960, on the other hand, Ross, Lord and Ley in Indianapolis reported significant increases in D_L with pressure suit inflation, provided that central venous pressure was elevated, alveolar volume (V_A) was controlled and no Valsalva maneuver was performed.[30] This increase in D_L was interpreted as a result of passive dilatation of the pulmonary vascular bed.

In 1961 Ross, Maddock and Ley further studied the effects of pressure suit inflation on D_L, Vc and D_M in 12 normal subjects.[6] The average increases in D_L, Vc and D_M over control values were 27, 33 and 21% respectively. These findings substantiated their early report that the pulmonary capillary bed could be passively dilated by increased intravascular pressure, but the data did not distinguish between the two possible responsible mechanisms—dilatation of open capillaries or opening of previously closed capillaries.

Subsequently, the two groups of investigators in Philadelphia and Indianapolis together restudied the problem in an attempt to reconcile the disagreement.[31] They reported that the discrepancy in their earlier studies appeared to have resulted from the construction of the two pressure suits used. The suit used in Philadelphia by Forster's group covered the entire body up to the nipple, whereas the suit used in Indianapolis by Ross' group extended only to the costal margin. In the former case the subject was likely to perform a Valsalva maneuver during the breath-holding, causing a smaller alveolar volume, and tending to reduce the D_L. When the Philadelphia pressure suit was rolled down to the costal margin, D_L increased, and results were similar to those obtained with the Indianapolis pressure suit. It was finally concluded by both groups that pressure suit inflation in man does produce an increase in D_L, probably by means of pulmonary congestion.

The Indianapolis group further demonstrated that pressure suit inflation reduced both the arterio-alveolar CO_2 gradient and the alveolar "dead space." These changes were interpreted as further evidence of acute pulmonary congestion associated with elevation of pulmonary vascular pressure and more even distribution of pulmonary perfusion and pulmonary capillary blood volume throughout the lungs.

Bondurant, Hickam and Isley observed that norepinephrine infusion produced greater elevation of central venous pressure and a decline in pulmonary compliance during inflation of the pressure suit.[28] On the other hand, hexamethonium infusion diminished the rise in central venous pressure which occurred with suit inflation, but did not affect the changes in compliance. They suggested that compliance changes depended partially on the degree of pulmonary vascular engorgement, which in turn was partly dependent on peripheral venous tone.

Daly, Ross and Behnke studied the effect of pretreatment with atropine on the acute pulmonary congestion produced by pressure suit inflation.[7] The increase in the right atrial pressure, pulmonary arterial pressure, D_L and Vc was less after atropine. This suggested that atropine caused a shift of blood out of the lungs into areas where it was not effectively mobilized by pressure suit inflation. This study demonstrated in man the dependence of D_L and Vc on pulmonary vascular pressure or volume, or both.

Positive or Negative Pressure Breathing

Positive Pressure Breathing. Utilizing teeter-board and plethysmographic methods, Fenn and co-workers showed movement of blood out of the thorax during positive pressure breathing.[32] They calculated that an increase in pulmonary pressure of 30 cm H_2O displaced 500 ml, about half the blood believed to be present in the lungs. They further estimated that about 30% of the displaced blood went to the limbs and the remainder to the abdomen. Our present estimate of the pulmonary blood volume in normal subjects is 271 ± 10 ml/M^2, so that the earlier figure was probably too high, although their percentage estimates of redistribution may be valid.

Daly, Ross and Behnke demonstrated a decrease in D_L and Vc during 10 mm Hg of positive pressure breathing (Table 14-3).[7] The mechanism was considered to be similar to that observed during the Valsalva maneuver.

Negative Pressure Breathing. Coates, Snidal and Shepard found variable effects of negative intraalveolar pressure on D_L and Vc.[33]

Steiner, Frayser and Ross reported the effects of negative pressure breathing (-26 and -52 cm H_2O) on D_L, V_A and V_C in normal subjects.[8] The results are summarized in Table 14-4. The increase in D_L and Vc was not due to the metabolic effects of muscular work, a decrease in alveolar oxygen tension, an increase in V_A, or an increase in pulmonary blood flow. The authors felt that the changes were attributable to an increase in the size

TABLE 14-3 Pulmonary Diffusing Capacity (D_L) and Pulmonary Capillary Blood Volume (V_C) during Positive Pressure Breathing (after Daly et al.)

Condition	*D_L*		*Vc*	
	Without Atropine	*With Atropine*	*Without Atropine*	*With Atropine*
Control	31.3 ± 7.3*	25.5 ± 7.3	112 ± 42	93 ± 34
Positive Pressure Breathing	27.9 ± 7.7	24.1 ± 9.1	88 ± 31	76 ± 29

D_L = ml/mm Hg/min
Vc = ml
* = mean $\pm$ S.D.
Eight normal subjects studied

TABLE 14-4   Pulmonary Diffusing Capacity (D$_L$), Alveolar Volume (V$_A$), and Pulmonary
             Capillary Blood Volume (Vc) during Negative Pressure Breathing (after
             Steiner et al.)

Negative Pressure Breathing	D$_L$ (8)	V$_A$ (8)	Vc (5)
−26 cm H$_2$O			
control	36.9 ± 5.2*	5.11 ± 0.82	93 ± 18
4 min.	47.4 ± 6.5	5.75 ± 0.73	99 ± 19
7 min.	49.7 ± 11.4	5.66 ± 0.76	116 ± 21
post 3 min.	39.2 ± 7.2	5.49 ± 0.71	95 ± 17
−52 cm H$_2$O			
control	34.6 ± 5.0	4.74 ± 0.67	92 ± 14
4 min.	48.2 ± 5.9	4.66 ± 0.98	113 ± 26
7 min.	46.2 ± 9.4	4.86 ± 0.94	108 ± 11
post 3 min.	39.0 ± 7.2	4.98 ± 1.07	88 ± 10

D$_L$ = ml CO per minute per mm Hg
V$_A$ = liters per breath
Vc = ml
Figures in parentheses denote number of subjects studied
* = mean ± S.D.

of the effectively ventilated pulmonary capillary bed resulting from distention of open capillaries or from the opening of previously closed capillaries. Two possible mechanisms were mentioned. The first was a mechanical consequence of the applied negative pressure with effective distending pressures considerably increased, inasmuch as the drop in vascular pressure was only about half that of the applied alveolar pressure. The second possible explanation was related to a more effective distribution of perfusion, inasmuch as negative pressure breathing probably abolished the postural blood flow gradient at the apices of the lung.

Zeckman and Mueller, on the other hand, demonstrated no significant change in steady state D$_L$ during negative pressure breathing.[34] They believed that any increase in intramural pressure was compromised by a decrease in the lung volume resulting in a decrease in the area of functional alveoli in contact with functional capillaries.

An increase in thoracic blood volume,[35-37] a decrease in central venous pressure,[38-40] and a decrease in pulmonary compliance[36] during negative pressure breathing were also observed by other workers.

The changes of D$_L$ and Vc described in relation to posture, pressure suit inflation and positive or negative pressure breathing agree with the results of animal experiments in which an increase in D$_L$ was observed in the isolated cat lung preparation during acute pulmonary congestion.[41,42] It was emphasized that the pressure across the walls of the pulmonary blood vessels was a primary factor in controlling the size of the pulmonary capillary bed as measured by D$_L$. In this regard, Lawson and co-workers considered the transmural pressure in the pulmonary veins more important than that in the pulmonary arteries.[43]

In a recent communication, Zeckman and associates studied the effects on D$_L$ and Vc of negative pressure (40 mm Hg) applied below the level of the iliac crests of 5 normal subjects.[44] There was a decrease in both D$_L$ and Vc. The factors contributing to the change may include (a) displacement of diaphragm, (b) compression of soft tissues, and (c) redistribution of blood to the lower body. Their study suggests that postural change in D_L may be more related to changes in Vc than alteration in distribution of flow.

Exercise

An increase in D_L with exercise was first observed by Krogh in 1915.[45] Subsequently, many investigators have reported an increase in D_L, D_{LO2} and Vc during exercise.[5,9,25,46-63] Roughton considered that the increase in D_L during exercise was in part due to an increase in Vc.[64] Riley and associates felt that during exercise an increase in the area of diffusing surface was associated with an increase in Vc resulting from the opening of previously closed capillaries or from enlargement in the caliber of those already patent.[47] Bjure found a direct correlation between D_L and stroke volume during exercise and a negative correlation between D_L and pulmonary vascular resistance.[65]

Extensive investigation, however, has failed to establish the exact mechanisms whereby exercise increases D_L and Vc. The physiologic parameters studied in this connection included the following:

Cardiac output augmented by

(1) intravenous infusion of 400 to 500 ml of 5% human serum albumin in normal saline solution,

(2) release of tourniquets which had occluded blood flow to the lower extremities for the preceding 15 minutes,

(3) drugs such as epinephrine or atropine plus norepinephrine.

Increasing cardiac output by these maneuvers did not increase either the steady state or breath-holding D_L.[53]

Increased Ventilation Rate. Hyperventilation induced voluntarily or by 5% CO_2 increased the steady state D_L, as did exercise sufficient to induce an equal rise in ventilation.[53,54,56] How-

ever, hyperventilation prior to single breath-holding D_L determinations did not increase breath-holding D_L.[53] On the other hand, D_L did increase during exercise when ventilation was voluntarily restrained to the resting level.[60] Thus, the increased ventilation from exercise, though increasing steady state D_L, could not be the only mechanism involved. It was suggested that the relationships among ventilation, perfusion, and diffusing surface during exercise became more uniform with both the steady state and breath-holding techniques; hence, the values of D_L with exercise determined by these two methods were comparable.[9] In other words, with increasing ventilation the pulmonary vascular bed is relatively larger with the steady state technique than with the breath-holding method.

Increased Pulmonary Vascular Pressure.

(1) Inflation of a pressure suit caused a rise in the central venous and pulmonary vascular pressures associated with a small but significant increase in steady-state and breath-holding D_L.[7,53] This could not be related to exercise in normal subjects in whom moderate exercise induced a much greater increase in D_L associated with minimal or no change in the pulmonary vascular pressures.[53,54,66-71]

(2) Alternate inflation and deflation of a pressure suit in the lower half of the body with increased ventilation caused the steady-state D_L to rise significantly, an effect which was attributed to the increase in ventilation.[53]

Johnson and co-workers stated that the behavior of the pulmonary capillary bed during exercise could not be explained entirely on the basis of passive compliance of small pulmonary blood vessels to changes in blood volume or changes in transmural pressure.[57]

Vc changed little under conditions where blood flow was increased transiently by the administration of epinephrine or by unilateral occlusion of a pulmonary artery, nor did it change consistently in patients with hyperthyroidism. Significant elevation of central venous and pulmonary vascular pressures was observed during pressure suit inflation, yet the Vc increased less than during exercise.[28,30,31,53] Further studies are needed to clarify the relationship between increase in D_L and change in pulmonary blood flow or pressure during exercise.

pH. Lowering of pH from anaerobic metabolism during exercise was simulated by release of arterial tourniquets after 15 minutes of occluding blood flow to the lower limbs, together with the oral ingestion of ammonium chloride, 20 grams daily. This maneuver did not increase D_L.[53] When lowering of pH during exercise was prevented by hyperventilation, the increase in D_L during exercise was not altered.[53]

Lowering of Oxygen Tension in Mixed Venous Blood. Breathing 10% oxygen for 10 minutes had no significant effect on breath-holding D_L.[53]

Changes in pCO_2. Mixed venous pCO_2 was found to rise with exercise. Forster and co-workers found only a slight increase in breath-holding D_L at rest when 6.0% CO_2 was included in the inspired mixture, but a 20% increase in breath-holding D_L at rest was observed in nine subjects after breathing 7.5% CO_2 for 10 minutes.[51,72]

Rankin and his colleagues measured D_L during hypercapnia in 9 normal subjects at rest.[73] When 10% CO_2 was added to the inspired mixture used in the measurement of D_L, CO disappeared more rapidly from the lung, and D_L increased only 5% on the average after 10 seconds of breath holding. Vc was measured in 2 subjects and was

increased approximately 46.5%. After the subjects breathed a gas mixture containing 7.5% CO_2 for 10 minutes, D_L was increased an average of 24% in all subjects, and Vc was increased 112% in the one subject in whom it was studied.

Reaction Rate of CO and Hemoglobin. The rate of formation of carboxyhemoglobin may be affected by changes in the mean pO_2 of pulmonary capillary blood.[74] The reduced pO_2 of mixed venous blood during exercise should not cause more than a negligible change in the reaction rate of CO and hemoglobin since the mean capillary pO_2 is usually less than 10 mm Hg lower during exercise than at rest.[53]

Increased Pulmonary Capillary Hematocrit. The pulmonary capillary hematocrit may increase during exercise, which may, in turn, increase the rate of CO transfer. The point is entirely speculative, however, inasmuch as no relevant evidence is available in human subjects.

Increase in Lung Volume. Barocroft suggested that increased lung volume is the mechanism by which exercise increases D_L.[75] Grape and Tyler found that the steady state D_L increased when the alveolar volume increased, but the amount of increase observed was not sufficient to account for the rise which usually occurs with exercise.[76] Increase in lung volume could not be the complete explanation because D_L expressed per liter of lung volume was still significantly increased with exercise. Cadigan *et al* have shown that the alveolar volume at which the breath is held may influence the measured D_L.[77]

Venous Pump. Daly and associates showed that passive motion of the lower extremities in upright normal men decreased pressure in the saphenous vein at the ankle, and increased breath-holding D_L.[78] This effect was present in the first 10 seconds of passive leg motion. They suggested, therefore, that the venous pump increased pulmonary capillary blood volume with exercise in the upright position. The effect was not observed, however, with passive leg motion in the supine position. Systemic venous venoconstriction and displacement of blood from the periphery toward the lungs cannot be excluded.

Thus, multiple factors may be involved in increasing D_L and Vc during exercise. The most important may include: (a) the opening of previously closed capillaries or the distention of already open capillaries or both caused by increased pulmonary blood flow; (b) increased transmural pulmonary capillary pressure resulting from a slight increase in pulmonary vascular pressure and a decline in the intrapleural pressure; (c) more even distribution of perfusion in relation to ventilation; (d) increased compliance of the pulmonary vascular bed; and (e) constriction of the systemic veins associated with displacement of blood toward the lungs.

The reactivity of the D_L during exercise has been recently shown by Krumholz and associates to be dependent upon at least two separate mechanisms.[79] The rise in D_L during the first 10 seconds of exercise was attentuated or altered by changing position from upright to supine. The same response was significantly decreased by intravenous atropine or by oral reserpine administration for 7 days. The elevation of D_L later in exercise was not influenced by body position, ganglionic blockade or atropine administration, but it was reduced somewhat by oral reserpine administration. These studies suggest that the immediate and the later rise in D_L with

exercise are produced by different mechanisms. The initial rise appeared to be volume-pressure dependent, perhaps subject to the effects of peripheral pooling of blood. The later rise was independent of the initial rise and was only partly modified by a peripheral vasodilating effect.

Krumholz, King and Ross determined D_L in normal subjects before, during and soon after a period of exercise with and without pressure suit inflation.[62] D_L was increased in resting subjects by suit inflation, but less than with exercise. Exercise with suit inflation did not increase D_L more than exercise alone. Suit inflation three minutes after exercise ended, however, increased D_L to higher levels than at any other time with suit inflation alone. The pulmonary capillary bed apparently was not further dilated by vascular engorgement during exercise beyond that caused by exercise alone. Soon after exercise, however, the pulmonary capillary bed appeared to become more susceptible to passive dilatation by vascular engorgement with suit inflation.

The apparent D_{LO_2} has been noted to approach a plateau or upper limit during exercise as work load increases.[47,52] A similar plateau for the diffusing capacity for carbon monoxide has been recently observed by Johnson and co-workers.[2] D_L increased during exercise, principally because of a twofold increase in Vc and a 20% increase in D_M. As the exercise work load increased beyond that causing maximal oxygen consumption, however, no further increase in either D_L or Vc was observed. In patients with mitral stenosis, Vc rose to the same level as in normal subjects during exercise but did not exceed the normal upper limit.

The results reported by Johnson and co-workers[2] are consistent with the hypothesis that the pulmonary capillary bed approaches its maximal potential volume at peak exercise and cannot be distended more significantly. by higher capillary pressure. The maximal Vc in normal subjects and in patients with mitral stenosis agrees closely with Weibel's anatomical estimates of the maximal capacity of the pulmonary capillary bed.[80]

Table 14-5 summarizes the changes in D_L, D_M and Vc during exercise as reported by various investigators.

Respiratory Gases

Alveolar Oxygen Tension. *High Oxygen Tension.* Nairn and associates measured D_L in five normal subjects in a hyperbaric pressure chamber at 1, 3.5 and 4.8 atmospheres respectively.[81] D_L was found to decrease progressively with rising oxygen tension, accompanied by a corresponding reduction in pulmonary capillary blood flow.

TABLE 14-5   Effects of Exercise on D_L, D_M and Vc

Year	Authors	Method	Subjects	No.	Condition	D_L C	D_L E	D_M C	D_M E	Vc C	Vc E
1954	Filley *et al.*	S.S.	Normal								
				7		16.9					
				11			36.3				
1955	Bates *et al.*	S.S.	Normal	18		17.7	31.3				
1958	Lewis *et al.*	B.H.	Normal	4				69.8	100.2	64.1	75.8
1959	Turino *et al.*	S.S.	Normal								
			Males	28		14.8					
				10			23.3				
			Females	8		11.5					
				5			20.1				
			RHD								
			Males	3		19.3	27.9				
			Females	10		13.2	17.5				
1959	Ross *et al.*	S.S.	Normal	6		25.4	39.8				
		B.H.	Normal			39.8	48.9				
1960	Bannister *et al.*	B.H.	Non-Athletes	11		31.3	40.8				
			Athletes	7		36.1	46.5				
1960	Johnson *et al.*	B.H.	Normal	4				36–91	48–117	56–108	96–182*
1960	MacNamara *et al.*	S.S.	ASD	9		30.0	38.0				
1962	Newman *et al.*	B.H.	Non-Athletes	9		36.7	51.9				
			Athletes	11		40.2	62.4				
1962	Bedell and Adams	B.H.	Normal	8		28.0	34.0				
			Pregnant Women	11		23.0	28.0				
			ASD	6		40.0	45.0				
			Lung Disease	10		19.0	20.0				
1963	Rotman and Woolf	S.S.	Normal								
			Males	20		26.3	33.6				
			Females	20		14.2	26.8				
			Total	40		22.1	30.2				
1966	Miller and Johnson	B.H.	Normal	5	At TLC			78.6	82.4	89.9	173
					At FRC			50.6	56.5	102.2	117
1966	Krumholz *et al.*	B.H.	Normal	16	First 10 Sec. of Exercise						
					Seated	40.6	43.9				
					Supine	42.0	44.0				
				9	2–3 Min. after Exerc.						
					Seated	33.0	46.0				
					Supine	37.0	47.0				

C   = Control
E   = Exercise
S.S. = Steady state
B.H. = Breath holding
RHD = Rheumatic heart disease

ASD = Atrial septal defect
D_L = ml/mm Hg/min
D_M = ml/mm Hg/min
Vc = ml
All figures are mean values except for* which denote range

With rising pO_2 in the erythrocytes, few unsaturated hemoglobin molecules are available for the formation of carboxyhemoglobin, which, in turn, might limit the rate of removal of CO from the alveolar gas, decreasing the diffusing capacity for CO.

The diffusing surface and gas exchange characteristics of vessels were not affected by breathing oxygen for 10 minutes at an alveolar oxygen tension of approximately 2600 mm Hg. D_L was not changed significantly by independent variations in the partial pressure of nitrogen between 30 and 2400 mm Hg at constant alveolar oxygen tension. The changes observed were considered to result from prolonged inactivity of the subjects in the chamber than to oxygen inhalation or to increased barometric pressure *per se.*

Low Oxygen Tension. Many workers have demonstrated pulmonary vasoconstriction during acute hypoxia,[82-88] attributed largely to local effects of low oxygen tension on the vascular wall. A number of animal experiments have directly or indirectly indicated that acute hypoxia elicits post-capillary constriction,[85,88-89] but strong recent evidence has suggested that the site of vasoconstriction is actually in the precapillary pulmonary vessels.[91,92] Bergofsky and co-workers demonstrated that a decrease in the oxygen tension of mixed venous blood elicited an increase in pulmonary arterial pressure and in pulmonary vascular resistance in dogs.[92] The pressor response was shown to be a direct effect of low oxygen tension on the precapillary pulmonary vessels.

In cattle and in dogs, acute hypoxia has been shown to induce a pressure gradient from the pulmonary wedge position to the left atrium as a consequence of sphincter contraction either within the pulmonary veins or at their junction with the left atrium.[93,94]

Utilizing a rapid freezing technique, Staub measured the diameter of the pulmonary arterioles in cats receiving 100% N_2 in one lung and 100% oxygen in the other.[92] The diameter of the pulmonary arterioles was smaller in the hypoxic lung in 6 of the 8 cats, consistent with hypoxic constriction on the arterial side.

In normal subjects and in patients with cardiopulmonary disease, inhalation of low oxygen concentrations usually induces a rise in pulmonary arterial pressure without significantly altering the pulmonary wedge or left atrial pressure.[95-102] The pulmonary blood flow may be slightly increased or remain unchanged. In most instances PVR increases. In cardiac patients we have reported an increase in the pulmonary distending pressure (average of the pulmonary arterial and left atrial mean pressures) during hypoxia, associated with a decrease or no change in the pulmonary blood volume.[102] The increase in the pulmonary distending pressure was mainly pulmonary arterial pressure, with no appreciable alteration in the left atrial pressure. The discordant change in the pulmonary vascular pressure and volume was interpreted as strong evidence of active vasoconstriction of the pulmonary vascular bed. Similar findings were observed subsequently in several normal subjects. In our studies the bulk of the evidence seemed to indicate that acute hypoxia produced most of its effect on pressure by its action proximal to the pulmonary capillaries. The results agreed with those obtained in animals by Berfosky and associates[91] and by Staub.[92]

Measurement of Vc by the method of CO diffusion at low alveolar pO_2 creates a difficult problem because of uncertainty regarding the accuracy of spectroscopic or photocolorimetric determination of CO at pO_2 tensions below 100 mm Hg, when large amounts of all three pigments, oxyhemoglobin, carboxyhemoglobin and reduced hemoglobin, are present. Since the first and last molecules of CO react with hemoglobin at a kinetic rate different from that of the middle two molecules, the curve for Θ at low pO_2 levels may be suspected to be nonlinear. Thus, reasonable estimates of D_L and V_c are almost impossible at low alveolar pO_2 tension. It may be assumed that V_c and D_L probably would be decreased during acute hypoxia inasmuch as constriction of pulmonary arterioles occurs with little change in the pulmonary venous pressure. This assumption, however, would be at variance with the observations of Aviado, Reid and their respective associates, who demonstrated an increase in pulmonary capillary blood volume in dogs during acute hypoxia, utilizing a technique of measuring radioactivity from the pleural surface.[103,104]

Alveolar CO_2 Tension. Rankin, McNeill and Forster found a rise in D_L in normal subjects breathing 7.5% CO_2 in air. The pulmonary arterial pressure changed little or not at all during exposure to 5% CO_2 inhalation.[73]

Hyde, Lawson and Forster studied the effects of CO_2 on isolated perfused cat lungs.[105] Ventilation with 5 to 10% CO_2 caused significant increases in D_L (20 to 26%) and PVR (70 to 90%), regardless of whether perfusion was forward (through pulmonary arteries) or reversed (through pulmonary veins). If either pulmonary arteries or veins were perfused with blood equilibrated with 7.5 to 10% CO_2 while ventilating with room air, only PVR increased with no significant change in D_L. These workers interpreted their findings to indicate (*a*) that when the pulmonary arteries and veins are directly exposed to blood equilibrated with increased

CO_2 tension, they can constrict independently, resulting in an increase in PVR; and (*b*) that if the capillaries and downstream vessels are exposed to elevated CO_2 tension, D_L is increased.

A number of possible mechanisms may be postulated for the rise in D_L. The increased CO_2 tension may (*a*) influence alveolar surface tension and change the surface area of the capillaries; (*b*) activate axon reflexes in the lungs, opening the pulmonary capillary bed; (*c*) exert direct vasodilating action on the capillaries; (*d*) accentuate uptake of CO by erythrocytes; and (*e*) cause constriction of vessels downstream from the capillaries, which, in turn, might raise the upstream transmural pressures in the capillaries and cause an increase in V_c. The last mechanism seems likely to be the most important, if not the only one responsible. However, in man there is no clear-cut evidence that a rise in D_L is primarily caused by an increased postcapillary CO_2 tension.

In excised dog lungs, Salem and co-workers found that alveolar CO_2 may act directly on the intrapulmonary arteries and veins to reduce their compliance.[106] This finding was compatible with most of the experimental observations of others that alveolar CO_2 exerts a vasoconstrictive effect on pulmonary vessels, mainly due to contraction of the smooth muscles. The changes related to CO_2 concentration may be partly or largely due to alteration in the concentration of H^+ ions.

Forced Respiration

Valsalva Maneuver. Ross, Lord and Ley observed that the Valsalva maneuver reduced the D_L both at rest and during pressure suit inflation.[30] The maneuver compresses the pulmonary capillary bed and decreases V_c as the intrathoracic pressure increases in relation to the intracapillary pressure, *i.e.*, as net transmural capillary pressure declines. The maneuver also produces an unfavorable pressure gradient for venous return to the right ventricle, diminishing capillary blood flow and contributing to the decrease in V_c.[57]

On the other hand, Daly and Roe demonstrated an increase in D_L immediately *following* the Valsalva maneuver, accompanied by an average increase of 25% for V_c.[107] This increase was probably not related to changes in alveolar O_2 tension, alveolar CO_2 tension, alveolar volume or breath-holding time. These authors concluded that the transient increase in trans-mural net pulmonary capillary pressure which immediately follows a Valsalva maneuver increases the dimensions of the normal pulmonary capillary bed. In addition, increased rate of blood flow would be expected to result from augmented venous return to the right heart.

Mueller Maneuver. Johnson and associates reported that D_L increased during the Mueller maneuver, a change which was interpreted as reflecting passive expansion of the capillary bed as efflux of blood from the capillaries was temporarily reduced.[57] During the maneuver the decrease in intrathoracic pressure exceeds that in intracapillary pressure, resulting in a net increase in the transmural capillary pressure.

Forward Acceleration

Arterial hypoxemia has been reported in animals and man during exposure to increased gravitational stress.[108-112] The extent of this change depends upon the magnitude of stress and the duration of exposure. Reed and co-workers observed a fall in arterial saturation to 81 to 87% after 1 minute

of acceleration at 8G,[112] and Steiner and Mueller reported reduction of arterial saturation to 75% after 3 minutes of acceleration at 8G.[108] In the latter instance, approximately 40% of the total pulmonary blood flow was calculated as shunting through non-ventilated regions of lung. Wood and co-workers[113,114] reported progressively greater arterial unsaturation with more intense and more extended forward acceleration and found that breathing a high concentration of oxygen did not entirely prevent the effect. Several workers have postulated that the decreased arterial oxygen saturation associated with forward acceleration may result from distortion of pulmonary membrane tissue resulting in significant perfusion through non-ventilated regions.[109,115,116] This postulation was consonant with radiographic studies suggesting that alveoli are collapsed and capillaries congested in dependent regions during acceleration, while capillaries are distended and relatively empty in the apical regions.[113,117] Pathologic changes of similar nature were also reported in dog lungs following intense and prolonged acceleration.[108,113]

Recent advances in the use of radioactive tracers in the inspired gas as well as in the blood may make possible more quantitative localization of uneven intrapulmonary distribution during acceleration.[116]

Lindberg and collaborators measured cardiac output, heart rate, mean aortic pressure, stroke volume, peripheral vascular pressure and right atrial pressure in 6 healthy subjects during forward acceleration.[115] Cardiac output, heart rate, mean aortic pressure and total peripheral resistance increased slightly, associated with a decrease in stroke volume. The most striking hemodynamic alteration was the increase in mean right atrial pressure, which averaged more than 20 mm Hg.

Zeckman and Mueller found a decrease in D_L during forward acceleration at 4G.[118] They explained the reduction in D_L on the basis of decreased lung volume and by an alteration in distribution of blood flow from front to back along the vector of the initial force. Power and associates measured D_L and effective pulmonary capillary blood flow ($\dot{Q}c$) simultaneously after forward acceleration in 4 subjects.[116] After 1 minute of forward acceleration at 8G, the average D_L had decreased 35% from a control value of 33.7 to 21.5 ml/min/mm Hg, and the average $\dot{Q}c$ had also decreased 35% from a control value of 12.9 to 8.2 liters/min. The changes in both parameters were statistically significant. D_L and $\dot{Q}c$ returned approximately to the initial levels within 8 minutes after cessation of acceleration in 3 of 4 subjects.

Pregnancy

Krumholz, Echt and Ross determined D_L and Vc in 11 women during early and late pregnancy.[119] The mean D_L and Vc in the third trimester were not different from corresponding mean values in the first trimester, despite the increased cardiac output and circulating blood volume in the last trimester. Such observations support the contention that Vc is more pressure-volume than flow dependent.

In our laboratory measurements of D_L and Vc were made in a series of 8 pregnant women. The data are summarized in Table 14-6. Although there was some decrease in both D_L and Vc during the third trimester as compared with those during the first trimester of pregnancy, the changes were statistically not significant.

Miscellaneous Conditions

Apprehension. Cinkotai, Thompson and Guyatt studied D_L in 10 students 1 hour before and 1 hour after announcement of a final examination.[120] After the results were known, the mean D_L fell 7.7% and the mean systolic blood pressure decreased 8.2%. The reduction in both D_L and blood pressure was thought to result from reduction in the release of epinephrine and possibly norepinephrine.

Diurnal Variation. Cinkotai and Thompson measured D_L in 24 normal subjects at 2-hour intervals from 9:30 a.m. to 9:30 p.m.[121] D_L declined progressively at a rate of 1.2% to 2.2%/hour.

TABLE 14-6 D_L, D_M and Vc in Eight Normal Women during Pregnancy and Two Months after Delivery

Condition		D_L per			D_M per			Vc per		
		$M^2(BSA)$	TLC	$Kg(BW)$	$M^2(BSA)$	TLC	$Kg(BW)$	$M^2(BSA)$	TLC	$Kg(BW)$
Pregnancy										
1st trimester	mean	15	5.2	0.45	46	15	1.28	35	12	0.98
	range	12–16	4.5–7.1	0.33–0.61	24–81	8–26	0.46–2.17	24–57	8–15	0.66–1.19
2nd trimester	mean	14	5.2	0.39	33	12	0.93	35	13	0.96
	range	12–17	4.5–6.1	0.33–0.46	19–53	7–16	0.50–1.48	26–43	8–16	0.73–1.14
3rd trimester	mean	13	4.7	0.33	33	12	0.85	31	12	0.80
	range	11–15	4.2–5.5	0.26–0.39	21–43	8–15	0.61–1.15	27–40	9–14	0.67–1.03
Two months	mean	15	5.2	0.43	33	12	0.99	37	13	1.03
post partum	range	12–17	4.6–5.9	0.31–0.54	24–43	10–16	0.79–1.24	32–44	11–15	0.79–1.34

BSA = Body surface area
TLC = Total lung capacity
BW = Body weight
Other symbols and abbreviations are identical to those used in Table 14-1

This result could not be explained by initial apprehension, difference in measurement technique or posture. The change in D_L appeared to be a diurnal rhythm resembling that in hematocrit and urinary catecholamine excretion. The authors suggested that fluctuation in the internal release of catecholamines might play a part in producing the hourly change in D_L.

Smoking. Chosy, Gee and Rankin studied the effects of cigarette smoking on D_L.[122] In 68 non-smokers the mean D_L was 31.1 ± 8.3, whereas in 58 smokers it was 25.9 ± 5.9. The difference was significant at the 1% level of confidence. In the absence of a corresponding difference in expiratory flow rates, the authors concluded that the reduction in D_L was physiologic evidence of pulmonary parenchymal change due to smoking.

Effects of Pharmacologic Agents

Numerous publications describe the actions of various pharmacologic agents on the pulmonary circulation in man and animals, but information concerning the effects of pharmacologic agents on either D_L or V_c is scanty. For more complete understanding of the pharmacology of pulmonary circulation, the reader is referred to Aviado's excellent recent treatise *The Lung Circulation*.[123]

5-Hydroxytryptamine (Serotonin). Many investigators have demonstrated that 5-hydroxytryptamine produces local pulmonary vasoconstriction in animals.[124-128] Gilbert and co-workers reported significant pulmonary arterial and venous constriction and increase in lung weight during infusion of 5-hydroxytryptamine.[125] The pulmonary venous constrictor effect was subsequently demonstrated by Aviado.[128] Other workers, however, considered the possibility of constriction at the junction between the pulmonary veins and the left atrium.[129,130] Duke and Stedeford were the first to study the effect of constant infusion of 5-hydroxytryptamine on diffusing capacity for oxygen in cats.[131] They found that D_{LO_2} fell during the infusion and continued to decline afterward. Recently, Young and co-workers studied 5-hydroxytryptamine infusion in dogs and reported an increase in V_c (average 29%) associated with an increase in pulmonary arterial pressure and no appreciable change in the systemic arterial and left atrial pressures.[132] Intrapleural and intrapulmonary pressures, airway resistance, lung volume, left ventricular diastolic pressure, and alveolar CO_2 tension were not significantly affected. Direct injury to the capillaries by the drug was unlikely inasmuch as V_c returned to control values after the infusion of 5-hydroxytryptamine was discontinued. The authors considered findings consistent with the hypothesis that 5-hydroxytryptamine produced constriction at some point in the pulmonary venous segment.

In man, the infusion of 5-hydroxytryptamine caused inconsistent effects on pulmonary arterial pressure, although vasoconstriction of the small pulmonary arteries could not be entirely excluded.[133,134]

Acetylcholine. In normal subjects and in patients with cardiopulmonary disease, acetylcholine infused into the right side of the heart or pulmonary artery has been found to cause a reduction in pulmonary arterial pressure accompanied by a slight increase or no appreciable change in pulmonary blood flow.[135-152] In patients with cardiac disease we have reported an increase in pulmonary blood volume accompanying the decline in pulmonary arterial

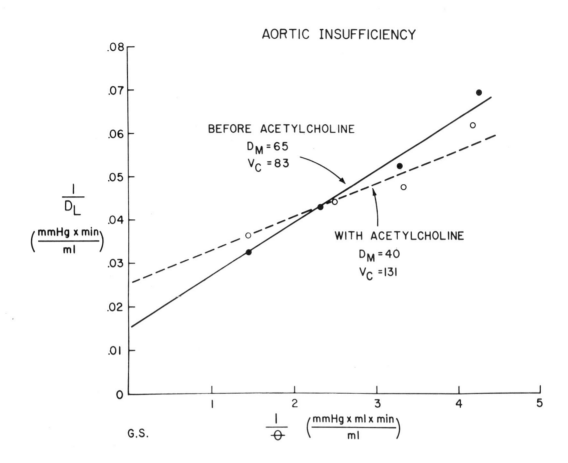

Figure 14-1. The effect of acetycholine infused into the main pulmonary artery of a patient with aortic insufficiency at a rate of 4 mg per minute. There was an increase in the pulmonary capillary blood volume (Vc), accompanied by a decrease in pulmonary arterial pressure.

pressure.[102,153] We have measured D_L, D_M, and Vc before and during infusion of acetylcholine in several such patients. While·the pulmonary arterial pressures decreased as expected, Vc increased moderately despite a smaller decline in D_M (Figure· 14-1).

The pulmonary vascular actions of acetylcholine in animals have not been conclusive. Pulmonary arterial pressure was reduced only if the dose of acetylcholine was large enough to slow the heart rate.[154,155] This reduction most likely resulted from a decrease in cardiac output similar to that produced

by vagal stimulation. On the other hand, if the dose injected was not large enough to slow the heart rate, pulmonary arterial and sometimes pulmonary venous pressure increased, probably as a result of pulmonary vasoconstriction.[155,156] Recently, Rudolph and Scarpelli reported ipsilateral pulmonary arterial constriction in unanesthetized dogs following administration of acetylcholine to one pulmonary artery.[157]

Atropine. Berry and Corten and their respective associates reported an increase in heart rate and cardiac index and a decrease in right atrial pressure and stroke index following administration of atropine in man.[158,159] Subsequently, Daly and co-workers confirmed these findings and also observed a decrease in pulmonary arterial pressure, D_L, Vc and pulmonary blood volume.[7,160] Inasmuch as atropine has been found not to affect the intrapleural pressure, a reduction in the transmural pulmonary capillary pressure would be expected.

Positive pressure breathing following atropine administration caused a further reduction in D_L and Vc, although the changes were small and not statistically significant. Inflation of the pressure suit after atropine increased the central vascular pressure, D_L and Vc much less than during inflation before atropine. These observations strongly suggested redistribution of blood away from the lung, probably into an area where it was not mobilized effectively by pressure suit inflation.[7]

Although an increase in anatomical dead space and a decrease in airway resistance were observed,[7,161] these changes were not due to altered distribution of ventilation or change in the lung volume. A specific effect of atropine on the pulmonary vasculature could not be ruled out, however, resulting in an increase in the compliance of the pulmonary vascular reservoir.

Trimethaphan (Arfonad). As mentioned in a previous section, Lewis and associates reported a decrease in Vc during head-up tilt in man.[17] Infusion of trimethaphan, a ganglionic blocking agent, also reduced Vc in the recumbent position and further accentuated the decrease in Vc during head-up tilt. D_M did not change significantly during these procedures. Krumholz and co-workers demonstrated a proportionate decrease in D_L at rest and during exercise after administration of trimethaphan.[79] Studies in our laboratory

supported these results by demonstrating a decrease in pulmonary blood volume and pulmonary distending pressure in patients with cardiac disease during the administration of hexamethonium, another ganglionic blocking agent.[153] This agent caused a striking decrease in Vc and pulmonary arterial and pulmonary wedge pressures in a patient with mitral stenosis and pulmonary hypertension (Figure 14-2).

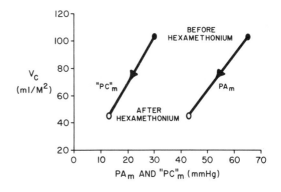

Figure 14-2. The effect of intravenous administation of 8 mg of hexamethonium in a patient with mitral stenosis and pulmonary hypertension. There was a decrease in pulmonary capillary blood volume (Vc), pulmonary arterial mean pressure (PAm), and pulmonary wedge mean pressure ("PC"m).

These changes were considered to be passive in nature, inasmuch as pulmonary vascular pressure and volume changed concordantly.[153] The underlying mechanism was most likely a movement of blood from the pulmonary vascular bed to the peripheral vessels secondary to peripheral venous dilatation.

Norepinephrine. In animals and in man pulmonary arterial and wedge pressures both increased following infusion of norepinephrine.[162-168] The drug may constrict the precapillary sphincters of the pulmonary vessels, although no convincing demonstration of this action has been reported.[169] Rudolph and Scarpelli observed local pulmonary vasoconstriction in unanesthetized dogs following administration of epinephrine.[157] During infusion of norepinephrine, blood volume changes in animal lungs have been inconsistent.[170,171]

According to Lewis and co-workers, infusion of norepinephrine in normal subjects did not change Vc in the recumbent position, although D_M increased.[17] The decrease in Vc usually observed during head-up tilt was almost entirely abolished by norepinephrine. These observations were interpreted as evidence of active vasomotion of the pulmonary arterioles and capillaries with a decrease in pulmonary capillary volume independent of change in transmural pressure.

Isoproterenol (Isuprel). Isoproterenol in man primarily causes pulmonary vasodilation, cardiac stimulation and bronchodilation.[123] In general, isoproterenol infusion results in a decrease in pulmonary arterial pressure and an increase in cardiac output in most normal subjects as well as in patients with cardiopulmonary disease.[176-181] An increase in pulmonary blood volume and a decrease in left ventricular diastolic, left atrial and pulmonary arterial pressures in most patients with cardiac disease have been reported from our laboratory.[182] We would expect D_L and Vc that would be increased during isoproterenol infusion.

Ross and Eller observed no further increase in Vc in isoproterenol infusion during pressure suit inflation.[183]

REFERENCES

1. McCredie, R.M., Lovejoy, F.W., and Yu, P.N.: Pulmonary diffusing capacity and pulmonary capillary blood volume in patients with intracardiac shunts. J. Lab. Clin. Med., *63*, 914, 1964.

2. Johnson, R.L., Taylor, H.F., and Lawson, W.H.: Maximal diffusing capacity of the lung for carbon monoxide. J. Clin. Invest., *44*, 349, 1965.

3. Roughton, F.J.W., and Forster, R.E.: Relative importance of diffusion and chemical reaction rates in determining rate of exchange of gases in the human lung, with special reference to true diffusing capacity of pulmonary membrane and volume of blood in the lung capillaries. J. Appl. Physiol., *11*, 290, 1957.

4. McNeill, R.S., Rankin, J., and Forster, R.E.: The diffusing capacity of the pulmonary membrane and the pulmonary capillary blood volume in cardiopulmonary disease. Clin. Sci., *17*, 465, 1958.

5. Lewis, B.M., Lin, T.H., Noe, F.E., and Komisaruk, R.: The measurement of pulmonary capillary blood volume and pulmonary membrane diffusing capacity in normal subjects; the effects of exercise and position. J. Clin. Invest., *37*, 1061, 1958.

6. Ross, J.C., Maddock, G.E., and Ley, G.D.: Effect of pressure suit inflation on pulmonary capillary blood volume. J. Appl. Physiol., *16*, 674, 1961.

7. Daly, W.J., Ross, J.C., and Behnke, R.H.: The effect of changes in the pulmonary vascular bed produced by atropine, pulmonary engorgement, and positive pressure breathing on diffusing and mechanical properties of the lung. J. Clin. Invest., *42*, 1083, 1963.

8. Steiner, S.H., Frayser, R., and Ross, J.C.: Alterations in pulmonary diffusing capacity and pulmonary capillary blood volume with negative pressure breathing. J. Clin. Invest., *44*, 1623, 1965.

9. Miller, J.M., and Johnson, R.L.: Effect of lung inflation on pulmonary diffusing capacity at rest and exercise. J. Clin. Invest., *45*, 493, 1966.

10. Flatley, F.J., Constantine, H., McCredie R.M., and Yu, P.N.: Pulmonary diffusing capacity and pulmonary capillary blood volume in normal subjects and in cardiac patients. Am. Heart J., *64*, 159, 1962.

11. Daly, W.J., Giammona, S.T., Ross, J.C., and Feigenbaum, H.: Effects of pulmonary vascular congestion on postural changes in the

perfusion and filling of pulmonary vascular bed. J. Clin. Invest., *43*, 68, 1964.

12. Daly, W.J., Giammona, S.T., and Ross, J.C.: The pressure-volume relationship of the normal pulmonary capillary bed. J. Clin. Invest., *44*, 1261, 1965.

13. Gazioglu, K., and Yu, P.N.: Pulmonary blood volume and pulmonary capillary blood volume in valvular heart disease. Circulation, *35*, 701, 1967.

14. Krumholz, R.A.: Pulmonary membrane diffusing capacity and pulmonary capillary blood volume. An appraisal of their clinical usefulness. Am. Rev. Resp. Dis., 94, 195, 1966.

15. Constantine, H., Flatley, F.J., Gazioglu, K., and Yu, P.N.: Unpublished data.

16. McCredie, R.M.: The diffusing characteristics and pressure volume relationships of the pulmonary capillary bed in mitral valve disease. J. Clin. Invest., *43*, 2279, 1964.

17. Lewis, B.M., McElroy, W.T., Hayford-Welsing, E.J., and Samberg, L.C.: The effects of body position, ganglionic blockage and norepinephrine on the pulmonary capillary bed. J. Clin. Invest., *39*, 1345, 1960.

18. Cohn, J.E., Carroll, D.J., Armstrong, B.W., Shepard, R.H., and Riley, R.L.: Maximal diffusing capacity of the lung in normal subjects of different ages. J. Appl. Physiol., *6*, 588, 1954.

19. Donevan, R.E., Palmer, W.H., Varvis, C.J., and Bates, D.V.: Influence of age on pulmonary diffusing capacity. J. Appl. Physiol., *14*, 483, 1959.

20. McGrath, M., and Thomson, M.L.: The effect of age, body size and lung volume change on alveolar-capillary permeability and diffusing capacity in man. J. Physiol., *146*, 572, 1959.

21. Rankin, J., Gee, J.B.L., and Chosy, L.W.: The influence of age and smoking on pulmonary diffusing capacity in healthy subjects. Med. Thorac., *22*, 366, 1965.

22. Hanson, J.J., and Tabakin, B.S.: Steady state carbon monoxide diffusing capacity in normal females. J. Appl. Physiol., *16*, 839, 1961.

23. Hamer, N.A.J.: The effect of age on the components of the pulmonary diffusing capacity. Clin. Sci., *23*, 85, 1962.

24. Bucci, G., Cook, C.D., and Barrie, H.: Studies of respiratory physiology in children. V. Total lung diffusion, diffusing capacity of pulmonary membrane and pulmonary capillary blood volume in normal subjects from 7 to 40 years of age. J. Pediatrics, *58*, 820, 1961.

25. Ogilvie, C.M., Forster, R.E., Blakemore, W.S., and Morton, J.W.: A standardized breath holding technique for the clinical measurement of the diffusing capacity of the lung for carbon monoxide. J. Clin. Invest., *36*, 1, 1957.

26. Bates, D.V., and Pearce, J.F.: The pulmonary diffusing capacity. A comparison of methods of measurement and a study of the effect of body position. J. Physiol., *132*, 232, 1956.

27. Newman, F.: The effect of change in posture on alveolar capillary diffusion and capillary-blood volume in the human lung. J. Physiol., *162*, 29, 1962.

28. Bondurant, S., Hickam, J.B., and Isley, J.K.: Pulmonary and circulatory effects of acute pulmonary vascular engorgement in normal subjects. J. Clin. Invest., *36*, 59, 1957.

29. Lewis, B.M., Forster, R.E., and Beckman, E.L.: Effect of inflation of a pressure suit on pulmonary diffusing capacity in man. J. Appl. Physiol., *12*, 57, 1958.

30. Ross, J.C., Lord, T.H., and Ley, G.D.: Effect of pressure-suit inflation on pulmonary diffusing capacity. J. Appl. Physiol., *15*, 843, 1960.

31. Ross, J.C., Ley, G.D., Coburn, R.F., Eller, J.L., and Forster, R.E.: Influence of pressure suit inflation on pulmonary diffusing capacity in man. J. Appl. Physiol., *17*, 259, 1962.

32. Fenn, W.O., Otis, A.B., Rahn, H., Chadwick, L.E., and Hegnauer, A.H.: Displacement of blood from the lungs by pressure breathing. Am. J. Physiol., *151*, 258, 1947.

33. Coates, J.E., Snidal, D.P., and Shepard, R.H.: Effect of negative intraalveolar pressure on pulmonary diffusing capacity. J. Appl. Physiol., *15*, 372, 1960.

34. Zeckman, F., and Mueller, G.: Effect of forward acceleration and negative pressure breathing on pulmonary diffusion. J. Appl. Physiol., *17*, 909, 1962.

35. Hubay, C.A., Waltz, R.C., Brecker, G.A., Praglin, J., and Hingson, R.A.: Circulatory dynamics of venous return during positive-negative pressure respiration. Anesthesiol., *15*, 445, 1954.

36. Ernsting, J.: The compliance of the human lungs during positive and negative pressure breathing. J. Physiol.(abstract), *144*, 14, 1958.

37. Kilburn, K.H., and Seiker, H.O.: Hemodynamic effects of continuous positive and negative pressure breathing in normal man. Circ. Res., *8*, 660, 1960.

38. Holt, J.P.: The effect of positive and negative intrathoracic pressure on cardiac output and venous pressure in the dog. Am. J. Physiol., *142*, 594, 1944.

39. Ting, E.Y., Hong, S.K., and Rahn, H.: Cardiovascular responses of man during negative pressure breathing. J. Appl. Physiol., *15*, 557, 1960.

40. Lenfant, C., and Howell, B.J.: Cardiovascular adjustments in dogs during continuous pressure breathing. J. Appl. Physiol., *15*, 425, 1960.

41. Rosenberg, E., and Forster, R.E.: Changes in diffusing capacity of isolated cat lungs with blood pressure and flow. J. Appl. Physiol., *15*, 883, 1960.

42. Duke, H.N., and Rouse, W.: Pulmonary diffusing capacity for CO and hemodynamic changes in isolated perfused cats' lungs. J. Appl. Physiol., *18*, 83, 1963.

43. Lawson, W.H., Duke, H.N., Hyde, R.W., and Forster, R.E.: Relationship of pulmonary arterial and venous pressure to diffusing capacity. J. Appl. Physiol., *19*, 381, 1964.

44. Zeckman, F.W., Musgrave, E.S., Mains, R.C., and Cohn, J.: Respiratory mechanism and pulmonary diffusing capacity with lower body negative pressure. J. Appl. Physiol., *22*, 247, 1967.

45. Krogh, M.: Diffusion of gases through the lungs of man. J. Physiol., *49*, 271, 1915.

46. Lilienthal, J.L., Riley, R.L., Proemmel, D.D., and Franke, R.E.: An experimental analysis in man of the oxygen pressure gradient from alveolar air to arterial blood during rest and exercise at sea level and at altitude. Am. J. Physiol., *147*, 199, 194.,

47. Riley, R.L., Shepard, R.H., Cohn, J.E., Carroll, D.G., and Armstrong, B.W.: Maximal diffusing capacity of the lungs. J. Appl. Physiol., *6*, 573, 1954.

48. Filley, G.F., MacIntosh, D.J., and Wright, G.W.: Carbon monoxide uptake and the pulmonary diffusion capacity in normal subjects at rest and during exercise. J. Clin. Invest., *33*, 530, 1954.

49. Bates, D.V., Boucot, N.G., and Dormer, A.E.: The pulmonary diffusing capacity in normal subjects. J. Physiol., *129*, 237, 1955.

50. Cugell, D.W., Marks, A., Ellicott, M.F., Badger, T.L., and Gaensler, E.A.: Carbon monoxide diffusing capacity during steady exercise. Comparison of physiologic and histologic findings in patients with pulmonary fibrosis and granulomatoses. Am. Rev. Tuberc., *74*, 317, 1956.

51. Forster, R.E.: Exchange of gases between alveolar air and pulmonary capillary blood: pulmonary diffusing capacity. Physiol. Rev., *37*, 391, 1957.

52. Shepard, R.H., Varnauskas, E., Martin, H.B., White, H.A., Permutt, S., Cotes, J.E., and Riley, R.L.: Relationship between cardiac output and apparent diffusing capacity of the lung in normal men during treadmill exercise. J. Appl. Physiol., *13*, 205, 1958.

53. Ross, J.C., Frayser, R., and Hickam, J.B.: A study of the mechanism by which exercise increases the pulmonary diffusing capacity for carbon monoxide. J. Clin. Invest., *38*, 916, 1959.

54. Turino, G.M., Brandfonbrener, M., and Fishman, A.P.: The effect of changes in ventilation and pulmonary blood flow on the diffusing capacity of the lungs. J. Clin. Invest., *38*, 1186, 1959.

55. Bannister, R.G., Cotes, J.E., Jones, R.S., and Meade, F.: Pulmonary diffusing capacity on exercise in athletes and nonathletic subjects. J. Physiol., *152*, 66, 1960.

56. MacNamara, J., Prime, F.J., and Sinclair, J.D.: The increase in diffusing capacity of the lungs on exercise. An experimental and clinical study. Lancet, *1*, 404, 1960.

57. Johnson, R.L., Spicer, W.S., Bishop, J.M., and Forster, R.E.: Pulmonary capillary blood volume flow and diffusing capacity during exercise. J. Appl. Physiol., *15*, 893, 1960.

58. Bedell, G.N., and Adams, R.W.: Pulmonary diffusing capacity during rest and exercise. A study of normal persons and persons with atrial septal defects, pregnancy and pulmonary disease. J. Clin. Invest., *41*, 1904, 1962.

59. Newman, F., Smalley, B.F., and Thomson, M.L.: Effect of exercise, body and lung size on CO diffusion in athletes and nonathletes. J. Appl. Physiol., *17*, 649, 1962.

60. Ross, J.C., Reinhart, R.W., Boxell, J.F., and King, L.H.: Relationship of increased breath-holding diffusing capacity to ventilation in exercise. J. Appl. Physiol., *18*, 794, 1963.

61. Rotman, H.H., and Woolf, C.R.: The diffusing capacity of the lungs at rest and on exercise in adults with atrial or ventricular septal defects. Dis. Chest, *43*, 613, 1963.

62. Krumholz, R.A., King, L.H., and Ross, J.C.: Effect of pulmonary vascular engorgement on D_L during and immediately after exercise. J. Appl. Physiol., *18*, 1180, 1963.

63. Krumholz, R.A., and Ross, J.C.: Effect of atropine and reserpine on pulmonary diffusing capacity during exercise in man. J. Appl. Physiol., *19*, 465, 1964.

64. Roughton, F.J.W.: The average time spent by the blood in the human lung capillary and its relation to the rates of CO uptake and elimination in man. Am. J. Physiol., *143*, 621. 1945.

65. Bjure, J.: Pulmonary diffusing capacity for carbon monoxide in relation to cardiac output

in man. Scand. J. Clin. Lab. Invest., *17*, Suppl. 81, 1965.

66. Riley, R.L., Himmelstein, A., Motley, H.L., Weiner, H.M., and Cournand, A.: Studies of pulmonary circulation at rest and during exercise in normal individuals and in patients with chronic pulmonary disease. Am. J. Physiol., *152*, 372, 1948.

67. Hickam, J.B., and Cargill, W.H.: Effect of exercise on cardiac output and pulmonary arterial pressure in normal persons and in patients with cardiovascular disease and pulmonary emphysema. J. Clin. Invest., *27*, 10, 1948.

68. Dexter, L., Whittenberger, J.L., Haynes, F.W., Goodale, W.T., Gorlin, R., and Sawyer, C.G.: Effect of exercise on circulatory dynamics of normal individuals. J. Appl. Physiol., *3, 439*, 1951.

69. Slonim, N.B., Ravin, A., Balchum, O.J., and Dressler, S.H.: The effect of mild exercise in the supine position on the pulmonary arterial pressure of five normal human subjects. J. Clin. Invest., *33*, 1022, 1954.

70. Donald, K.W., Bishop, J.M., Cumming, G., and Wade, O.L.: The effect of exercise on the cardiac output and circulatory dynamics of normal subjects. Clin. Sci., *14*, 37, 1955.

71. Sancetta, S. M., and Rakita, L.: Response of pulmonary artery pressure and total pulmonary resistance of untrained, convalescent man to prolonged mild steady state exercise. J. Clin. Invest., *36*, 1138, 1957.

72. Forster, R.E., Fowlar, W.S., Bates, D.V., and Van Lingen, B.: The absorption of carbon monoxide by the lungs during breath holding. J. Clin. Invest., *33*, 1135, 1954.

73. Rankin, J., McNeill, R.S., and Forster, R.E.: Influence of increased alveolar CO_2 tension on pulmonary diffusing capacity for CO in man. J. Appl. Physiol., *15*, 543, 1960.

74. Forster, R.E., Roughton, F.J.W., Cander, L., Briscoe, W.A., and Kreuzer, F.: Apparent pulmonary diffusing capacity for CO at varying alveolar O_2 tension. J. Appl. Physiol., *11*, 277, 1957.

75. Barcroft, J.: *Features in the Architecture of Physiological Function,* London, Cambridge University Press, 1938.

76. Grape, B., and Tyler, J.: The effect of altering lung volume and pulmonary diffusing of carbon monoxide. Clin. Res., *6*, 313, 1958.

77. Cadigan, J.B., Marks, A., Ellicott, M.F., Jones, R.H., and Gaensler, E.A.: An analysis of factors affecting the measurement of pulmonary diffusing capacity by the single breath method. J. Clin. Invest., *40*, 1495, 1961.

78. Daly, W.J., Krumholz, R.A., and Ross, J.C.: The venous pump in the legs as a determinant of pulmonary capillary filling. J. Clin. Invest., *44*, 271, 1965.

79. Krumholz, R.A., Brashear, R.E., Daly, W.J., and Ross, J.C.: Physiological alterations in the pulmonary capillary bed at rest and during exercise. The effect of body position and trimethaphan camphorsulfonate. Circulation, *33*, 872, 1966.

80. Weibel, E.R.; *Morphometry of the Human Lung,* New York, Academic Press, Inc., 1963. p. 86.

81. Nairn, J.R., Power, G.G., Hyde, R.W., Forster, R.E., Lembertsen, C.J., and Dickson, J.: Diffusing capacity and pulmonary capillary blood flow at hyperbaric pressures. J. Clin. Invest., *44*, 1591, 1965.

82. Von Euler, U.S. and Liljestrand, G.: Observations on the pulmonary arterial blood pressure in the cat. Acta Physiol. Scand., *12*, 301, 1946.

83. Logaros, G.: Further studies of the pulmonary arterial blood pressure. Acta Physiol. Scand., *14*, 120, 1947,

84. Duke, H. N.: Pulmonary vasomotor responses of isolated perfused cat lungs to anoxia and hypercapnia. Quart. J. Exp. Physiol., *36*, 75, 1951.

85. Nisell, O.I.: The influence of blood gases on the pulmonary vessels of the cat. Acta Physiol. Scand., *23*, 85, 1951.

86. Stroud, R.C., and Rahn, H.: Effect of O_2 and CO_2 tensions upon the resistance pulmonary blood vessels. Am. J. Physiol., *172*, 211, 1953.

87. Rahn, H., and Bahnson, H.T.: Effect of unilateral hypoxia on gas exchange and calculated pulmonary blood flow in each lung. J. Appl. Physiol., *6*, 105, 1953.

88. Lloyd, T.C.: Effect of alveolar hypoxia on pulmonary vascular resistance. J. Appl. Physiol., *19*, 1086, 1964.

89. Duke, H.N., and Killick, E.M.: Pulmonary vasoconstriction to anoxia: its site of action. J. Physiol., *117*, 78, 1952.

90. Fishman, A.P.: Respiratory gases in the regulation of the pulmonary circulation. Physiol. Rev., *41*, 214, 1961.

91. Bergofsky, E.II., Bass, B.G., Ferretti, R., and Fishman, A.P.: Pulmonary vasoconstriction in response to precapillary hypoxemia. J. Clin. Invest., *42*, 1201, 1963.

92. Staub, N.C.: Site of action of hypoxia on the pulmonary vasculature. Fed. Proc., *22*, 463, 1963.

93. Rivera-Estrada, C., Saltzman, P.W,. Singer, D., and Katz, L.N.: Action of hypoxia on pulmonary vasculature. Circ. Res., 6, 10, 1958.

94. Tsagaris, T.J., Kuida, H., and Hecht, H.H.: Evidence for pulmonary vaso-constriction in Brisket disease. Fed. Proc., 21, 108, 1962.

95. Motley, H.L., Cournand, A., Werkö, L., Himmelstein, A., and Dresdale, D.: Influence of short periods of induced acute anoxia upon pulmonary artery pressures in man. Am. J. Physiol., 150, 315, 1947.

96. Westcott, R.N., Fowler, N.O., Scott, R.C., Hauenstein, V.D., and McGuire, J.: Anoxia and pulmonary vascular resistance. J. Clin. Invest., 30, 957, 1951.

97. Doyle, J.T., Wilson, J.S., and Warren, J.V.: Pulmonary vascular responses to short-time hypoxia in human subjects. Circulation, 5, 263, 1952.

98. Fishman, A.P., McClement, J., Himmelstein, A., and Cournand, A.: Effects of acute anoxia on the circulation and respiration in patients with chronic pulmonary disease studied during the "steady state." J. Clin. Invest., 31, 770, 1952.

99. Siebens, A.A., Smith, R.E., and Storey, C.F.: Effect of hypoxia on pulmonary vessels in man. Am. J. Physiol., 180, 428, 1955.

100. Yu, P.N., Beatty, D.C., Lovejoy, F.W., Nye, R.E., and Joos, H.A.: Hemodynamic effects of acute hypoxia in patients with mitral stenosis. Am. Heart J., 52, 683, 1956.

101. Fishman, A.P., Fritts, H.W., and Cournand, A.: Effects of acute hypoxia and exercise in the pulmonary circulation. Circulation, 22, 204, 1960.

102. Yu, P.N., Glick, G., Schreiner, B.F., and Murphy, G.W.: Effects of acute hypoxia on the pulmonary vascular bed of patients with acquired heart disease. With special reference to the demonstration of active vasomotion. Circulation, 27, 541, 1963.

103. Reid, A.: Cited from Jekines. M.T., Jones, R.F., Wilson, B., and Moyer, C.A,: Congestive atelectasis—a complication of the intravenous infusion of fluids. Ann. Surg., 132, 342, 1950.

104. Aviado, D.M., Cerletti, A., Alanis, J., Bulle, P.H., and Schmidt, C.F.: Effects of anoxia on pressure, resistance and blood (P^{32}) volume of pulmonary vessels. Am. J. Physiol., 169, 460, 1962.

105. Hyde, R.W., Lawson, W.H., and Forster, R.E.: Influence of carbon dioxide on pulmonary vasculature. J. Appl. Physiol., 19, 734, 1964.

106. Salem, E.S., Permutt, S., Riley, R.L., and Johnson, J.W.C.: Effect of respiratory gases on compliance of intrapulmonary arteries and veins. J. Appl. Physiol., 19, 1202, 1964.

107. Daly, J.J., and Roe, J.W.: The effect of a Valsalva maneuver on the pulmonary diffusing capacity for carbon monoxide in man. Clin. Sci., 23, 405. 1962.

108. Steiner, S.H., and Mueller, G.C.E.: Pulmonary arterial shunting in man during forward acceleration. J. Appl. Physiol., 16, 1081, 1961.

109. Wood, E.H., Sutterer, W.F., Marshall, H.W., Lindberg, E.F., and Headley, R.N.: Effect of headward and forward acceleration on the cardiovascular system. Wright Air Develop. Div. Tech. Report, AM RL-TDR-60-634, 1961.

110. Barr, P.O.: Hypoxemia in man induced by prolonged acceleration. Acta Physiol. Scand. 54, 128, 1962.

111. Nolan, C.A., Marshall, H.W., Cronin, L., and Wood, E.H.: The effect of forward acceleration on arterial oxygen saturation. Physiologist, 4, 83, 1961.

112. Reed, J.H., Burgess, B.F., and Sandler, H.: Effects on arterial oxygen saturation of positive pressure breathing acceleration. Aerospace Med., 35, 238, 1964.

113. Wood, E.H., Nolan, A.C., Marshall, H.W., Cronin, L., and Sutterer, W.F.: Decreases in arterial oxygen saturation as an indicator of the stress imposed on the cardiorespiratory system by forward acceleration. Wright Air Develop. Div. Tech. Report, AM-RL-RDR-63-104, 1963.

114. Wood, E.H., Nolan, A.C., Donald, E.E., and Cronin, L.: Influence of acceleration on pulmonary physiology. Fed. Proc., 22, 1024, 1963.

115. Lindberg, E.F., Marshall, H.W., Sutterer, W.F., McQuire, T.F., and Wood, E.H.: Studies of cardic output and circulatory pressures in human beings during forward acceleration. Aerospace Med., 33, 81, 1962.

116. Power, G.G., Hyde, R.W., Sever, R.J., Hoppin, F.G., and Nairn, J.R.: Pulmonary diffusing capacity and capillary blood flow during forward acceleration. J. Appl. Pysiol., 20, 1199, 1965.

117. Hershgold, E.J.: Roentgenographic study of human subjects during transverse acceleration. Aerospace Med., 31, 213, 1960.

118. Zechman, F.W., Cherniack, N.S., and Hyde, A.S.: Ventilation response to forward acceleration. J. Appl. Physiol., 15, 907, 1960.

119. Krumholz, R.A., Echt, E.R., and Ross, J.C.: Pulmonary diffusing capacity, capillary blood volume, lung volumes and mechanics of ventilation in early and late pregnancy. J. Lab. Clin. Med., 63, 648, 1964.

120. Cinkotai, F.F., Thompson, M.L., and Guyatt, A.R.: Effect of apprehension on pulmonary diffusing capacity in man. J. Appl. Physiol., *21*, 534, 1966.

121. Cinkotai, F.F., and Thompson, M.L.: Diurnal variation in pulmonary diffusing capacity for carbon monoxide. J. Appl. Physiol., *21*, 539, 1966.

122. Chosy, L., Gee, J.B.L., and Rankin, J.L.: The effects of cigarette smoking on the pulmonary diffusing capacity. Clin. Res., *11*, 301, 1963.

123. Aviado, D.M.: *The Lung Circulation*, vols. I and II, London & New York, Pergamon Press, 1965.

124. Gaddum, J.H., Hebb, C.O., Silver, A., and Swan, A.A.: 5-Hydroxytryptamine. Pharmacological action and destruction in perfused lungs. Quart. J. Exp. Physiol., *38*, 255, 1953.

125. Gilbert, R.P., Hinshaw, L.B., Kuida, H., and Visscher, M.B.: Effects of histamine, 5-hydroxytryptamine and epinephrine on pulmonary hemodynamics with particular reference to arterial and venous segment resistances. Am. J. Physiol., *194*, 165, 1958.

126. Rose, J.C., and Lazaro, E.J.: Pulmonary vascular responses to serotonin and effects of certain serotonin antagonists. Circ. Res., *6*, 283, 1958.

127. Rudolph, A.M., and Auld, P.A.M.: Physical factors affecting normal and serotonin-constricted pulmonary vessels. Am. J. Physiol., *198*, 864, 1960.

128. Aviado, D.M.: Pulmonary vascular responses to anoxia, 5-hydroxytryptamine and histamine. Am. J. Physiol., *198*, 1032, 1960.

129. Kabins, S.A., Molina, C., and Katz, L.N.: Pulmonary vascular effects of serotonin (5-OH tryptamine) in dogs: Its role in causing pulmonary edema. Am. J. Physiol., *197*, 955, 1959.

130. Rudolph, A.M.: Pulmonary venomotor activity. Med. Thorac., *19*, 184, 1962.

131. Duke, H.N., and Stedeford, R.D.: O_2 diffusion in lung of the anesthetized cat. J. Appl. Physiol., *14*, 917, 1959.

132. Young, R.C., Nagano, H., Vaughn, T.R., and Staub, N.C.: Pulmonary capillary blood volume in dog: Effects of 5-hydroxytryptamine. J. Appl. Physiol., *18*, 264, 1963.

133. Harris, P., Fritts, H.W., and Cournand, A.: Some circulatory effects of 5-hydroxytryptamine in man. Circulation, *21*, 1132, 1960.

134. Stone, H.H., and Nemir, P.: Study of the role of 5-hydroxytryptamine (serotonin) and histamine in the pathogenesis of pulmonary embolism in man. Ann. Surg., *152*, 890, 1960.

135. Cournand, A., Fritts, H.W., Harris, P., and Himmelstein, A.: Preliminary observations on the effects in man of continuous perfusion with acetylcholine of one branch of the pulmonary artery upon the homolateral pulmonary blood flow. Trans. Ass. Am. Phys., *69*, 163, 1956.

136. Harris, P.: Influence of acetylcholine on the pulmonary arterial pressure. Brit. Heart J., *19*, 272, 1957.

137. Wood, P., Besterman, E.M., Towers, M.K., and McIlroy, M.B.: The effect of acetylcholine on vascular resistance and left atrial pressure in mitral stenosis. Brit. Heart J., *19*, 279, 1957.

138. Fritts, H.W., Harris, P., Clauss, R.H., Odell, J.E., and Cournand, A.: The effect of acetylcholine on the human pulmonary circulation under normal and hypoxic conditions. J. Clin. Invest., *37*, 99, 1958.

139. Sheperd, J.T., Semler, H.J., Helmholz, H.F., and Wood, E.H.: Effects of infusion of acetylcholine on pulmonary vascular resistance in patients with pulmonary hypertension and congenital heart disease. Circulation, *20*, 381, 1959.

140. Marshall, R.J., Helmholz, H.F., and Sheperd, J.T.: Effect of acetylcholine on pulmonary vascular resistance in a patient with idiopathic pulmonary hypertension. Circulation, *20*, 391, 1959.

141. Söderholm, B., and Werkö, L.: Acetylcholine and the pulmonary circulation in mitral valvular disease. Brit. Heart J., *21*, 1, 1959.

142. Crittenden, I.H., Adams, F.H., and Latta, H.: Preoperative evaluation of the pulmonary vascular bed in patients with pulmonary hypertension associated with left to right shunts. I. Effects of acetylcholine. Preliminary report. Pediatrics, *24*, 448, 1959.

143. Chidsey, C.A., Fritts, H.W., Zocche, R., Himmelstein, A., and Cournand, A.: Effect of acetylcholine on the distribution of pulmonary blood flow in patients with chronic pulmonary emphysema. Mal. Cardiovasc., *1*, 15, 1960.

144. Samet, P., Bernstein, W.H., and Widrich, J.: Intracardiac infusion of acetylcholine in primary pulmonary hypertension. Am. Heart J., *60*, 433, 1960.

145. Charms, B.L.: Primary pulmonary hypertension. Effect of unilateral pulmonary artery occlusion and infusion of acetylcholine. Am. J. Cardiol., *8*, 94, 1961.

146. Samet, P., Bernstein, W.H., and Litwak, R.S.: Intracardiac acetylcholine infusion and left heart dynamics in rheumatic heart disease. Brit. Heart J., *23*, 616, 1961.

147. Stanfield, C.A., Finlayson, J.K., Luria, M.N., Constantine, H., Flatley, F.J., and Yu, P.N.: Effects of acetylcholine on hemodynamics and blood oxygen saturation in mitral stenosis. Circulation, 24, 1164, 1961.

148. Bateman, M., Davidson, L.A.G., Donald, K.W., and Harris, P.: A comparison of the effect of acetylcholine and 100 per cent oxygen on the pulmonary circulation in patients with mitral stenosis. Clin. Sci., 22, 223, 1962.

149. Charms, B.L., Givertz, B., and Toshihiko, I.: Effect of acetylcholine on the pulmonary circulation in patients with chronic pulmonary disease. Circulation, 25, 814, 1962.

150. Samet, P., Bernstein, W.H., Fernandez, L., and Victoria, W. de: The effects of intracardiac acetylcholine infusion upon right heart dynamics in patients with rheumatic heart disease studied at rest. Am. J. Cardiol., 9, 32, 1962.

151. Schlant, R.C., Tsagaris, T.J., Robertson, R.J., Winter, T.S., and Edwards, F.K.: The effect of acetylcholine upon arterial saturation. Am. Heart J., 64, 512, 1962.

152. Behnke, R.H., Williams, J.F., and White, D.H.: The effect of acetylcholine infusion upon cardiac dynamics in patients with pulmonary emphysema. Am. Rev. Resp. Dis., 87, 57, 1963.

153. Oakley, C., Glick, G., Luria, M.N., Schreiner, B.F., and Yu, P.N.: Some regulatory mechanisms of the human pulmonary vascular bed. Circulation, 26, 917, 1962.

154. Johnson, V., Hamilton, W.F., Katz, L.N., and Weinstein, W.: Studies on the dynamics of the pulmonary circulation. Am. J. Physiol., 120, 624, 1937.

155. Jiménez-Vargas, J., and Vidal-Sivilla, S.: Efectos de sustancias vasoconstrictoras y vasodilatadoras sobre la circulación pulmonar. Rev. exp. Fisiol., 5, 19, 1949.

156. Eliakim, M., Rosenberg, S.Z., and Braun, K.: Effect of acetylcholine on the pulmonary artery pressure in anesthetized dogs. Arch. int. Pharmacodyn., 113, 169, 1957.

157. Rudolph, A.M., and Scarpelli, E.M.: Drug action on pulmonary circulation of unanesthetized dogs. Am. J. Physiol., 206, 1201, 1964.

158. Berry, J.N., Thompson, H.K., Miller, D.E., and McIntosh, H.D.: Changes in cardiac output, stroke volume and central venous pressure induced by atropine in man. Am. Heart J., 58, 204, 1959.

159. Corten, R., Gunnells, J.C., Weissler, A.M., and Stead, E.A.: Effects of atropine and isoproterenol on cardiac output, central venous pressure and mean transit time of indicators placed at three different sites in the venous system. Circ. Res., 9, 979, 1961.

160. Daly, W.J., and Behnke, R.H.: The behavior of the venous reservoir as affected by atropine. Trans. Ass. Am. Phys., 75, 277, 1962.

161. Severinghaus, J.W., and Stupel, M.: Respiratory dead space increase following atropine in man, and atropine, vagal or ganglionic blockade and hypothermia in dogs. J. Appl. Physiol., 8, 1055, 1955.

162. Goldenberg, M., Pines, K.L., Baldwin, E., de F., Greene, D.G., and Roh, C.E.: The hemodynamic response of man to norepinephrine and epinephrine and its relation to the problem of hypertension. Am. J. Med., 5, 792, 1948.

163. Fowler, N.O., Westcott, R.N., Scott, R.C., and McQuire, J.: The effect of norepinephrine upon pulmonary arteriolar resistance in man. J. Clin. Invest., 30, 517, 1951.

164. Barcroft, H., and Starr, I.: Comparison of the actions of adrenaline and noradrenaline on the cardiac output in man. Clin. Sci., 10, 295, 1951.

165. Witham, A.C., and Fleming, J.W.: The effect of epinephrine on the pulmonary circulation in man. J. Clin. Invest., 30, 707, 1951.

166. Borst, H.G., Berglund, E., and McGregor, M.: The effects of pharmacologic agents on pulmonary circulation in the dog. Studies on epinephrine, norepinephrine, 5-hydroxytryptamine, acetylcholine, histamine and aminophylline. J. Clin. Invest., 36, 669, 1957.

167. Patel, D.J., Lange, R.L., and Hecht, H.H.: Some evidence for active constriction in the human pulmonary vascular bed. Circulation, 18, 19, 1958.

168. Bousvaros, G.A.: Effects of norepinephrine on human pulmonary circulation. Brit. Heart J., 24, 738, 1962.

169. Zweifach, C.B.: General principles governing behavior of the microcirculation. Am. J. Med., 23, 684, 1957.

170. Konzett, H., and Hebb, C.O.: Vaso- and bronchomotor actions of noradrenaline (arterenol) and adrenaline in isolated perfused lungs of dogs. Arch. int. Pharmacodyn., 78, 210, 1949.

171. Shadle, O.W., Moore, J.C., and Billig, D.M.: Effect of 1-arterenol infusion on "central blood volume" in the dog. Circ. Res., 3, 385, 1955.

172. Nathanson, M.H., and Miller, H.: Clinical observations on a new epinephrine-like

compound, methoxamine. Am. J. Med. Sci., *223*, 270, 1952.

173. Goldberg, L.I., Cotton, M., de V., Darby, T.D., and Howell, E.V.: Comparative heart contractile force effects of equipressor doses of several sympathomimetic amines. J. Pharmacol. & Exp. Ther., *108*, 177, 1953.

174. Stanfield, C.A., and Yu, P.N.: Hemodynamic effects of methoxamine in mitral valve disease. Circ. Res., *8*, 859, 1960.

175. Brewster, W.R., Osgood, P.F., Isaacs, J.P., and Goldberg, L.I.: Hemodynamic effects of a pressor amine (Methoxamine) with predominant vasoconstrictor activity. Circ. Res., *8*, 980, 1960.

176. Kaufman, J., Iglauer, A., and Herwitz, G.K.: Effect of Isuprel (isopropylepinephrine) on circulation of normal man. Am. J. Med., *11*, 442, 1951.

177. Weissler, A.M., Leonard, J.J., and Warren, J.V.: The hemodynamic effects of isoproterenol in man. J. Lab & Clin. Med., *53*, 921, 1959.

178. Dodge, H.T., Lord, J.D., and Sandler, H.: Cardiovascular effects of isoproterenol in normal subjects and subjects with congestive heart failure. Am. Heart J., *60*, 94, 1960.

179. Lee, T.D., Roveti, G.C., and Ross, R.S.: The hemodynamic effects of isoproterenol on pulmonary hypertension in man. Am. Heart J., *65*, 361, 1963.

190. McGaff, C.J., Roveti, G.C., Glassman, E., and Milnor, W.R.: The pulmonary blood volume in rheumatic heart disease and its alteration by isoproterenol. Circulation, *27*, 77, 1963.

181. Whalen, R.E., Cohen, A.I., Sumner, R.G., and McIntosh, H.D.: Hemodynamic effects of isoproterenol infusion in patients with normal and diseased mitral valves. Circulation, *27*, 512, 1963.

182. Schreiner, B.F., Murphy, G.W., James, D.H., and Yu, P.N.: The effects of isoproterenol upon the pulmonary blood volume in patients with valvular heart disease and primary myocardial disease. Circulation, *37*, 220, 1968.

183. Ross, J.C., and Eller, J.L.: Effect of isuprel infusion on the increase in pulmonary diffusing capacity for CO (D_L) produced by pressure suit inflation. Fed. Proc., *20*, 425, 1961.

CHAPTER 15

Pulmonary Capillary Blood Volume in Disease*

Valvular Heart Disease

Predominant Mitral Valve Disease. In patients with valvular heart disease pulmonary capillary blood volume (Vc) is influenced by many factors. These include pulmonary arterial and venous pressures, pulmonary blood flow, pulmonary vascular resistance, structural and functional state of the vessels, the extent and patency of bronchopulmonary arterial anastomoses, obstruction of airway passages and the co-existence of chronic pulmonary disease.

Table 15-1 presents the estimated Vc and other parameters in a series of 69 patients with predominant mitral valve disease studied in our laboratory. The data on some of these patients were reported previously.[1] The mean values of Vc for the three classes (II, III and IV) of patients were, respectively, 49 ml/M², 49 ml/M² and 26 ml/M². Vc was increased in only 9% of these patients and was normal or reduced in the remaining 91%, regardless of the functional classification. Pulmonary diffusing capacity (D_L) and membrane diffusing capacity (D_M) declined progressively in patients from class II to class IV. D_L was significantly lower for the group as a whole

than in normal subjects ($p < 0.01$). In certain patients, particularly those with moderate pulmonary hypertension, increased pulmonary blood volume (PBV) may be associated with a normal Vc. This implies that the pulmonary vascular bed in these patients is abnormally and chronically dilated and that the increased blood volume is in the pulmonary veins and arteries. A negative correlation was observed between Vc and total pulmonary resistance (TPR) ($p < 0.02$). Even though no significant correlation was observed between Vc and PBV in any individual class of patients, a positive correlation between the two variables ($p < 0.01$) was found in the group of 69 patients as a whole.

Hamer reported the D_L and Vc in 40 patients with mitral valve disease.[2] In 38% of 29 patients with mitral stenosis, Vc was increased, while in 41% D_M was decreased. His findings were consistent with increase in the size and number of pulmonary capillaries and thickening of alveolar walls. He stated that the increase in Vc tends to counteract the effect of the reduction in D_M so that the measurements of D_L are often normal in mitral valve disease. In the majority of patients, however, Vc was normal or decreased.

Daly and associates reported studies of D_L, Vc and D_M in a group of ten

---

*Much of the work presented in this chapter was done by my colleague, Dr. Kuddusi Gazioglu.

TABLE 15-1 Pulmonary Capillary Blood Volume in Patients with Predominant Mitral Valve Disease

F.C.	No. of Cases	CI	SI	PAm	LAm	TPR	PVR	PBV	Vc	D_L	D_M
II	11	2.6*	31	26	15	480	200	295	49	16	39
		±.15	±2.9	±2.6	±1.5	±41	±32	±16	±3.4	±1.3	±9.2
III	45	2.2	28	32	21	726	284	310	49	13	28
		±0.1	±1.3	±1.4	±0.9	±47	±28	±11	±2.8	±0.7	±2.3
IV	13	1.5	18	49	26	1807	855	232	26	8	21
		±0.1	±1.5	±3.3	±1.4	±304	±175	±10	±2.3	±0.7	±3.4
Total	69	2.1	27	34	21	891	378	293	44	13	28
		±0.1	±1.1	±1.5	±0.8	±84	±46	±9	±2.2	±0.6	±2.2

F.C. = Functional classification
CI = Cardiac index (L/min/M²)
SI = Stroke index (ml/beat/M²)
PAm = Pulmonary arterial mean pressure (mm Hg)
LAm = Left atrial mean pressure (mm Hg)
TPR = Total pulmonary resistance (dynes·sec/cm⁵)
PVR = Pulmonary vascular resistance (dynes·sec/cm⁵)
PBV = Pulmonary blood volume (ml/M²)
Vc = Pulmonary capillary blood volume (ml/M²)
D_L = Pulmonary diffusing capacity (ml/mm Hg/min/M²)
D_M = Membrane diffusing capacity (ml/mm Hg/min/M²)
* = Mean ± S.E.,

patients with mitral stenosis and pulmonary hypertension.[3] Compared with similar measurements in 10 normal subjects in the recumbent position, both D_L and D_M were significantly reduced, but Vc was not appreciably different. Although Vc was not increased absolutely, the ratio Vc/V$_A$ was substantially greater in patients with mitral stenosis. This means that V$_C$ was consistently and considerably increased in these patients for a given alveolar volume. The reduction in V$_A$ was probably a reflection of the decrease in vital capacity known to occur in patients with pulmonary hypertension and chronic pulmonary congestion.

McCredie also found a significant reduction in D_L and D_M in a group of 31 patients with mitral valve disease.[4,5] The mean value of Vc (44 ml/M²) in those patients was lower than that (52 ml/M²) in a group of normal subjects, but the difference was not statistically significant.

Previous studies by Flatley et al in our laboratory, however, demonstrated an appreciable increase in Vc in some class III and class IV patients with mitral stenosis.[6] Palmer and associates also found that Vc was considerably increased in many of their class III patients with mitral stenosis.[7]

In the later stage of the disease, when pulmonary arterial pressure and vascular resistance have increased considerably, the blood volume in the pulmonary vascular bed may return to normal. Such a reduction is probably secondary to structural change in the pulmonary vessels and to vasoconstriction resulting from hypoxia. When appreciable parenchymal change occurs in the lungs, the pulmonary vascular bed may be restricted as manifested by a reduction in both Vc and D_M. Thus, in 13 class IV mitral stenosis patients studied in our laboratory, the mean values of both PBV and Vc were significantly lower than similar measurements in normal subjects. In this regard, the negative correlations between the pulmonary vascular resistance and PBV as well as Vc might be expected, with restriction of the pulmonary vascular bed leading to significantly elevated pulmonary vascular resistance. Such structural changes may include (*a*) thickening of the walls of pulmonary arteries and veins with intimal proliferation and muscular hypertrophy; (*b*) multiple thrombi or emboli in both pulmonary arteries and veins; (*c*) thickening of the alveolar capillary membrane; and (*d*) destruction of some capillaries and dilatation of others.[8-10]

Many workers have reported reduction in D_L in patients with mitral valve disease, particularly in those with associated pulmonary hypertension,[11,17] while others have found no significant change in D_L in most of these patients.[18,19] Recently, Aber and Campbell measured D_L in 79 patients with mitral stenosis and compared the results with histologic observations in lung biopsies obtained at operation.[20] They found that reduction in D_L was usually associated with intimal thickening in the small vessels in the lungs and with elevated pulmonary vascular resistance.

McCredie suggested that the association of diminished Vc with increasing pulmonary vascular pressure and resistance could be explained by nonuniform distribution of capillary blood volume as well as by a true reduction of capillary blood volume resulting from constriction or partial obliteration of the pulmonary capillary bed.[4,5] He also observed that Vc was inversely related to the intravascular pressures and he noted that the reduction in Vc was more closely related to the pulmonary arterial mean pressure (PAm) than to the left atrial mean pressure (LAm). The association of reduced Vc with markedly increased PAm (more than 50 mm Hg) also has been previously reported from our laboratory, although we found no linear relationship between Vc and PAm when

the latter was less than 50 mm Hg.

Daly and associates reported that tilting decreased D_L and Vc in normal subjects but not in patients with mitral valve disease and pulmonary hypertension.[3]

Palmer and associates found that Vc increased significantly with exercise in moderately disabled patients with mitral disease and that the magnitude of increase in Vc on exercise was less in patients with severe disease.[7]

Riley and co-workers studied the D_{LO2} in 14 patients with incapacitating mitral stenosis after mitral valve surgery.[21] About half their patients showed an increase in postoperative D_L during exercise. These patients presumably did not have extensive structural changes in the pulmonary membrane. Six patients whose D_L was low at rest preoperatively were greatly improved after mitral valve surgery. Two patients with very low values of D_L probably had extensive changes in the pulmonary vascular bed.

Reid and Stevenson reported pulmonary function studies in 40 patients with mitral stenosis before and after mitral commissurotomy.[22] In mild cases, the D_L was virtually normal before operation and was almost identical afterwards. In more severe cases, particularly in those with pulmonary hypertension, D_L was impaired befoer operation and little change was observed postoperatively. They explained these observations principally by irreversible lung damage from pulmonary endarteritis and from thickening of the alveolar membrane. McCredie also observed no significant change in D_L, D_M, or Vc up to 8 months after surgery in 11 patients who underwent mitral valvotomy.[5]

In our laboratory we have measured D_L, D_M, and Vc in 7 patients before and 8 to 25 months after replacement

TABLE 15-2   D$_L$, D$_M$ and Vc in Patients before and after Replacement of the Mitral Valve (Starr-Edwards)

Patient	Sex	Status	Age	BSA	D$_L$	D$_M$	Vc
C.C.	M	A	43	1.82	23	35	97
		B (19 mo.)	45	1.74	11	17	32
P.A.	F	A	29	1.46	19	30	65
		B (18 mo.)	31	1.50	24	30	100
B.E.	F	A	27	1.42	11	15	50
		B (8 mo.)	28	1.50	15	23	46
C.L.	F	A	29	1.46	19	30	50
		B (25 mo.)	31	1.50	24	30	58
L.L.	M	A	43	1.57	16	29	47
		B (23 mo.)	45	1.72	15	24	47
H.M.	F	A	61	1.64	10	19	28
		B (21 mo.)	62	1.60	10	18	25
C.Ca.	F	A	54	1.44	10	—	9
		B (12 mo.)	56	1.42	15	24	62

A = Preoperative
B = Postoperative
The symbols and abbreviations are identical to those used in Table 15-1

of the mitral valve with a Starr-Edwards prosthesis. The data are presented in Table 15-2. In 4 patients (B.E., H.M., L.L. and C.L.), D$_L$ and Vc showed no appreciable change. The D$_L$ and Vc of 2 patients (C.Ca. and P.A) increased, and one patient (C.C.) showed a significant reduction in D$_L$ and Vc. The postoperative increase in D$_L$ and Vc in patient C.Ca. might be explained by reversible vasoconstriction and structural abnormality, whereas the mechanism of similar increase in patient P.A. remained obscure. The significant reduction in D$_L$ and Vc in patient C.C. probably resulted from relief of the mitral valve obstruction and decrease in left atrial and pulmonary venous pressures.

Predominant Aortic Valve Disease. Few studies of Vc and related parameters have been reported in patients with predominant aortic valve disease. In a series of 48 such patients studied in our laboratory, the mean Vc was normal in the group as a whole, and varied from 46 to 54 ml/M² with an overall average value of 50 ml/M². The data on some of these patients were reported previously.[1] Table 15-3 shows

no difference in Vc and related parameters in three classes (I, II and III) of these patients. Vc exceeded the upper normal limit (66 ml/M²) in 6 patients and was less than the lower normal limit (39 ml/M²) in 13 patients. Furthermore, the mean values of Vc for the three classes did not differ significantly from that observed in normal subjects. The mean values of D$_M$ and D$_L$ were also normal for the three classes of patients. Vc and PBV correlated positively for the group of aortic patients as a whole (p < 0.02). In class III patients, an even more significant correlation was found between these two variables (p < 0.01). Further statistical study revealed a significant negative correlation between Vc and TPR (p < 0.02) and between Vc and PVR in these patients (p < 0.02).

In patients with predominant aortic disease, CI and SI were usually within normal limits and PAm, LAm and PVR were normal or only slightly elevated. Since pulmonary venous and arterial hypertension is less frequent in these patients than in patients with mitral disease, structural change in the pulmo-

TABLE 15-3   Pulmonary Capillary Blood Volume in Patients with Predominant Aortic Valve Disease

F.C.	No. of Cases	CI	SI	PAm	LAm	TPR	PVR	PBV	Vc	D_L	D_M
I	5	3.6	43	16	8	144	73	250	54	18	35
		±0.25	±2.9	±1.5	±1.0	±54	±26	±31	±7.8	±3.4	±7.2
II	14	2.9	38	19	13	342	109	255	46	17	27
		±0.29	±3.6	±1.8	±1.5	±66	±25	±16	±4.3	±1.6	±4.7
III	29	2.5	35	21	13	425	178	299	51	15	41
		±0.12	±1.7	±1.6	±1.2	±50	±24	±14	±5.4	±1.1	±6.9
Total	48	2.8	37	20	13	371	147	281	50	16	36
		±0.12	±1.5	±1.1	±0.9	±38	±18	±11	±3.6	±0.9	±4.5

The symbols and abbreviations are identical to those used in Table 15-1

nary vessels and hypoxemia would be expected to be less severe. The normal D_M and D_L and normal lung volumes strongly support the absence or minimal extent of structural or functional derangement in the alveolo-capillary membrane. If the LAm and PAm of these patients had been higher, an elevated Vc and reduced D_L and D_M might have been expected. It is also possible that class IV patients with aortic disease might show a normal or reduced PBV, associated with a decreased Vc.

McCredie recently reported D_L, D_M and Vc in 6 patients with predominant aortic valve disease.[5] Compared with data from normal subjects, D_L and D_M were reduced significantly, but the mean values of Vc were almost identical (53 vs. 52 ml/M²).

We have studied D_L, D_M and Vc in 8 patients with aortic valve disease before and 6 to 29 months after replacement of the aortic valve with a Starr-Edwards prosthesis. The data are presented in Table 15-4.

In general, the alterations in D_L were insignificant and the changes in Vc were small and inconsistent. In 4 patients Vc increased slightly, in 3 patients Vc decreased slightly, and in

TABLE 15-4 D_L, D_M and Vc in Patients before and after Replacement of the Aortic Valve (Starr-Edwards)

Patient	Sex	Status	Age	BSA	D_L	D_M	Vc
R.S.	M	A	45	1.82	13	16	96
		B (12 mo.)	47	1.75	13	26	33
J.S.	M	A	27	2.17	24	46	75
		B (19 mo.)	29	2.13	17	33	45
S.T.	M	A	32	2.04	16	31	63
		B (7 mo.)	34	2.04	16	25	55
D.C.	M	A	52	1.90	25	68	55
		B (18 mo.)	54	1.87	24	43	71
C.B.	M	A	39	1.90	16	29	52
		B (19 mo.)	41	1.95	17	28	42
L.Z.	M	A	53	1.90	18	36	45
		B (17 mo.)	55	1.80	19	39	47
J.B.	M	A	34	1.93	19	43	43
		B (6 mo.)	35	1.85	18	29	72
C.L.	M	A	42	1.93	18	38	40
		B (18 mo.)	44	1.94	17	32	51
J.A.	F	A	57	1.78	10	27	24
		B (29 mo.)	60	1.68	17	26	66

The symbols and abbreviations are identical to those used in Tables 15-1 and 15-2 one patient no change was discernible. Values of Vc were normal for all but one patient prior to the valve replacement, suggesting that the small and inconsistent changes postoperatively were probably of no consequence.

Congenital Cardiovascular Malformations

In 1962 Flatley and co-workers in our laboratory reported an increase in Vc in 10 patients with atrial septal defect (ASD) in the recumbent position.[6] The mean value was 88.3 ml/M[2] with a range from 53 to 162 ml/M[2], in contrast to a mean value of 43 ml/M[2] (range from 27 to 72 ml/M[2]) in 13 normal subjects. They found no significant correlation between Vc and pulmonary blood flow, pulmonary arterial pressure or pulmonary wedge pressure in patients with ASD. Recently we measured Vc in another 10 patients with ASD and in 23 normal subjects in the recumbent position. The mean value of Vc for the former group was 69 ml/M[2] and for the latter group 54 ml/M[2] (Table 15-5).

In 1964 McCredie and associates in our laboratory estimated Vc in 9 patients with ASD in the standing position and compared the results with those from 16 normal subjects.[23] The mean value of Vc in patients with ASD was 72 ml/M[2], compared with 31 ml/M[2] in the normal subjects (Table 15-5). The standing position undoubtedly exaggerates the difference between values for Vc in patients with

ASD and normals, compared with measurements in the recumbent position. The Vc of patients with ASD is about the same in both positions, but the Vc of normal subjects declines appreciably from the recumbent to the standing position. This difference may be attributed largely to altered distribution of pulmonary blood flow in the upper and lower lobes of the lung in the two positions. Recent isotope studies have shown a reduction in perfusion in the upper zones of the lung in the standing position in normal subjects, a discrepancy which disappears in the recumbent position.[24-26] In patients with ASD no difference in the perfusion of upper and lower zones is found in the standing or recumbent positions.[27]

McCredie and associates also observed an increase in Vc in patients with ventricular septal defect (VSD), but the values were distinctly lower than those associated with ASD[23] (Table 15-6). They felt that the difference between the two groups was probably related to the difference in magnitude of pulmonary blood flow, inasmuch as the intravascular pressure in the two groups did not differ significantly. Similarly, they found no significant correlation between Vc and pulmonary arterial pressure in patients with either ASD or VSD. They concluded that the increased Vc in patients with left to right intracardiac shunts is related to pulmonary blood flow and is independent of intravascular pressure. The situation is similar to that in normal

TABLE 15-5 DL, DM and Vc in Patients with Atrial Septal Defect (ASD)

Author	Diagnosis	No. of Cases	Age (Mean)	BSA (Mean)	Position	D_L Mean	Range	D_M Mean	Range	Vc Mean	Range
McCredie	Normal	16	30	1.82	Standing	14	9–22	43	24–89	31	24–48
et al.	ASD	9	25	1.69	Standing	22	16–33	45	31–62	72	52–107
Gazioglu	Normal	23	25	1.79	Supine	18	12–21	38	25–62	54	39–66
and Yu	ASD	10	25	1.70	Supine	23	17–28	49	31–87	69	51–135

The symbols and abbreviations are identical to those used in Table 15-1

TABLE 15-6 D_L, D_M and V_C in Patients with Ventricular Septal Defect or Patent
             Ductus Arteriosus

Author	Diagnosis	No. of Patients	Position	D_L Mean	D_L Range	D_M Mean	D_M Range	V_C Mean	V_C Range
McCredie et al.	VSD with L to R	8	Standing	18	13–25	54	23–99	48	36–65
	VSD with R to L	2	Standing	15	15–15	66	41–91	29	22–36
Gazioglu and Yu	VSD with L to R	4	Supine	22	15–26	37	23–49	80	45–110
Gazioglu and Yu	PDA with L to R	5	Supine	20	10–28	35	20–56	66	21–107

VSD   = Ventricular septal defect
PDA   = Patent ductus arteriosus
L to R = Left to right shunt
R to L = Right to left shunt
Other symbols and abbreviations are identical to those used in Table 15–1

subjects during exercise. The mechanism for the flow dependency of V_C in these two situations is unexplained but contrasts sharply to other high flow conditions such as hyperthyroidism and anemia where V_C is independent of flow. The increase in D_L in patients with left to right shunts is presumably largely a result of the increase in V_C. However, in contrast to D_L and V_C, the variability of D_M is so great that definite conclusions concerning D_M are not possible in the groups studied.

Table 15–6 includes estimates of D_L, D_M, and V_C in patients with VSD and in those with patent ductus arteriosus (PDA) studied in our laboratory. In 12 patients with VSD and left to right shunt, the V_C was either normal or subnormal. In 3 of 5 patients with PDA the V_C was elevated, in 1 patient it was normal, and in another patient it was subnormal. The reason for the low V_C in this patient was obscure.

Many workers have reported that D_L and V_C are usually increased in patients with left to right intracardiac shunts.[15,28-32] More than 10 years ago, Rankin and Callies found increased D_L in 12 patients with ASD or VSD.[28] In the absence of pulmonary hypertension, D_L was increased 11 to 92% with D_M

and V_C increasing proportionately. In those with pulmonary hypertension and elevated pulmonary vascular resistance, D_L was decreased because of a disproportionate reduction in D_M.

Auchincloss and associates also reported significantly elevated D_L in 10 of 16 patients with intracardiac septal defects.[15] Pulmonary blood flow was increased in 9 of these 10 patients.

Bucci and co-workers reported a mean V_C of 57 ml/M^2 in 3 patients with VSD, 38 ml/M^2 in 4 patients with pulmonary stenosis, 50 ml/M^2 in 1 patient with tricuspid atresia, and 39 ml/M^2 in 4 patients with tetralogy of Fallot.[30] They considered the increase in V_C in most patients with left to right shunts to be secondary to an increase in pulmonary blood flow, occasionally exaggerated by elevated capillary pressure. The passive regulating function of the pulmonary capillary pressure is emphasized by the observation that patients with the greatest increase in V_C also have the highest wedge pressure. These workers further suggested that failure of the wedge pressure to correlate more exactly with V_C is probably due to variability in the measurement and lability of the circulation and pulmonary function. Murao and associates also observed an increased Vc in patients with intra-cardiac shunts and high pulmonary arterial pressure.[32]

McCredie and co-workers analyzed the mean capillary transit time in patients with intracardiac defects and found no significant differences between patients with ASD and those with VSD.[23] The interpretation of transit time was subject to the same limitations in rela-tion to the accuracy and comparability of pulmonary blood flow. Despite such limitations, however, they found that increasing Vc accompanied increasing pulmonary blood flow and progressive shortening of mean transit time. This was consistent with the finding of a shortened appearance time in indicator-dilution curves in patients with left to right shunts.[33] The shortest calculated mean transit time in their series was 0.25 second. These findings are probably explained by the intracardiac shunt itself rather than by other pulmonary or circulatory changes. The classical Bohr integration technique for estima-ting oxygen diffusion gradients suggests the possibility that the short transit time could exaggerate the alveolar arterial oxygen difference and con-tribute to the arterial desaturation so commonly found in patients with large ASD. The work of Staub, Bishop and Forster on the reaction rate between oxygen and Hb, however, suggests that reduction of mean transit time even to

one third of the normal value of 0.75 second is not likely to cause significant arterial desaturation in end-capillary blood.[34,35] Mixing of desaturated blood in the "common" atrial chamber, which has been clearly demonstrated, is more likely to be the major cause of arterial desaturation in ASD.

MacNamara, Prime and Sinclair found less increase in D_L during exer-cise in patients with ASD than in normal subjects.[36] This may indicate that the area of blood-gas interface is substantially greater at rest in patients with ASD than in normal subjects and that increase in the area of interface during exercise is much smaller.

One patient in the series reported by Bucci and co-workers responded to exercise with a 32% increase in Vc, suggesting that the capillary bed may increase in size even after years of increased pulmonary blood flow.[30] Rotman and Woolf also reported an increase in D_L during exercise in patients with either ASD or VSD.[31]

Bucci and co-workers reported diffusion studies in 10 patients at least 3 months after surgical correction of their cardiac malformations.[30] In 8 patients with ASD or VSD, D_L, D_M, and Vc decreased to normal on the average, indicating that the changes were reversible at least in most cases. They observed no significant changes in Vc in 2 patients after surgery for

TABLE 15-7 D_L, D_M and Vc in Patients with ASD before and after Surgical Correction

Patient	Sex	Status	Age	BSA	D_L	D_M	Vc
S.M.	F	A	21	1.86	26	34	135
		B (12 mo.)	22	1.80	18	36	52
P.L.	M	A	39	1.93	30	43	121
		B (5 mo.)	39	1.98	23	39	80
V.DiG.	M	A	23	1.74	27	53	77
		B (8 mo.)	24	1.76	24	56	55
I.B.	F	A	16	1.68	23	31	76
		B (12 mo.)	17	1.71	17	31	47
F.G.	M	A	61	1.56	20	32	66
		B (3 mo.)	61	1.58	22	32	87

The symbols and abbreviations are identical to those used in Tables 15–1, 15–2 and 15–5.

pulmonic stenosis, although D_L and D_M decreased slightly. Reversibility of elevation of Vc after surgical repair of ASD was also observed by Murao and associates.[32]

We have studied changes in Vc and D_L in 5 patients with ASD following surgical repair of the defect, and the data are included in Table 15-7. In 4 of these patients Vc decreased after successful closure of the defect. In 1 patient (F.G.) the postoperative Vc increased. This patient was a 60-year-old man who had a large atrial septal defect demonstrated at operation. The

defect was closed by intermittent silk sutures and no patch was used. Postoperative studies showed evidence of an uncorrected atrial septal defect, including persistence of the fixed splitting of the pulmonary second sound. It was assumed that the sutures were torn apart after the operation.

Chronic Pulmonary Disease

The data of D_L, D_M and Vc on 27 patients with chronic pulmonary disease studied in our laboratory are summarized in Table 15-8. In 3 patients

TABLE 15-8 D_L, D_M and Vc in Patients with Chronic Pulmonary Disease

Patient	Diagnosis	Position	Age	Sex	BSA	Vc	D_L	D_M	Vc	Remarks
D.H.	Asthma	S	24	F	1.58	2.03	19	56	38	
A.C.	Asthma	S	57	M	2.00	2.10	20	32	63	
H.B.	Asthma	R	59	F	1.74	1.00	27	66	57	
L.S.	Emphysema	S	30	F	1.51	2.00	14	47	25	
J.H.	Emphysema	R	56	M	1.92	1.70	9	22	20	
J.G.	Emphysema	R	61	M	2.15	2.50	16	28	46	
S.S.	Emphysema	R	40	F	1.70	1.10	18	30	55	
H.S.	Emphysema	R	54	M	1.85	3.20	21	45	54	
E.C.	Sarcoidosis	S	33	F	1.63	2.00	13	28	43	Pregnant
A.A.	Sarcoidosis	S	27	F	1.77	1.40	8	32	15	Pregnant
E.T.	Interstitial	R	48	M	1.86	1.47	8	16	23	Control
	Fibrosis	R	48	M	1.95	1.82	10	25	24	6 months after steroid therapy
C.H.	Scoliosis	S	45	M	1.49	0.95	10	16	36	Severe kyphosis
K.B.	Scoliosis	S	13	F	1.52	1.88	19	46	44	
A.L.	Scoliosis	S	44	M	1.85	1.81	17	36	44	
G.W.	Scoliosis	S	14	F	1.50	1.97	15	27	48	
F.S.	Scoliosis	S	14	F	1.54	1.06	10	21	25	
S.M.	Scoliosis	S	14	F	1.46	1.71	14	28	43	
L.M.	Scoliosis	S	20	F	1.30	1.02	10	22	32	
S.K.	Scoliosis	S	20	F	1.54	1.27	12	29	27	
S.K.	Scoliosis	R	20	F	1.54	1.23	12	30	39	
R.D.	Scoliosis	R	49	M	2.36	1.74	11	19	34	
C.F.	Scoliosis	R	15	F	1.45	2.19	20	37	57	
D.P.	Scoliosis	R	18	F	1.54	2.72	22	59	52	
L.F.	Alveolar Proteinosis	R	28	M	1.70	1.70	8	12	32	
L.S.	Alveolar Proteinosis	R	39	M	1.79	2.50	16	31	45	
		R	39	M	1.70	2.60	15	39	63	After treatment
S.S.	Goodpasture Syndrome	R	22	M	1.95	2.40	15	26	48	
L.F.	"Pickwickian Syndrome"	S	61	M	2.12	1.70	15	27	44	Weighing 101 kg
I.K.	"Pickwickian Syndrome"	S	45	M	3.10	0.90	10	12	54	Weighing 196 kg

S = Sitting
R = Recumbent
VC = Vital capacity in liters
Other symbols and abbreviations are identical to those used in Table 15-1

with bronchial asthma the values of both D_L and V_c were normal. In 5 patients with pulmonary emphysema the D_L and V_c were either normal or decreased. The D_L and V_c were reduced in 1 of 2 patients with sarcoidosis and in 2 patients with interstitial fibrosis. In 9 of 12 patients with scoliosis the V_c was normal, and in the remaining 3 patients it was decreased. The value of D_L was either normal or slightly decreased. The D_L and V_c were significantly decreased in 1 of 2 patients with alveolar proteinosis. In 1 patient with Goodpasture syndrome and in 2 patients with alveolar hypoventilation associated with obesity ("Pickwickian syndrome"), the V_c was normal and the D_L slightly reduced.

McNeill, Rankin and Forster measured V_c, D_M and D_L in 8 patients with various chronic pulmonary diseases.[37] V_c was normal in 3 of 5 patients with diffuse interstitial fibrosis and reduced in 2. Most significant was the decrease in D_M and D_L in all 5 patients. The V_c in 3 patients with chronic obstructive emphysema was normal.

Bates and associates measured V_c in 4 patients with diffuse pulmonary interstitial fibrosis and in 2 with sarcoidosis.[38] They found that V_c was reduced in 4 patients and normal in 2 (one with diffuse fibrosis, another with sarcoidosis). Both D_M and D_L were reduced in these patients, except for 1 patient with sarcoidosis whose D_M was normal.

Bedell and Eggers reported consistent reduction in D_L, D_M and V_c in 7 patients with pulmonary fibrosis and in 7 patients with pulmonary emphysema.[39] The reduction in D_L was comparable in both groups, but the reduction in V_c in patients with pulmonary emphysema was significantly greater than in patients with pulmonary fibrosis ($p < 0.05$). They concluded that the reduction in D_L was produced primarily by a reduction in D_M in pulmonary fibrosis and represents involvement of alveolar walls by the fibrotic process. In contrast, in patients with pulmonary emphysema, destruction of the pulmonary capillary bed was manifested by a disproportionate reduction in V_c, compared to the reduction in D_L. Williams and Zohman found that D_L was reduced in most patients with pulmonary emphysema and usually normal in those with bronchial asthma.[40] MacNamara and associates also found a decrease in D_L in patients with pulmonary emphysema.[41]

In pulmonary sarcoidosis, diffusing capacity for both oxygen and carbon monoxide is usually reduced.[42-48] Hamer measured D_L, D_M and V_c in 30 patients with pulmonary sarcoidosis: (a) those with normal D_L, (b) those with impaired D_M only, and (c) those with impaired D_M and V_c.[48] No diffusion abnormality was found in patients with pulmonary infiltration of short duration. After 1 to 3 years of disease, D_M was impaired. In patients with long-standing disease and radiographic changes for 5 years or more, both D_M and V_c were usually reduced. Changes in diffusing capacity were considered most likely a result of diffuse pulmonary fibrosis. In these patients the improvement in diffusing capacity after steroid therapy was either moderate or not impressive.[44,45,49,50]

The low V_c in chronic pulmonary disease results from a combination of anatomical and functional factors. For example, in diffuse interstitial diseases of the lung (e.g. alveolo-capillary block), anatomic changes in pulmonary vessels and parenchyma impair diffusion across the alveolo-capillary membrane. A low V_c in this condition may also represent a structural vascular alteration, associated with an altered ventilation-perfusion ratio simulating a shunt effect. Alveolar ventilation is preserved and perfusion is reduced causing a functional decrease in Vc. On the other hand, in the alveolar hypoventilation associated with extreme obesity, respiratory paralysis, kyphoscoliosis, hypoxia or respiratory acidosis, the resulting pulmonary hypertension may cause a decrease in Vc. In pulmonary emphysema and chronic bronchitis, a combination of anatomic changes and functional derangement (hypercapnia, respiratory acidosis) may be present. Destruction of alveolar capillaries restricts the pulmonary vascular bed, usually without evoking pulmonary hypertension. Finally, disturbances of alveolar ventilation and perfusion occur, usually incidental to acute bronchitis which superimposes hypoxic vasoconstriction and respiratory acidosis on the structural changes. Polycythemia, secondary to hypoxia in pulmonary emphysema, may cause thromboembolic damage to the pulmonary capillary bed, resulting in a subnormal Vc.

Cardiomyopathy

In our laboratory we have estimated D_L, D_M, and Vc in 10 patients with cardiomyopathy or primary myocardial disease. The results are summarized in Table 15-9.

All patients but one (A.L.) were compensated at the time of study. The D_L was either normal or reduced. The Vc was normal in all but 2 patients (T. McI. and B.S.), both of whom were diagnosed as having idiopathic non-obstructive cardiomyopathy. In these two patients the Vc was, respectively, 64 ml/M² and 76 ml/M². The PBV was normal in 5 of the 6 patients in whom it was determined. The patient whose PBV was elevated (370 ml/M²) had an obstructive cardiomyopathy proved by hemodynamic and angiographic studies, as well as at operation.

The literature is scanty concerning measurements of D_L, D_M and Vc in patients with cardiomyopathy. McCredie recently reported D_L, D_M and Vc in 5 patients with primary myocardial disease, including 3 with idiopathic hypertrophic subaortic stenosis and 2 with left ventricular failure of unknown etiology.[5] The mean values of D_L, D_M and Vc respectively were as follows: 9.2 ml/min/mm Hg/M², 13 ml/min/mm Hg/M², and 55 ml/M². Although both D_L and D_M were significantly lower than those observed in normal subjects, Vc was within normal limits.

Changes in the pulmonary capillary bed in these patients are undoubtedly related to the effects of disturbed myocardial function on pulmonary venous and arterial pressures. Normal D_L and Vc would be expected when

TABLE 15-9 D_L, D_M and Vc in Patients with Cardiomyopathy

Patient	Age	Sex	BSA	D_L	D_M	Vc	PBV
V.L.	61	M	2.04	12	30	30	280
D.P.	45	F	1.42	14	49	31	272
E.C.	42	F	1.88	10	15	42	—
P.C.	39	M	2.12	19	42	43	370
H.H.	52	F	1.75	14	19	43	240
A.M.	48	F	1.48	15	23	49	—
L.G.	20	M	1.86	19	30	54	301
A.L.	58	M	2.00	16	27	57	273
T.McI.	17	M	1.72	23	49	64	—
B.S.	36	M	1.74	13	20	76	—

The symbols and abbreviations are identical to those used in Table 15-1

left ventricular function is fully compensated and pulmonary hypertension is absent. With left ventricular decompensation and associated elevation of pulmonary venous and arterial pressures, Vc may be increased, with or without an accompanying increase in D_L. If decompensation and pulmonary hypertension have persisted for a long period, structural changes such as these associated with chronic mitral stenosis may ensue and a normal or reduced Vc may be expected. We have reported normal PBV in patients with cardiomyopathy and long-standing cardiac decompensation.[51,52]

Idiopathic or Thromboembolic Pulmonary Hypertension

Vc and related parameters in 8 patients with idiopathic or thromboembolic pulmonary hypertension determined in our laboratory are presented in Table 15-10. D_L was moderately or markedly decreased in all 8 patients. Vc was 31 ml/M^2 or less in 6 of the 8. In the remaining 2 patients (R.D. and S.S.) the Vc was low normal. Thus, the pulmonary capillary bed was greatly reduced as a result of thromboembolism and/or marked pulmonary hypertension.

McNeill, Rankin and Forster measured Vc and related parameters in 2 patients with pulmonary hypertension of unknown etiology.[37] D_L was less than the predicted normal in both patients, but was reduced more than twice the standard error of the estimate (8 ml/min/mm Hg) in only one. Both D_M and Vc were also reduced. They concluded that the parallel decrease in D_M and Vc could be explained either by increased pulmonary vascular resistance from an increase in precapillary resistance with a decrease in the size of the perfused capillary bed, or by partial destruction of the capillary bed itself.

McCredie reported D_L, D_M and Vc in two patients with idiopathic pulmonary hypertension.[5] D_L and D_M were significantly reduced, but the value of Vc was within normal limits.

Bates and Christie pointed out that idiopathic pulmonary hypertension, although often associated with exertional dyspnea, is not accompanied by impaired ventilation or by significant reduction in diffusing capacity.[53] They emphasized that the consequences of mitral valve stenosis, in which the pulmonary capillary bed is located between the stenosed orifice and the

TABLE 15-10 D_L, D_M and Vc in Patients with Idiopathic or Thromboembolic Pulmonary Hypertension

Patient	Age	Sex	Pressures (mm Hg) PAm	LAm	D_L	D_M	Vc	Remarks
			Idiopathic Pulmonary Hypertension					
J.H.	35	M	74	10	12	39	27	
M.R.	30	F	67	7	14	54	26	
			Thromboembolic Pulmonary Hypertension					
S.S.	18	M	57	6	18	32	49	lung biopsy
C.K.	64	M	45	10	9	15	31	autopsy
J.Ha.	56	M	—	—	9	39	20	autopsy
J.G.	63	M	—	—	4	5	22	lung biopsy
H.N.	58	M	—	—	14	—	21	
R.D.	49	M	—	—	11	17	34	

PAm = Pulmonary arterial mean pressure
LAm = Left atrial mean pressure
Other symbols and abbreviations are identical to those used in Table 15-1

right ventricle, and in which pulmonary venous and pulmonary arterial hypertension co-exist, are likely to be very different from those of thrombotic obliteration of the arterial bed, in which pulmonary venous hypertension is absent.

Colp and Williams observed that D_L was usually normal or only slightly reduced in patients several weeks following pulmonary embolization.[54] Dunér and associates mentioned that 3 months after recovery from a clinically severe pulmonary embolism normal cardiopulmonary functions may be observed, including normal exercise D_L, normal cardiac output and pulmonary arterial pressure, and an entirely normal working capacity.[55] In this regard the observations of Marshall and associates were of unusual interest.[56,57] They found that embolization with autologous clots less than a millimeter in diameter reduced D_L in dogs. Unilateral pulmonary embolization in dogs with autologous clots large enough to occlude major branches of the pulmonary arteries also produced a decrease in D_L. A striking finding was that the occluded lung regained most of its function by 2 weeks after embolization, even though thrombi were still found at necropsy. On the other hand, embolization in dogs with glass beads of 60 micra in diameter did not lead to a significant fall in steady state D_L, although peripheral blood pressure fell and pulmonary arterial pressure rose. Diffuse damage to the capillary bed must be overwhelming before it affects D_L, but localized occlusion of a relatively small portion of the lung will lower D_L, suggesting the importance of uneven distribution.

The recent report of Nadel and co-workers concerning pulmonary function tests in 3 patients with dyspnea of unknown origin is of special interest.[58] Decreased D_L and V_c, increased physiologic dead space and increased difference between arterial and end-expired pCO_2 were suggestive of the presence of pulmonary vascular obstruction. All 3 patients had similar lesions in the small pulmonary arteries, characterized histologically by intimal hyperplasia, chronic perivascular and interstitial inflammation, and the presence of macrophages. Other organs were not involved, but serum globulin was increased, suggesting the possibility of an abnormal immune process.

In normal animals and man, almost two-thirds of the lungs must be removed before pulmonary arterial pressure rises significantly. Many pulmonary diseases, however, gradually and inconspicuously reduce the number and caliber of small pulmonary vessels and modify the distensibility of the remaining vessels, so that even normal pulmonary blood flow is associated with marked pulmonary hypertension. Examples of such diseases include pulmonary emboli, pulmonary arteritis, interstitial fibrosis and granuloma, bullous emphysema, and idiopathic pulmonary hypertension. Abnormal architecture of the thorax, such as may occur with severe kyphoscoliosis, may also limit the capacity and expansibility of the pulmonary vascular bed, predisposing to pulmonary hypertension.

The diagnosis of minimal or moderate idiopathic or thromboembolic pulmonary hypertension may be notoriously difficult when pulmonary vascular obstruction is insufficient to cause clinically manifest physiologic abnormalities. The clinical, physiologic and pathologic features of idiopathic pulmonary hypertension have been described by many workers. In 1958, the author reviewed 54 reported cases of idiopathic or primary pulmonary hypertension.[59] Pharmacodynamic responses and histologic examination in 6 patients studied by the author suggested that pulmonary hypertension in these patients was a result of structural pulmonary vascular change, and that functional pulmonary vasoconstriction was no more than a minor contributing factor. As reported in Chapter 12, recent studies of 5 such additional patients again showed failure to respond to an infusion of acetylcholine into the main pulmonary artery, substantiating the original postulation. In this sense, these patients appear to closely resemble those with severe thromboembolic pulmonary hypertension. On the other hand, other workers have reported significant reduction of pulmonary arterial pressure in patients with idiopathic pulmonary hypertension after the administration of certain pharmacologic agents, indicating that functional vasoconstriction was an important factor in the pulmonary vascular restriction of the patients studied.[60-62]

In pulmonary embolism, the gas-exchange functions of the lung are impaired. Robin and associates listed three major abnormalities resulting from reduced gas exchange:[63,64] (a) arterial oxygen unsaturation from venoarterial shunting, decreased diffusing capacity of the lung and relative alveolar hypoventilation; (b) hyperventilation which improves arterialization of pulmonary capillary blood; and (c) significant differences between pCO_2 of arterial blood and end-tidal air, because of dilution of alveolar air by the newly formed dead space. These authors particularly emphasized that significant arterial desaturation is a feature of patients who had just suffered a major pulmonary infarction, and suggested that this observation may be useful in considering the differential diagnosis. They felt that diminution of D_L appeared to be the major

cause of the anoxemia in some patients, and that significant venoarterial shunting must have been responsible for the anoxemia in others, since full saturation could not be achieved during pure oxygen breathing.

Complete pulmonary function tests may give much additional information concerning the presence or absence of other physiologic respiratory abnormalities in addition to the direct effects of vascular obstruction. In the presence of previously existing cardiorespiratory abnormalities, disturbances in gas exchange may not have specific diagnostic value. Pulmonary arteritis, primary alveolar hypoventilation, diffuse pulmonary interstitial fibrosis and particularly pulmonary emphysema may all cause similar abnormalities. As suggested by Severinghaus and Stuppel, in the absence of these complicating diseases, the increased physiologic dead space and the increased arterio-alveolar pCO_2 gradient can be explained by obstruction of pulmonary blood vessels in areas of the lungs in which ventilation persists.[65] The reduction in D_L and in Vc is consistent with the expected decrease in the number of patent pulmonary capillaries in these patients. These specific pulmonary function tests may yield results which would be diagnostic of pulmonary vascular obstruction at a time when the results of other studies are within normal limits. It should be emphasized, however, that even a wide variety of pulmonary function tests sometimes may fail to yield specific diagnostic information in cases of pulmonary vascular obstruction.

Other Diseases

Hyperthyroidism. Stein, Kimmel and Johnson found that D_L, D_M and Vc were essentially normal in 13 patients with hyperthyroidism, despite elevation of pulmonary capillary blood flow to approximately 2 to 3 times normal.[66] Reduction in pulmonary blood flow following antithyroid therapy was not associated with appreciable change in D_L, D_M and Vc. These observations support the contention that Vc is independent of the magnitude of pulmonary blood flow.

Polycythemia Vera. In 1927, Harrop and Heath, using Krogh's original CO method, reported subnormal D_L in 7 patients with polycythemia vera.[67] Newman, Feltman and Devlin reported normal alveolo-arterial oxygen differences in 4 of 5 patients with polycythemia vera.[68] Forster, in his review, briefly mentioned that D_L, D_M and Vc were normal in polycythemia vera.[69]

In 1963 Burgess and Bishop[70] reported D_L, D_M and Vc in 10 patients with polycythemia vera before and after treatment with repeated phlebotomies or with P^{32}. D_L was greater than normal in all patients before treatment and declined to normal or below normal after treatment. Vc, corrected for hemoglobin concentration, was less than normal before treatment and was not affected by treatment. D_M varied widely both before and after treatment. The increased D_L before treatment was considered to be a consequence of the increased hemoglobin concentration and the reduced Vc, a possible result of thrombosis of small pulmonary arteries.

Bjure also observed a fall in D_L after phlebotomy in patients with polycythemia vera, despite assumed improvement in the ventilation to perfusion ratio and a rise in cardiac output and stroke volume.[71] The result strongly suggests the dominant role of available pulmonary capillary hemoglobin in determining the level of D_L.

Anemia. Rankin, McNeill and Forster found reduced D_L in 5 patients with chronic iron deficiency due to blood loss.[72] As the anemia was corrected, D_L rose in proportion to the hematocrit. Vc was unchanged, and the results regarding D_M were not conclusive.

Jouasset-Strieder and associates determined D_L, D_M and Vc in dogs made anemic by replacing whole blood with plasma.[73] The mean arterial hemoglobin concentration declined from 14.3 to 6.6 grams %. D_L and D_M were proportional to the decline in hemoglobin concentration and to the volume of red blood cells in the pulmonary capillaries (VRBC). These results suggest that VRBC may be an estimate of the useful area of alveolo-capillary membrane, and that D_M/VRBC should vary with changes in the thickness of the membrane. The latter was not altered by anemia. The effect of anemia on D_L in dogs has been studied by several groups of investigators, utilizing various techniques. D_L and blood hemoglobin concentration changed proportionately, but measurements of Vc and D_M were not reported.[74-76]

Recently, Femi-Pearse and associates in our laboratory studied D_L, D_M and Vc in 10 patients with sickle cell disease.[77] Six patients had SS-hemoglobin disease and 4 had SC-hemoglobin disease. The D_L and Vc were normal in 6 patients with SS-hemoglobin disease and in 3 of 4 patients with SC-hemoglobin disease. D_L and Vc were subnormal in the remaining patient with SC-hemoglobin disease. The D_L in patients with SS-hemoglobin disease, however, was disproportionately high compared with their hemoglobin level. The disproportionately high D_L might have been due to (a) a relatively high pulmonary capillary hematocrit, (b) a relative increase in

Vc, or (c) a selective increase in D_M.

Hemorrhagic Shock. Burrows and Niden reported that hemorrhagic shock induced a marked fall in D_L in the dog, and that D_L failed to return completely to normal levels when blood was replaced.[76] The authors cautioned that a meaningful calculation of overall D_L is impossible during severe shock from any diffusion method which is inaccurate in the presence of D_L/V_A or D_L/ventilation inequalities.

Jouasset-Strieder, Cahill and Byrne studied changes of D_L and Vc in dogs during acute hemorrhagic shock produced by arterial bleeding.[78] During acute hemorrhagic shock D_L fell to 63% and Vc to 53% of the respective mean control values. When transfusion was given after 30 minutes of hemorrhagic hypotension, both D_L and Vc returned almost to control levels, and the difference was not significant. In normovolemic, irreversible shock after delayed transfusion, D_L rose to 84% of normal but the mean Vc remained at its low hypovolemic shock level. Changes in the pulmonary circulation with persistent narrowing of the vascular bed induced by hypovolemic shock were thought to have caused persistent reduction of Vc.

REFERENCES

1. Gazioglu, K., and Yu, P.N.: Pulmonary blood volume and pulmonary capillary blood volume in valvular heart disease. Circulation, *35*, 701, 1967.

2. Hamer, J.: The pulmonary capillary bed in mitral valve disease. Brit. Heart J., *27*, 319, 1965.

3. Daly, W.J., Giammona, S.T., Ross, J.C., and Feigenbaum, H.: Effects of pulmonary vascular congestion on postural changes in the perfusion and filling of the pulmonary vascular bed. J. Clin. Invest., *43*, 68, 1964.

4. McCredie, R.M.: Diffusing characteristics and pressure-volume relationships of the pulmonary capillary bed in mitral valve disease. J. Clin. Invest., *43*, 2279, 1964.

5. McCredie, R.M.: The pulmonary capillary bed in various forms of pulmonary hypertension. Circulation, *33*, 854, 1966.

6. Flatley, F.J., Constantine, H., McCredie, R.M., and Yu, P.N.: Pulmonary diffusing capacity and pulmonary capillary blood volume in normal subjects and in cardiac patients. Am. Heart J., *64*, 159, 1962.

7. Palmer, W.H., Gee, J.B.L., Mills, F.C., and Bates, D.V.: Disturbances of pulmonary function in mitral valve disease. Canad. Med. Ass. J., *89*, 744, 1963.

8. Parker, F., and Weiss, S.: The nature and significance of the structural changes in the lungs in mitral stenosis. Am. J. Pathol., *12*, 573, 1936.

9. Heath, D., and Edwards, J.E.: Histological changes in the lung in diseases associated with pulmonary venous hypertension. Brit. J. Dis. Chest, *53*, 8, 1959.

10. Short, D.S.: The arterial bed of the lung in pulmonary hypertension. Lancet, *2*, 12, 1957.

11. Carroll, D., Cohn, J., and Riley, R.L.: Pulmonary function in mitral valve disease: Distribution and diffusion characteristics in resting patients. J. Clin. Invest., *32*, 510, 1953.

12. Williams, M.H.: Pulmonary function studies in mitral stenosis before and after commissurotomy. J. Clin. Invest., *32*, 1094, 1953.

13. MacIntosh, D.J., Sinnot, J.C., Milne, I.G., and Reid, E.A.S.: Some aspects of disordered pulmonary function in mitral stenosis. Ann. Int. Med., *49*, 1294, 1958.

14. Dogliotti, G.C., Angelino, P.F., Brusca, A., Garbagni, R., Gavosto, F., Magri, G., and Minetto, E.: Pulmonary function in mitral valve disease. Hemodynamic and ventilatory studies. Am. J. Cardiol., *3*, 28, 1959.

15. Auchincloss, J.H., Gilbert, R., and Eich, R.H.: The pulmonary diffusing capacity in congenital and rheumatic heart disease. Circulation, *19*, 232, 1959.

16. Friedman, B.L., Macios, de J., and Yu, P.N.: Pulmonary function studies in patients with mitral stenosis. Am. Rev. Tuberc. & Resp. Dis., *79*, 265, 1959.

17. Burrows, B., Kasik, J. E., Niden, A.H., and Barclay, W.R.: Clinical usefulness of the single breath pulmonary diffusing capacity test. Am. Rev. Resp. Dis., *84*, 789, 1961.

18. Driscoll, J.F., Cugell, D.W., and Tobin, J.R.: Carbon monoxide diffusing capacity in mitral stenosis. Circulation, *28*, 713, 1963.

19. Reid, J.M., and Stevenson, J.G.: Pulmonary diffusing capacity in mitral valve disease. Brit. Heart J., *25*, 741, 1963.

20. Aber, C.P., and Campbell, J.A.: Significance of changes in the pulmonary diffusing capacity in mitral stenosis. Thorax, *20*, 135, 1965.

21. Riley, R.L., Johns, C.J., Cohen, G., Cohn, J.E., Carroll, D.G., and Shepard, R.H.: The diffusing capacity of the lungs in patients with mitral stenosis studied postoperatively. J. Clin. Invest., *35*, 1008, 1956.

22. Reid, J.M., and Stevenson, J.G.: The pulmonary diffusing capacity and ventilatory capacity before and after mitral valvotomy. Brit. Heart J., *26*, 649, 1964.

23. McCredie, R.M., Lovejoy, F.W., and Yu, P.N.: Pulmonary diffusing capacity and pulmonary capillary blood volume in patients with intracardiac shunts. J. Lab. Clin. Med., *63*, 914, 1964.

24. West, J.B., and Dollery, C.T.: Distribution of blood flow and ventilation perfusion ratio in the lung, measured with radioactive CO_2. J. Appl. Physiol., *15*, 405, 1960.

25. West, J.B.: Regional differences in gas exchange in the lung of erect man. J. Appl. Physiol., *17*, 893, 1962.

26. Dollery, C.T., Dyson, N.A., and Sinclair, J.D.: Regional variations in uptake of radioactive CO_2 in the normal lung. J. Appl. Physiol., *15*, 411, 1960.

27. Dollery, C.T., West, J.B., Wilcken, D.E.L., Goodwin, J.F., and Hughes-John, P.: Regional pulmonary blood flow in patients with circulatory shunts. Brit. Heart J., *23*, 225, 1961.

28. Rankin, J., and Callies, Q.C.: Diffusing characteristics of the human lung in congenital and acquired heart disease. Circulation, *18*, 768, 1958.

29. Bedell, G.N.: Comparison of pulmonary diffusing capacity in normal subjects and in patients with intracardiac septal defects. J. Lab. Clin. Med., *57*, 269, 1961.

30. Bucci, G., and Cook, C.D.: Studies on respiratory physiology in children. VI. Lung diffusing capacity, diffusing capacity of the pulmonary membrane and pulmonary capillary blood volume in congenital heart disease. J. Clin. Invest., *40*, 1431, 1961.

31. Rotman, H.H., and Woolf, C.R.: The diffusing capacity of the lungs at rest and on exercise in adults with atrial or ventricular septal defect. Dis. Chest, *43*, 6, 1963.

32. Murao, M., Momose, T., Hatano, S., Koike, S., Shiraishi, T., Uzawa, T., and Fukasu, S.: Studies of pulmonary diffusion. III. The measurement of pulmonary capillary blood volume and pulmonary membrane diffusing capacity in cardiac patients. Jap. Circ. J., *27*, 746, 1963.

33. McDonald, L., Emanuel, R., and Towers, M.: Aspects of pulmonary blood flow in atrial septal defect. Brit. Heart J., *21*, 279, 1959.

34. Staub, N.C., Bishop, J.M., and Forster, R.E.: Importance of diffusion and chemical reaction rates in O_2 uptake in the lung. J. Appl. Physiol., *17*, 21, 1962.

35. Staub, N.C.: Alveolar-arterial oxygen tension gradient due to diffusion. J. Appl. Physiol., *18*, 673, 1963.

36. MacNamara, J., Prime, F.J., and Sinclair, J.D.: The increase in diffusing capacity of the lungs on exercise. An experimental and clinical study. Lancet, *1*, 404, 1960.

37. McNeill, R.S., Rankin, J., and Forster, R.E.: The diffusing capacity of the pulmonary membrane and the pulmonary capillary blood volume in cardiopulmonary disease. Clin. Sci., *17*, 465, 1958.

38. Bates, D.V., Varvis, C.J., Donovan, R.E., and Christie, R.V.: Variation in the pulmonary capillary blood volume and membrane diffusion component in health and disease. J. Clin. Invest., *39*, 1401, 1960.

39. Bedell, G.N., and Eggers, R.L.: Pulmonary capillary blood volume and diffusing capacity of the pulmonary membrane. Findings in men with emphysema contrasted with those in men with fibrosis. J. Clin. Invest., *43*, 1245, 1964.

40. Williams, M.H., and Zohman, L.R.: Cardiopulmonary function in bronchial asthma: A comparison with chronic pulmonary emphysema. Am. Rev. Resp. Dis., *81*, 173, 1960.

41. MacNamara, J., Prime, F.J., and Sinclair, J.D.: An assessment of the steady-state carbon monoxide method for estimating pulmonary diffusing capacity. Thorax, *14*, 166, 1959.

42. Austrian, R., McClement, J.H., Renzetti, A.D., Donald, K.W., Riley, R.L., and Cournand, A.: Clinical and physiologic features of some types of pulmonary diseases with impairment of alveolar-capillary diffusion: The syndrome of "alveolar-capillary block." Am. J. Med., *11*, 667, 1951.

43. Williams, M.H.: Pulmonary function in Boeck's sarcoid. J. Clin. Invest., *32*, 909, 1953.

44. Riley, R.L., Riley, M.C., and Hill, H. McD.: Diffuse pulmonary sarcoidosis: Diffusing

capacity during exercise and other lung function studies in relation to ACTH therapy. Bull. Johns Hopkins Hosp., *91*, 345, 1952.

45. Stone, D.J., Schwartz, A., Feltman, J.A., and Lovelock, F.J.: Pulmonary function in sarcoidosis: Results with cortisone therapy. Am. J. Med., *15*, 468, 1953.

46. Marshall, R., Smellie, H., Baylis, J.H., Hoyle, C., and Bates, D.V.: Pulmonary function in sarcoidosis. Thorax, *13*, 48, 1958.

47. Bates, D.V.: The measurement of the pulmonary diffusing capacity in the presence of lung disease. J. Clin. Invest., *37*, 591, 1958.

48. Hamer, N.A.J.: Changes in the components of the diffusing capacity in pulmonary sarcoidosis. Thorax, *18*, 275, 1963.

49. McClement, J.H., Renzetti, A.D., Himmelstein, A., and Cournand, A.: Cardiopulmonary function in the pulmonary form of Boeck's sarcoid and its modification by cortisone therapy. Am. Rev. Tuberc., *67*, 154, 1953.

50. Smellie, H., Apthorp, G.H., and Marshall, R.: The effect of corticosteroid treatment on pulmonary function in sarcoidosis. Thorax, *16*, 87, 1961.

51. Schreiner, B.F., Murphy, G.W., and Yu, P.N.: Pulmonary blood volume in congestive heart failure. Circulation, *34*, 249, 1966.

52. Yu, P.N., Schreiner, B.F., Cohen, J., and Murphy, G.W.: Idiopathic cardiomyopathy. A study of left ventricular function and pulmonary circulation in 15 patients. Am. Heart J., *71*, 330, 1966.

53. Bates, D.V., and Christie, R.V.: *Respiratory Function in Disease*, Philadelphia, W.B. Saunders Co, 1964.

54. Colp, C.R., and Williams, M.H.: Pulmonary function following pulmonary embolization. Am. Rev. Resp. Dis., *85*, 799, 1962.

55. Dunér, H., Pernow, B., and Rignér, K.G: The prognosis of pulmonary embolism. A medical and physiological follow-up examination of patients treated at the Departments of Medicine and Surgery, Karolinsha Sjukuset in 1952-58. Acta med Scand., *168*, 381, 1960.

56. Marshall, R., and Allison, P.R.: Pulmonary embolism by small blood clots. Physiological responses in the anesthetized dog. Thorax, *17*, 289, 1962.

57. Marshall, R., Sabiston, D.C., Allison, P.R., Bosman, A.R., and Dunnill, M.S.: Immediate and late effects of pulmonary embolism by large thrombi in dogs. Thorax, *18*, 1, 1963.

58. Nadel, J.A., Gold, W.M., Jennings, D.B., Wright, R.R., and Fundenberg, H.H.: Unusual disease of pulmonary arteries with dyspnea. Am. J. Med., *41*, 440, 1966.

59. Yu, P.N.: Primary pulmonary hypertension. Report of six cases and review of literature. Ann. Int. Med., *49*, 1138, 1958.

60. Dresdale, D.T., Schultz, M., and Michton, R.J.: Primary pulmonary hypertension. I. Clinical and hemodynamic study. Am. J. Med., *11*, 686, 1951.

61. Marshall, R.J., Helmholz, H.F., and Shephard, J.T.: Effect of acetylcholine on pulmonary vascular resistance in a patient with idiopathic pulmonary hypertension. Circulation, *20*, 391, 1959.

62. Wood, P.: Pulmonary hypertension, with special reference to the vasoconstrictive factor. Brit. Heart J., *20*,557, 1958.

63. Robin, E.D., Julian, D.G., Travis, D.M., and Crump, C.H.: A physiologic approach to the diagnosis of acute pulmonary embolism. New Engl. J. Med., *260*, 586, 1959.

64. Robin, E.D., Forkner, C.E., Bromberg, P.A., Croteau, J.R., and Travis, D.H.: Alveolar gas exchange in clinical pulmonary embolism. New Engl. J. Med., *262*, 283, 1960.

65. Severinghaus, J.W., and Stuppel, M.: Alveolar dead space as an index of distribution of blood flow in pulmonary capillaries. J. Appl. Physiol., *10*, 335, 1957.

66. Stein, M., Kimbel, P., and Johnson, R.L.: Pulmonary function in hyperthyroidism. J. Clin. Med., *40*, 348, 1961.

67. Harrop, G.A., and Heath, E.H.: Pulmonary gas diffusion in polycythemia vera. J. Clin. Invest., *4*, 53, 1927.

68. Newman, J., Feldman, J.A., and Devlin, B.: Pulmonary function studies in polycythemia vera. Results in five probable cases. Am. J. Med., *11*, 706, 1951.

69. Forster, R.E.: Exchange of gases between alveolar air and pulmonary capillary blood: Pulmonary diffusing capacity. Physiol. Rev., *37*, 391, 1957.

70. Burgess, J.H., and Bishop, J.M.: Pulmonary diffusing capacity and its subdivisions in polycythemia vera. J. Clin. Invest., *42*, 997, 1963.

71. Bjure, J.: Pulmonary diffusing capacity for carbon monoxide in relation to cardiac output in man. Scand. J. Clin. Lab. Invest., *17*, Suppl. 81, 1965.

72. Rankin, J., McNeill, R.S., and Forster, R.E.: The effect of anemia on the alveolar capillary exchange of carbon monoxide in man. J. Clin Invest., *40*, 1323, 1961.

73. Jouasset-Strieder, D., Cahill, J.M., Byrne, J.J., and Gaensler, E.A.: Pulmonary diffusing capacity and capillary blood volume in nor-

mal and anemic dogs, J. Appl. Physiol., *20*, 113, 1965.

74. Mochizuki, M.T., Anso, T., Goto, H., Hammamoto, A., and Makigughi, Y.: The dependency of the diffusing capacity on the HbO$_2$ saturation of the capillary blood and on anemia. Jap. J. Physiol., *8*, 225, 1958.

75. Kilburn, K.H.: Ventilation dead space and hemoglobin level as modifiers of the steady state method for diffusing capacity for carbon monoxide. Am. Rev. Resp. Dis., *81*, 945, 1961.

76. Burrows, B., and Niden, A.H.: Effects of anemia and hemorrhagic shock on pulmonary diffusing capacity in the dog lung. J. Appl. Physiol., *18*, 123, 1963.

77. Femi-Pearse, D., Gazioglu, K., and Yu, P.N.: Pulmonary diffusing capacity and capillary blood volume in sickle cell disease. To be published.

78. Jouasset-Strieder, D., Cahill, J.M., and Byrne, J.J: Pulmonary capillary blood volume in dogs during shock and after retransfusion. J. Appl. Physiol., *21*, 365, 1966.

Section IV

CHAPTER 16

Vasomotion of the Pulmonary Vascular Bed

In a comprehensive treatise on the pulmonary circulation of the dog, Plumier stated in 1904 that pulmonary vasoconstriction may be provoked by sympathetic stimulation and by asphyxia.[1] In 1946 Euler and Liljestrand demonstrated a rise of the pulmonary arterial pressure in the hypoxic cat and suggested that this effect resulted from the direct action of hypoxia on the pulmonary vessels because it was not abolished by stellate ganglionectomy or by vagotomy.[2] They also proposed the concept that local hypoxia from local hypoventilation may cause local vasoconstriction with consequent diversion of blood to better ventilated alveoli. During the past 15 years Daly, Duke and associates have provided convincing evidence for the presence of pulmonary vasomotor fibers in both isolated lung preparations and intact animals.[2-7] They believed that the pulmonary vasoconstrictor fibers demonstrated in the cervical vagosympathetic nerves were sympathetic in origin.[4,8] The existence of parasympathetic pulmonary vasomotor fibers, however, was less generally accepted, although many experiments have demonstrated cholinergic dilator activity.[4]

The importance of the carotid chemoreceptors and baroreceptors in regulating pulmonary hemodynamic responses has been emphasized by Daly and Daly.[9,10] They felt that reflex responses of the pulmonary vascular bed in the dog produced by stimulation of the carotid baroreceptors or chemoreceptors are mediated by efferent fibers of the upper thoracic sympathetic outflow.

As emphasized by Daly and Hebb in their monograph, "The demonstration of an active response of the lesser circulation to any stimulus demands experimental conditions that exclude the participation of passive effects which simulate or in any way modify a direct action on the vessels."[11] Factors potentially able to affect the pulmonary vascular bed passively or mechanically include the following: (*a*) cardiac output and contractile force of the myocardium, (*b*) systemic arterial pressure, (*c*) bronchial blood flow, (*d*) ventilation, (*e*) bronchomotor activity, and (*f*) release of hormones (*i.e.*, catecholamines) into the circulation.

Identification of active vasomotion in the pulmonary vessels requires physiologic or pharmacologic interventions which will alter flow-pressure-volume relationships in the pulmonary vascular bed without influencing cardiac function, systemic or bronchial circulation, bronchial muscles or ventilation. Under these conditions, and if experiments are conducted with pulmonary blood volume controlled or

269

unaltered, an increase in calculated pulmonary vascular resistance indicates active vasoconstriction; and a decrease in resistance reflects active vasodilatation. Indeed, if the pulmonary blood flow can be adequately controlled, any discordant changes in the pulmonary vascular pressure-volume relationship may be considered evidence of active vasomotion.[12,13] Thus, vasoconstriction is manifested by an increase in pulmonary vascular pressure associated with a decrease in pulmonary vascular volume, while vasodilatation is indicated by a decrease in pulmonary vascular pressure accompanied by augmented volume. Since the transmural pressure is the difference between intravascular pressure and tissue pressure,[14] such a conclusion is valid only when the tissue pressure remains constant.

Active pulmonary vasomotion in man has been demonstrated extensively by the use of two agents, low oxygen and acetylcholine.[12,13,15-26] The evidence is convincing in both animals and man that acute hypoxia causes active vasoconstriction and acetylcholine infusion produces active vasodilatation.

In our laboratory, pulmonary circulatory dynamics were studied during inhalation of low oxygen in 18 patients, including 7 with mitral valve disease, 9 with aortic valve disease, and 2 with idiopathic cardiomyopathy (Chapter 11 and Table 11-13).

During acute hypoxia the cardiac index increased slightly in most patients, largely due to a more rapid heart rate since no consistent change was observed in the stroke volume. Pulmonary arterial and distending pressures rose in the large majority of cases, while the left atrial pressure remained essentially unchanged. The pulmonary blood volume declined in 13 of 18 cases, increased slightly in 2 cases

and failed to change in the remaining 3. Left atrial pressure rose in 4 of the 5 patients in whom the pulmonary blood volume was either increased or unchanged. This increase in left atrial pressure may have caused sufficient passive distention of the pulmonary vascular bed to neutralize the decrease in volume which would otherwise have resulted from acute hypoxia.

When changes in pulmonary distending pressure and pulmonary blood volume are both considered, increased pulmonary distending pressure during acute hypoxia was accompanied by significantly decreased or unchanged pulmonary blood volume in 10 patients with cardiac disease (Figures 16-1 and 16 2). In 7 patients, pulmonary blood volume declined without change in pulmonary distending pressure. The remaining patient showed no significant change in either pressure or volume. Elevated pulmonary distending pressure together with decreased or unchanged pulmonary blood volume is

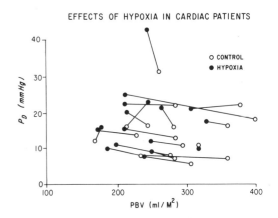

EFFECTS OF HYPOXIA IN CARDIAC PATIENTS

Figure 16-1. Pulmonary distending pressures (P_d) plotted against pulmonary blood volume (PBV) in cardiac patients during acute hypoxia. In most cases P_d increased with a decrease or no change in PBV. These discordant changes are highly suggestive of active vasoconstriction.

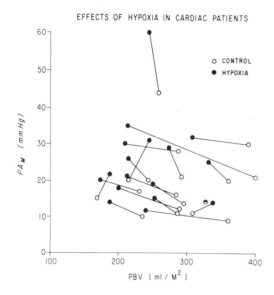

Figure 16-2. Pulmonary arterial mean pressure (PAm) plotted against pulmonary blood volume (PBV) in cardiac patients during acute hypoxia. The changes were similar to those observed between P_d and PBV as shown in Figure 16-1. The rise of pressure was predominantly in the pulmonary arterial segment, locating the active vasoconstriction proximal to the pulmonary capillaries.

strong evidence for active pulmonary vasoconstriction.

Inasmuch as most of our patients had valvular heart disease and pulmonary vascular abnormality, the possibility remains that increased pulmonary blood flow during acute hypoxia may contribute to the augmentation of pulmonary arterial pressure. This possibility is partly supported by the observation that the rise in the pulmonary arterial pressure of patients with significant pulmonary hypertension was usually greater than in patients with normal resting pressure. However, arguments against the significance of increased flow were (*a*) the relatively small increase in cardiac index; (*b*) absence of change in the left atrial pressure in most patients; and (*c*) as will be shown in a later section, demonstration of similar pulmonary vascular pressure-volume responses to hypoxia in a normal subject.

Liljestrand demonstrated persistence of the pulmonary pressor response after atropine and ergotamine, suggesting a direct rather than a reflex action of hypoxia.[27] Although direct action of low oxygen on vessel walls has been strongly suspected, the possibility of local release of catecholamines during acute hypoxia cannot be excluded. [28-30] Catecholamines might be released either from adrenergic nerve endings in the lung by direct or reflex stimulation, or from local chromaffin tissue.[31] Goldring and associates, however, reported no detectable rise in circulating catecholamines in 13 normal subjects during the inhalation of 11% O_2.[32] They found further that a rather large infusion of catecholamine into the pulmonary artery was required to reproduce the effects of low oxygen. Furthermore, while acute hypoxia caused the pulmonary arterial pressure to rise without affecting the pulmonary wedge pressure, the infusion of catecholamine raised both pulmonary arterial and wedge pressures.

Which segment of the pulmonary vascular bed is the site of active vasoconstriction is not certain. Pulmonary capillaries are probably not contractile, since they lack a muscular component.[33] The absence of a pressure gradient from the pulmonary wedge position to the left atrium, as previously reported from our laboratory, is strong evidence against significant sphincter action of the pulmonary vein in man.[12,13] Nevertheless, since the pulmonary veins probably contain 35 to 50% of the blood in the pulmonary vascular bed,[34-36] acute hypoxic constriction of the pulmonary veins might reduce the pulmonary blood volume appreciably without a demonstrable change in the venous pressure. In dogs and in cattle, however, hypoxia may indeed induce a pressure gradient between the pulmonary wedge position and the left atrium, resulting from a sphincter mechanism located within the pulmonary veins or at their junction with the left atrium.[37,38]

Inasmuch as pressure in the left atrium and in the pulmonary wedge position was not affected by acute hypoxia in our study, the evidence indicates that the pressor effect results from responses occurring proximal to the pulmonary capillaries. The increase in pulmonary arterial and distending pressures was generally greater in those patients who had pre-existing pulmonary hypertension than in those with normal pressure. In patients with pulmonary hypertension some degree of pulmonary vasoconstriction probably was already present. During acute hypoxia, additional constriction of the pulmonary arterioles would result in a disproportionately greater increase in pressure and resistance than in those patients without pre-existing pulmonary hypertension.

The postulation that hypoxia affects pulmonary arteries and arterioles predominantly is supported by two recent experimental studies. First, Staub and Kato observed reduction in the caliber of the precapillary vessels in rat lung, when it was rapidly frozen during nitrogen inhalation.[39,40] Second, Sackner and associates studied simultaneous changes in pulmonary vascular resistance and pulmonary arterial capacity in the hypoxic lung of the dog.[41] They found that during acute hypoxia the pulmonary arterial pressure and vascular resistance rose and the pulmonary arterial capacity declined. Such findings strongly suggest constriction of the pulmonary arterial system with a hypoxic stimulus.

Opposite to the effects of acute hypoxia, infusion of acetylcholine into the right side of the heart or main pulmonary artery of man usually causes a fall in pulmonary arterial and distending pressures and an augmentation of pulmonary blood volume.[12,13] The response is generally more pronounced in patients with moderate pulmonary hypertension than in normal subjects, although the hypotensive effect is greater in normal subjects when hypoxic pulmonary hypertension is induced first.

As reported in Chapter 12, we have studied the effects of acetylcholine infusion in 14 patients with predominant mitral stenosis, where mean pulmonary arterial pressure was 28 mm Hg or greater. Pulmonary arterial and distending pressures were consistently reduced in all patients. The fall in pressures was accompanied by an increase in pulmonary blood volume in 10 patients and no change in volume in 4. Cardiac index increased slightly in most patients, and changes in heart rate and systemic arterial pressure were insignificant. The left atrial pressure of half of the patients declined slightly. The discordant decrease in pulmonary vascular pressure and increase in pulmonary vascular volume reflect active vasodilatation (Figure 12-1). The slight increase in cardiac index was probably not important because augmented pulmonary blood flow would have tended to increase the pulmonary arterial and left atrial pres-

TABLE 16-1 Effects of Acetylcholine on Pulmonary Circulation during Acute Hypoxia

| Patient | Diagnosis | Age | Sex | BSA | Condition | Sa_{O_2} | CI | SI | Pressures (mm Hg) | | | | PA-BA | Tm (sec.) | | Blood Volume (mL/M²) | |
									PAm	LAm	P_d	BAm	PA-BA	LA-BA	PA-LA	CBV	PBV
R.D.	N	27	M	1.77	A	93.0	3.31	44	14	4	9.0	80	10.4	5.4	5.0	575	276
					B	76.5	3.35	45	23	4	13.5	82	9.3	5.1	4.2	526	234
					C	—	3.38	38	19	4	11.5	85	9.1	5.1	4.0	510	232
					D	—	—	—	14	4	9.0	85	—	—	—	—	—
P.H.	MS	37	F	1.57	A	92.9	2.56	39	10	6	8.0	80	12.8	7.3	5.5	546	234
					B	69.5	3.11	41	14	6	10.0	131	10.0	6.4	3.6	516	186
					C	79.8	2.87	36	8	5	6.5	53	11.9	6.5	5.4	568	256
					D	—	—	—	10	6	8.0	—	—	—	—	—	—
M.B.	MS TS	29	F	1.86	A	96.7	1.83	23	20	13	16.5	94	18.8	10.8	8.0	575	245
					B	81.3	2.08	21	26	14	20.0	96	16.3	10.1	6.2	565	215
					C	—	2.00	20	16	11	13.5	—	20.2	11.0	9.2	680	305
					D	—	—	—	22	10	16.0	—	—	—	—	—	—
C.M.	AS	47	M	1.98	A	—	3.06	41	30	12	21.0	92	14.6	6.9	7.7	742	378
					B	—	3.22	43	32	10	21.0	92	13.4	7.5	5.9	720	306
					C	—	3.70	45	21	8	14.5	84	12.3	7.4	4.9	765	300
B.M.	MS	26	M	1.68	A	88.3	1.60	21	44	18	31.0	68	21.8	12.1	9.7	580	258
					B	76.6	1.57	18	60	24	42.0	64	22.5	13.3	9.2	590	242
					C	59.2	2.38	20	52	24	38.0	78	15.4	7.4	8.0	610	330

N = Normal subject

A = Control period

B = Period of acute hypoxia

C = Period of acute hypoxia and acetylcholine infusion

D = Recovery period

Other symbols and abbreviations are identical to those used in Tables 11-1 and 11-13 sures, not reduce them. In the absence of appreciable change in systemic arterial pressure, heart rate and ventilation in nearly all the patients, passive or mechanical effects from bronchoconstriction and systemic vasodilatation may be safely ruled out. The possibility of augmented bronchial blood flow or local release of catecholamines has not been eliminated, but these factors probably would have been expected to cause a rise instead of a fall in the pulmonary arterial and distending pressures.

We have confirmed the reports by Fritts and co-workers that infusion of acetylcholine counteracts the pulmonary hypertension induced by acute hypoxia.[25] Table 16-1 and Figure 16-3 show a significant rise in pulmonary arterial and distending pressures associated with a decrease or no change in pulmonary blood volume in a normal subject and in 4 patients during hypoxia. Infusion of acetylcholine into the main pulmonary artery during the period of acute hypoxia caused a definite reduction of pulmonary arterial and distending pressures, accompanied by an increase or no change in pulmonary blood volume. These results clearly demonstrate that the augmented tone of the pulmonary vessels (principally arteries and arterioles) induced by acute hypoxia was counteracted by active vasodilatation during acetylcholine infusion.

Thus, the evidence strongly favors active vasomotion in the pulmonary vascular bed of man. It is uncertain which of the three compartments (arteries, capillaries and veins) actively participate, but the available data indicate that the pulmonary arteries are at least more actively involved than the pulmonary capillaries or veins. However, simultaneous opposite changes in two compartments have not

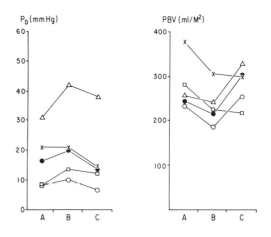

Figure 16-3.   Changes in pulmonary distending pressure (P_d) and pulmonary blood volume (PBV) in a normal subject (O) and four patients with valvular heart disease (• ✕) during control period (A), during inhalation of 12% oxygen (B), and during acute hypoxia and acetylcholine infusion (C). When the subjects were breathing low oxygen, P_d rose or did not change, and PBV declined. During this hypoxic period infusion of acetylcholine into the main pulmonary artery caused a definite decrease in P_d associated with an increase or no change in PBV. These changes clearly demonstrated that the augmented tone of the pulmonary vessels (principally precapillary in location) induced by acute hypoxia was counteracted by acute vasodilatation as a result of acetylcholine infusion.

been excluded, such as constriction of one segment (pulmonary arteries) and dilatation of another (pulmonary veins). The direction of the pressure changes, however, makes this possibility unlikely. Nevertheless, until a simple and reliable method is developed to measure pressures and volume in the consecutive vascular segments, active vasomotion in the pulmonary circulation must be interpreted on the basis of a total and somewhat ill-defined vascular bed.

REFERENCES

1. Plumier, L.: La circulation pulmonaire chez le chien. Arch. Int. de Physiol., *1*, 176, 1904.

2. Euler, U.S.V., and Liljestrand, G.: Observations on the pulmonary arterial pressure in the cat. Acta Physiol. Scand., *12*, 301, 1946.

3. Daly, I. de B., and Duke, H.: Note on a method for the demonstration of pulmonary vasomotor fibres. Quart. J. Exp. Physiol., *34*, 151, 1948.

4. Daly, I. de B., Duke, H., Hebb, C.O., and Weatherall, J.: Pulmonary vasomotor fibres in the sympathetic chain and its associated ganglia in the dog. Quart. J. Exp. Physiol., *34*, 285, 1948.

5. Daly, I. de B., and Hebb, C.: Pulmonary vasomotor fibres in the cervical vago-sympathetic nerve of the dog. Quart. J. Exp. Physiol., *37*, 19, 1952.

6. Daly, I. de B., Duke, H.M., Linzell, J.L., and Weatherall, J.: Pulmonary vasomotor nerve activity. Quart. J. Exp. Physiol., *37*, 149, 1952.

7. Daly, I. de B.: Intrinsic mechanisms of the lung. Quart. J. Exp. Physiol., *43*, 2, 1958.

8. Daly, M. de B., and Mount, L.E.: The origin, course and nature of bronchomotor fibers in the cervical sympathetic nerve of the cat. J. Physiol., *113*, 43, 1951.

9. Daly, I. de B., and Daly, M. de B.: The effects of stimulation of the carotid body chemoreceptors on pulmonary vascular resistance in the dog. J. Physiol., *137*, 436, 1957.

10. Daly, I. de B., and Daly, M. de B.: The effects of stimulation of the carotid sinus baroreceptors on the pulmonary vascular bed in the dog. J. Physiol., *148*, 220, 1959.

11. Daly, I. de B., and Hebb, C.: *Pulmonary and Bronchial Vascular Systems.* Baltimore, Williams & Wilkins Co., 1966, p. 158.

12. Oakley, C., Glick, G., Luria, M.N., Schreiner, B.F., and Yu, P.N.: Some regulatory mechanisms of the human pulmonary vascular bed. Circulation, *25*, 917, 1962.

13. Yu, P.N., Glick, G., Schreiner, B.F., and Murphy, G.W.: Effects of acute hypoxia on the pulmonary vascular bed of patients with acquired heart disease, with special reference to the demonstration of active vasomotion. Circulation, *27*, 541, 1963.

14. Burton, A.C.: *Physiology and Biophysics of the Circulation.* Chapter 8, Chicago, Year Book Medical Publishers, Inc., 1965.

15. Motley, H.L., Cournand, A., Werkö, L., Himmelstein, A., and Dresdale, D.: Influence of short periods of induced acute anoxia upon pulmonary artery pressures in man. Am. J. Physiol., *150*, 315, 1947.

16. Westcott, R.N., Fowler, N.O., Scott, R.C., Hanenstein, V.D., and McQuire, J.: Anoxia and pulmonary vascular resistance. J. Clin. Invest., *30*, 957, 1951.

17. Doyle, J.T., Wilson, J.S., and Warren, J.V.: Pulmonary vascular responses to short-time hypoxia in human subjects. Circulation, *5*, 263, 1952.

18. Cournand, A.F.: Pulmonary circulation. Its control in man, with some remarks on methodology. Am. Heart J., *54*, 172, 1957.

19. Himmelstein, A., Harris, P., Fritts, H.W., and Cournand, A.: Effect of severe unilateral hypoxia on the partition of pulmonary blood volume in man. J. Thorac. Surg., *36*, 369, 1958.

20. Siebens, A.A., Smith, R.E., and Storey, C.F.: Effect of hypoxia on pulmonary vessels in man. Am. J. Physiol., *180*, 428, 1955.

21. Fishman, A.P., Fritts, H.W., and Cournand, A.: Effects of acute hypoxia and exercise on the pulmonary circulation. Circulation, *22*, 204, 1960.

22. Fishman, A.P.: Respiratory gases in the regulation of the pulmonary circulation. Physiol. Rev., *41*, 214, 1961.

23. Harris, P.: Influence of acetylcholine on the pulmonary arterial pressure. Brit. Heart J., *19*, 272, 1957.

24. Wood, P., Besterman, E.M., Towers, M.K., and McIlroy, M.B.: The effect of acetylcholine on pulmonary vascular resistance and left atrial pressure in mitral stenosis. Brit. Heart J., *19*, 279, 1957.

25. Fritts, H.W., Harris P., Clauss, R.H., Odell, J.E., and Cournand, A.: Effect of acetylcholine on the human pulmonary circulation under normal and hypoxic conditions. J. Clin. Invest., *37*, 99, 1958.

26. Shepherd. J.T., Semler, H.J., Helmholz, H.F., and Wood, E.H.: Effects of infusion of acetylcholine on pulmonary vascular resistance in patients with pulmonary hypertension and congenital heart disease. Circulation, *20*, 381, 1959.

27. Liljestrand, G.: Regulation of pulmonary arterial blood pressure. Arch. Int. Med., *81*, 162, 1948.

28. Aviado, D.M., Cerletti, A., Alanis, J., Bulle, P.H., and Schmidt, C.F.: Effects of anoxia on pressure, resistance and blood volume (p^{32}) of pulmonary vessels. Am. J. Physiol., *169*, 460, 1952.

29. Hurlimann, A., and Wiggers, C.J.: Effects of progressive general anoxia on the pulmonary circulation. Circ. Res., *1*, 230, 1953.

30. Brutsaert, D.: Influence of reserpine and of adrenolytic agents on the pulmonary arterial pressor response to hypoxia and catecholamines. Arch. Int. Physiol., *72*, 395, 1964.

31. Daly, I. de B., and Hebb, C.: *Pulmonary and Bronchial Vascular Systems*. Baltimore, Williams & Wilkins Co., 1966, p. 345.

32. Goldring, R.M., Turino, G.M., Cohen, G., Jameson, A.G., Bass, B.G., and Fishman, A.P.: The catecholamines in pulmonary arterial pressor response to acute hypoxia. J. Clin. Invest., *41*, 1211, 1962.

33. Fishman, A.P.: Dynamics of the pulmonary circulation. *In Handbook of Physiology*. Section 2, Circulation, Vol. 2, p. 1675, Washington, D.C., American Physiological Society, 1963.

34. Green, H.D.: Circulation system: Physical principles. *In* O. Glasser (ed), *Medical Physics*, Vol. 2, p. 228, Chicago, Year Book Publishers, Inc., 1950.

35. Landis, E.M., and Hortenstine, J.C.: Functional significance of venous blood pressure. Physiol. Rev., *30*, 1, 1950.

36. Piiper, J.: Grosse des Arterien, des Capillar, und des Venevolumens in der isolierten Hundelunge. Pflueger's Arch fur die Ges. Physiol., *269*, 182, 1959.

37. Rivera-Estrada, C., Saltzman, P.W., Singer, D., and Katz, L.N.: Action of hypoxia on the pulmonary vasculature. Circ. Res., *6*, 10, 1958.

38. Tsagaris, T.J., Kuida, H., and Hecht, H.H.: Evidence for pulmonary venoconstriction in Brisket disease. Fed. Proc., *21*, 108, 1962.

39. Staub, N.C.: Site of action of hypoxia on the pulmonary vasculature. Fed. Proc., *22*, 453, 1963.

40. Kato, M., and Staub, N.C.: Site of effect of hypoxia and hypercapnia on peripheral pulmonary vasculature. Physiologist, *7*, 174, 1964.

41. Sackner, M.A., Will, D.H., and DuBois, A.B.: The site of pulmonary vasomotor activity during hypoxia or serotonin administration. Physiologist, *7*, 243, 1964.

CHAPTER 17

Distensibility Characteristics of the Pulmonary Vascular Bed

Elasticity may be defined as the property of materials which enables them to resist deformation by the development of a resisting force or tension.[1] In other words, it is the force which tends to restore the size and shape of a body which has been deformed. Extensibility of a vessel denotes the amount of lengthening which can be achieved short of rupture, whereas distensibility is the possible increase in its volume. The latter two terms are reciprocal functions of vascular elasticity.

Experiments have shown that the extensibility of the various tissues which comprise the blood vessels is not uniform.[1-4] Muscle, for example, is more extensible than elastic tissue which, in turn, is more extensible than collagen. Such differences may explain why, as an arterial vessel wall is stretched, it increasingly resists further stretching. When the distending pressure in an arterial vessel is low, the response to stretch has been suggested to be primarily that of elastic tissues, the collagen fibers remaining unstretched. According to this explanation, as distending pressure increases further, extension of the vessel wall invokes response of the less extensible collagen fibers. Thus, increased resistance to stretching is a predictable consequence of further increase in distending pressure.

The distending or transmural pressure in a blood vessel is the difference between the intravascular pressure and the surrounding tissue pressure. The intravascular pressure in pulmonary vessels is easily measured, but the tissue pressure is usually unknown. The latter probably lies between the atmospheric pressure and the subatmospheric intrapleural pressure. Thus, the true transmural pressure may be slightly higher than the conventionally measured intravascular pressure.

Pressure within a blood vessel is closely related to the tension in its wall. Laplace's law states that tension in the wall of a vessel is equal to the distending pressure multiplied by the radius of the vessel.[3,4]

$$T = Pr$$

Thus, the volume and pressure in a blood vessel can be related to its circumferential length and the tension in its wall. If tension is plotted along the ordinate and circumferential length along the abscissa, as pressure increases the line of relationship between circumferential length and tension bends toward the tension axis. This non-linear relationship again illustrates the decreasing extensibility of the wall of the vessel as it is stretched. Forces opposing the tension in the wall of a blood vessel may include (a) elastic recoil resistance to stretch of the muscles, elastic tissues and collagen fibers; (b) constriction of smooth muscles in the media of the vessel; and (c) surface tension between the endothelium and blood.[3-5]

The pulmonary trunk and its two main branches conduct blood and store it during right ventricular ejection. Since pressure in the pulmonary arteries is much lower than that in the aorta, the wall of the pulmonary arteries is much thinner than that of the aorta, and tension in the wall of the pulmonary trunk may be only one-tenth that in the aorta. The pulmonary trunk is, therefore, more extensible than the aorta.

The distensibility of the pulmonary vascular bed has been studied in dogs by Sarnoff and Berglund.[6] They measured the pulmonary vascular volume and pressure simultaneouly during stepwise infusion and withdrawal of blood and then constructed injection and relaxation pressure-volume curves. At low pressure, substantial increase or decrease in volume affected the pressure only slightly;but at high pressure, a small change in volume changed the pressure significantly. Similar results were reported by Frasher and Sobin who studied responses to stretch of the proximal segment of the pulmonary arteries of swine.[7]

Many workers have attempted to estimate the distensibility of the pulmonary vessels in man during life and after death. Meyer and Schollmeyer measured the static distensibility of the human pulmonary trunk and its two main branches after death.[8] They found volume distensibility coefficients varying from 1.6 to 1.1 ml/mm Hg in patients between 30 and 70 years of age. As pressure was increased from 10 to 25 mm Hg, the percentage increase in volume decreased progressively in older patients.

Deuchar and Knebel estimated the distensibility of the pulmonary arteries in young children during life.[9] Distensibility was 0.7 ml/mm Hg at the age of 5, 1.1 ml/mm Hg at the age of 10, and 1.9 ml/mm Hg at the age of 20 years.

An increase of 38% in the volume of the pulmonary artery during systole was reported in a study of measurements on chest roentgenograms.[10] An electrokymographic study of pulse wave velocity in the pulmonary arteries demonstrated a 48% increase in pulmonary arterial volume during systole.[11]

Measuring instantaneous pulmonary capillary blood flow in a normal subject, DuBois and associates reported a change of 20 ml and 3.5 mm Hg during diastole, a calculated distensibility of the pulmonary arterial system of 5.7ml/mm Hg.[12]

Lasser and Amram demonstrated a decrease in the distensibility of pulmonary arteries during exercise in 10 patients with predominant mitral stenosis.[13] This was manifested by a significant rise in the mean pulmonary artery pressure associated with a fall in the stroke volume. Furthermore, a greater decrease in distensibility was found in patients with higher pulmonary arterial pressures than in those with lower pressures. They postulated a probable increase in the blood volume in the pulmonary arteries during exercise and felt that the disproportionate rise in the pulmonary arterial pressure and the decrease in distensibility might be a passive consequence of an increase in volume and diameter of the pulmonary arteries and the expected altered elastic properties of the stretched vessel wall.

When the technique of measuring pulmonary blood volume (PBV) in man became available, it was possible to relate PBV to the pulmonary vascular pressure, both at rest and during physiologic and pharmacologic interventions. Thus, Milnor and associates attempted to estimate the relative compliance or distensibility of the human pulmonary vascular bed by dividing PBV in ml by mean pulmonary distending pressure (P_d) in mm Hg at rest.[14] P_d was the average of pulmonary arterial (PAm) and left atrial (LAm) mean pressures. They considered that this relative compliance might be directly related to true compliance or distensibility, $\triangle V/\triangle P$, if (a) vessel lumen diameter depends only on net transmural pressure and the elasticity of the vessel wall; (b) P_d is an accurate measurement of net transmural pressure; and (c) vessel length is constant, so that PBV is an index of average lumen diameter.

Milnor and associates observed a decrease in relative compliance or distensibility in patients with valvular heart disease and high pulmonary vascular resistance (PVR) compared to normal.[14] In some patients elevated PVR associated with a relatively low PBV may be attributed to widespread decrease in pulmonary vascular distensibility. However, large changes in PVR might occur as a result of constriction at a well-localized level of the vascular bed, such as the small arteries or arterioles. Under this circumstance, the change in PBV would be either minimal or undetectable. Therefore, as discussed in Chapter 10, no consistent relation between PVR and PBV would be expected. Freitas and co-workers reported relative compliance of 34 ± 16 ml/mm Hg in patients with normal pulmonary arterial mean pressure, and 13 ± 9 ml/mm Hg in patients with pulmonary hypertension.[15] The difference was statistically significant.

As mentioned by Fishman, pulmonary vascular distensibility is a composite term.[16] It includes not only the effects of the elastic properties of the vascular wall, but also effects resulting from the tone of their smooth muscles, the perivascular air pressure, the alveolar surface tension, the presence or absence of excessive interstitial fluid and the presence or absence of mechanical distortions of adjacent pulmonary tissue.

A vessel is more distensible when it is thin and the components of the vessel wall are normal. Significant thickening and fibrosis of the vessel wall decrease its distensibility. Stretching a vessel also reduces its distensibility. Thus, the distensibility of a pulmonary artery is reduced in the presence of pulmonary hypertension. Other factors such as tissue pressure, interstitial fluid, alveolar surface tension and mechanical distortions are difficult to assess. In this regard the recent finding by McCredie of increased tissue fluid in patients with elevated pulmonary vascular pressures is of special interest.[17]

We have studied the distensibility characteristics of the pulmonary vessels as reflected by the pressure-volume response to exercise in a group of 4 normal subjects and in 48 patients with organic heart disease. Preliminary data in some of these patients have been previously reported.[18] By comparing nearly simultaneous changes in the distending pressure (P_d) and PBV during exercise, it is possible to estimate the approximate distensibility of the pulmonary vascular bed.

The patients studied were divided into six groups.

Group 1. Four subjects, each of whom had a grade 1-2/6 systolic murmur along the left sternal border, belonged to this group. No abnormality was demonstrated by routine electrocardiogram, fluoroscopy and roentgenogram of the chest, right and left heart catheterization, indicator-dilution curves and selective angiocardiogram. These patients are hereafter referred to as normal subjects.

Group II. Six patients with predominant aortic regurgitation.

Group III. Eight patients with predominant aortic stenosis.

Group IV. Nine patients with predominant mitral regurgitation.

Group V. Nineteen patients with predominant mitral stenosis.

Group VI. Six patients with primary myocardial disease, one with pericardial effusion and one with constrictive pericarditis.

These diagnoses were based upon clinical, hemodynamic, angiocardiographic and, in most cases, operative findings.

Oxygen uptake, pulmonary blood flow, pressures and volumes were measured at rest and between the sixth and tenth minutes of exercise. Ten patients performed leg exercise for a second time after a recovery period of 15 to 20 minutes. The work load was increased during the second exercise period in order to ascertain whether the PBV could be further augmented.

Relationships between volume-pressure in the vessels at rest and during exercise were evaluated using the formulas for absolute volume distensibility and coefficient of distensibility as described by Burton, and Harris and Heath.[19,20]

$$DV = \frac{\triangle V}{\triangle P} \text{ and}$$

$$DC = \frac{1}{V} \cdot \frac{\triangle V}{\triangle P}$$

Where DV = absolute volume distensibility in ml/M²/mm Hg

$\triangle V$ = difference between PBV during exercise and PBV at rest in ml/M²

$\triangle P$ = difference between P_d during exercise and P_d at rest in mm Hg

DC = coefficient of distensibility

V = PBV at rest in ml/M²

Meaningful coefficients of distensibility could not be calculated in three normal subjects with data derived from the first exercise period, because the P_d or the PBV or both remained unchanged or decreased during exercise. During the second exercise period (Exercise II), however, the change in PBV and P_D was sufficient for this calculation in all three. Repeat exercise was also performed by two patients with predominant aortic regurgitation, four with predominant aortic stenosis and one with predominant mitral stenosis. Data obtained during repeat exercise in these patients were also included.

Tables 17-1 to 17-6 present respectively the values for P_d and PBV at

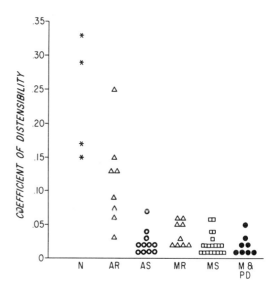

Figure 17-1. Coefficients of distensibility in six groups of patients. The coefficient of distensibility was 0.15 or greater in normal subjects (N), varied between 0.03 and 0.25 in patients with predominant aortic regurgitation (AR), and was 0.07 or smaller in patients with predominant aortic stenosis (AS), predominant mitral regurgitation (MR), predominant mitral stenosis (MS), or primary myocardial or pericardial disease. (M & PD).

TABLE 17-1 Coefficient *nf* Distensibility of Pulmonary Vascular Bed in Normal Patients

Patient	Control PAm	Control P_d	$\triangle P_d$	Control PBV	$\triangle$PBV	$\dfrac{\triangle PBV}{\triangle P_d}$	$\dfrac{1}{V} \cdot \dfrac{\triangle V}{\triangle P}$	Remgrks
R.C.	10	8.0	2.5	361	155	62.0	0.17	Exercise II
J.B.	13	11.5	1.5	272	62	41.5	1.15	Exercise II
G.G.	15	12.5	2.0	269	159	80.0	0.29	
D.G.	18	15.5	0.5	306	51	102.0	0.33	Exercise II
Mean	14	11.9	1.6	302	107	71.5	0.23	

PAm = Pulmonary arterial mean pressure (mm Hg)
P_d = Pulmonary distending pressure (mm Hg)
$\triangle P_d$ = Increase in pulmonary distending pressure (mm Hg)
PBV = Pulmonary blood volume (ml/M²)
$\triangle$PBV = Increase in pulmonary blood volume (ml/M²)
V = PBV
$\triangle$V = $\triangle$PBV
$\triangle$P = $\triangle P_d$

rest, the differences in P_d and PBV between the exercise and control periods, the absolute volume distensibility and the coefficient of distensibility in the six groups of patients during the first and second exercise periods. The coefficients of distensibility in the various groups of patients are also plotted in Figure 17-1.

Table 17-1 shows that the $\triangle P_d$ of normal subjects varied from 0.5 to 2.5 mm Hg with a mean value of 1.6 mm Hg between exercise and control periods; and the $\triangle$PBV varied between 51 and 159 ml/M² with a mean value of 107 ml/M². The absolute volume distensibility averaged 71.5 ml/M³/mm Hg (range 41.5 to 102.5 ml/M²/mm Hg), and the coefficient of distensibility averaged 0.23 (range 0.15 to 0.33). In

patient R.C., the control PBV before the first exercise period was 296 ml/M², but it rose to 361 ml/M² before the second exercise period. The greater than normal volume before the repeat exercise period was probably related to slow return of the augmented PBV to normal after the first exercise. Normal subjects appear to be able to achieve a much larger increase in PBV per mm Hg during exercise than has been previously reported under static conditions. The large increase in PBV is also in keeping with the substantial increase in pulmonary capillary blood volume observed in normal subjects during exercise.

In patients with aortic regurgitation the $\triangle P_d$ ranged from 1.5 to 11.5 mm Hg with an average value of 4.0 mm

TABLE 17-2 Coefficient of Distensibility of Pulmonary Vascular Bed in Patients with Predominant Aortic Regurgitation

Patient	Control PAm	Control P_d	$\triangle P_d$	Control PBV	$\triangle$PBV	$\dfrac{\triangle PBV}{\triangle P_d}$	$\dfrac{1}{V} \cdot \dfrac{\triangle V}{\triangle P}$	Remarks
S.S.	8	7.5	3.0	330	96	31.0	0.09	
R.Ha.	15	11.0	1.5	364	86	57.0	0.15	
	10	7.0	4.5	270	72	16.0	0.06	Exercise II
J.G.	16	11.0	1.5	208	80	53.0	0.25	
R.V.	16	13.0	6.0	375	180	30.0	0.08	
D.K.	17	15.0	1.5	321	64	42.5	0.13	
	14	12.0	2.5	308	99	39.5	0.13	Exercise II
T.M.	32	26.5	11.5	330	100	8.7	0.03	
Mean	16	12.8	4.0	313	97	34.7	0.12	

Symbols and abbreviations are the same as those used in Table 17-1

Hg, while the $\triangle$PBV varied between 64 and 180 ml/M² with an average value of 97 ml/M² (Table 17-2). The average absolute distensibility was 34.7 ml/M²/mm Hg (range 8.7 to 57.0), and the coefficient of distensibility averaged 0.12 with a range from 0.06 to 0.15. In all but one patient (T.M.) the coefficient of distensibility was 0.06 or greater during both first and second exercise periods. In patient T.M. the LAm and the PAm were both significantly elevated at rest, 21 and 32 mm Hg respectively. With exercise, the LAm rose to 29 and the PAm to 47 mm Hg, resulting in an increase in P_d of 11.5 mm Hg. In this regard, the response of patient T.M. resembled that observed

in most of the patients with predominant aortic stenosis.

In patients with predominant aortic stenosis, the $\triangle P_d$ averaged 11.7 mm Hg (range 2.5 to 27.0 mm Hg) and the $\triangle$PBV varied from 7 to 210 ml/M² with a mean of 69 ml/M² (Table 17-3). A significant decrease in the absolute volume distensibility was observed, with a range of 0.6 to 19.1 and an average of 6.3 ml/M² mm Hg. The coefficient of distensibility was uniformly low, varying between 0.01 and 0.07 with an average of 0.03, during both exercise periods.

As summarized in Table 17-4, the $\triangle P_d$ in patients with predominant mitral regurgitation varied from 6.0 to

TABLE 17-3 Coefficient of Distensibility of Pulmonary Vascular Bed in Patients with Predominant Aortic Stenosis

Patient	Control PAm	Control P_d	$\triangle P_d$	Control PBV	$\triangle PBV$	$\dfrac{\triangle PBV}{\triangle P_d}$	$\dfrac{1}{V} \cdot \dfrac{\triangle V}{\triangle P}$	Remarks
W.S.	7	5.0	6.0	202	84	14.0	0.07	
F.W.	10	8.0	6.5	230	17	2.6	0.01	
J.S.	13	9.5	9.0	401	22	2.4	0.01	
	12	10.0	14.0	370	98	7.0	0.02	Exercise II
A.Bu.	16	14.0	11.0	349	210	19.1	0.05	
	16	14.0	9.0	378	63	7.0	0.02	Exercise II
C.W.	18	15.0	13.5	198	58	4.3	0.02	
	18	16.0	26.0	168	163	6.2	0.04	
V.M.	21	16.0	27.0	414	16	0.6	0.01	
R.Hu.	21	17.0	2.5	234	11	4.4	0.02	
	16	12.0	3.0	228	7	2.3	0.01	Exercise II
W.L.	23	18.5	13.0	230	80	6.1	0.03	
Mean	15.9	12.9	11.7	284	69	6.3	0.03	

Symbols and abbreviations are the same as those used in Table 17-1

TABLE 17-4 Coefficient of Distensibility of Pulmonary Vascular Bed in Patients with Predominant Mitral Regurgitation

Patient	Control PAm	Control P_d	$\triangle P_d$	Control PBV	$\triangle PBV$	$\dfrac{\triangle PBV}{\triangle P_d}$	$\dfrac{1}{V} \cdot \dfrac{\triangle V}{\triangle P}$
S.C.	12	10.0	7.0	369	69	9.8	0.03
D.B.	13	10.0	6.0	211	75	12.5	0.06
E.McK.	17	12.0	9.0	230	106	11.8	0.05
E.P.	18	14.0	22.0	226	227	10.3	0.05
J.R.	22	18.0	17.0	248	97	5.7	0.02
F.W.	23	18.5	9.5	254	132	14.0	0.06
K.G.	23	19.0	15.0	372	128	8.5	0.02
H.F.	35	26.5	16.5	226	82	5.0	0.02
B.A.	42	35.0	16.0	290	106	6.0	0.02
Mean	22.8	18.1	13.1	270	114	9.3	0.04

Symbols and abbreviations are the same as those used in Table 17-1

22.0 mm Hg with an average value of 13.1 mm Hg. The average $\triangle$PBV was 114 ml/M² with a range from 69 to 227 ml/M². Absolute volume distensibility and coefficient of distensibility were both strikingly decreased. The former averaged 9.3 ml/M²/mm Hg, ranging from 5.0 to 14.0 ml/M²/mm Hg, and the latter averaged 0.04 with a range of 0.02 to 0.06.

In patient with predominant mitral stenosis the changes in $\triangle P_d$ and $\triangle$PBV were similar to those observed in patients with mitral regurgitation, although the distensibility was generally even more impaired (Table 17-5). The $\triangle P_d$ ranged between 4.0 and 44.0 with an average of 16.0 mm Hg, ten times that observed in normal subjects. Great variation in $\triangle$PBV was observed, ranging from 10 to 265 ml/M². The average $\triangle$PBV was 86 ml/M². The absolute volume distensibility varied from 1.4 to 14.8 ml/M²/mm Hg with an average value of 6.1 ml/M²/mm Hg. The average coefficient of disten-

sibility was only 0.02 (range from 0.01 to 0.06). In all but two patients (M.B. and C.C.) the absolute volume distensibility was less than 10 ml/M²/mm Hg and the coefficient of distensibility was less than 0.05.

In patients with myocardial or pericardial disease the average $\triangle P_d$ was 8.4 mm Hg, ranging from 3.0 to 17.5 mm Hg, and the $\triangle$PBV varied from 6 to 106 ml/M², with an average of 37 ml/M² (Table 17-6). These values were lower than those observed in other groups. The explanation for this difference may be that less work was imposed on these patients than on patients in other groups, as suggested by substantially less oxygen uptake during exercise. The average absolute volume distensibility was the lowest of all the groups, being only 5.5 ml/M²/mm Hg (range 1.6 to 17.6). The coefficient of distensibility was correspondingly markedly decreased in each case, with a range from 0.01 to 0.05 and an average of 0.02.

TABLE 17-5 Coefficient of Distensibility of Pulmonary Vascular Bed in Patients with Predominant Mitral Stenosis

Patient	Control PAm	Control P_d	$\triangle P_d$	Control PBV	$\triangle$PBV	$\dfrac{\triangle PBV}{\triangle P_d}$	$\dfrac{1}{V} \cdot \dfrac{\triangle V}{\triangle P}$	Remarks
J.I.	14	10.5	4.5	192	10	2.2	0.01	
M.T.	14	11.0	15.0	275	77	5.2	0.02	
G.B.	16	13.0	12.0	222	106	8.8	0.04	
M.B.	17	14.5	4.0	224	50	12.5	0.06	
C.C.	20	16.5	8.5	246	126	14.8	0.06	
S.F.	20	17.5	12.5	336	34	2.7	0.01	
G.C.	22	19.0	28.5	349	92	3.2	0.01	
E.C.	24	19.5	12.0	330	56	4.7	0.01	
M.P.	25	23.5	12.5	236	66	5.3	0.02	
H.C.	26	23.0	23.5	275	113	4.8	0.02	
J.Sm.	27	22.5	17.0	272	25	1.4	0.01	
G.H.	27	25.5	3.5	292	33	9.5	0.03	
E.G.	28	23.0	11.5	345	41	3.5	0.01	
J.Ra.	30	21.0	14.5	325	121	8.3	0.02	
G.F.	32	23.0	24.0	300	31	1.3	0.01	
A.B.	32	24.5	27.0	354	180	6.7	0.02	
R.H.	34	27.0	28.0	398	160	5.7	0.01	
	36	30.0	44.0	315	265	6.0	0.02	Exercise II
N.G.	35	30.0	8.0	252	46	5.8	0.02	
M.Ti.	40	34.0	9.5	243	86	9.0	0.04	
Mean	26	21.4	16.0	289	86	6.1	0.02	

Symbols and abbreviations are the same as those used in Table 17-1

TABLE 17-6   Coefficient of Distensibility of Pulmonary Vascular Bed in Patients with Myocardial or Pericardial Disease

Patient	Control PAm	Control P_d	$\triangle P_d$	Control PBV	$\triangle PBV$	$\dfrac{\triangle PBV}{\triangle P_d}$	$\dfrac{1}{V} \cdot \dfrac{\triangle V}{\triangle P}$
H.C.	15	11.0	3.0	232	12	4.0	0.02
A.O.	17	11.5	7.5	225	60	8.0	0.03
M.De.	17	13.0	12.0	400	6	2.0	0.01
H.Be.	19	16.0	6.0	332	106	17.6	0.05
M.A.	20	17.0	6.0	308	10	1.6	0.01
R.F.	28	26.0	17.5	312	49	2.8	0.01
L.V.	18	13.0	5.5	254	29	5.3	0.02
I.K.	21	18.5	9.5	298	27	2.8	0.01
Mean	19.3	15.7	8.4	295	37	5.5	0.02

Symbols and abbreviations are the same as those used in Table 17-1

It is important to emphasize that the absolute volume distensibility and the coefficient of distensibility as calculated in this study refer to the pulmonary circulation in general and cannot be used with reference to particular segments of the pulmonary vascular tree. For example, in patients with idiopathic or thromboembolic pulmonary hypertension, the pulmonary arteries may be severely diseased, without significant involvement of the pulmonary venous system. The P_d, as calculated, would be greatly increased and the absolute volume distensibility and the coefficient of distensibility may both be abnormally low. In these cases structural damage undoubtedly seriously compromises the distensibility of the pulmonary arteries, but the status of pulmonary venous distensibility cannot be accurately ascertained.

The average of pulmonary arterial and left atrial pressures may not represent true pulmonary distending or transmural pressure, because tissue or intrathoracic pressure was not measured. As mentioned previously, the tissue pressure is probably slightly subatmospheric, intermediate between the intrapleural pressure and atmospheric pressure. Inasmuch as intrapleural pressure has been reported as more negative during exercise, the pulmonary distending or transmural pressure might be expected to be even greater during exercise.[21,22] Thus, both the absolute volume distensibility and the coefficient of distensibility would be even more reduced had we been able to measure intrapleural pressure for the calculation of pulmonary distending pressure.

Limitations must be recognized in the interpretation of distensibility of the pulmonary vascular bed based upon estimation of PBV and distending pressure during exercise because of the influence of many neurohumoral and metabolic factors. For instance, in the mixed venous blood an appreciable decrease of the oxygen tension and pH is usually associated with an increase in carbon dioxide tension. There is a substantial increase in both tissue and blood lactic acid. Augmented production of catecholamines and kinins is probably also important.

When changes in either P_d or PBV are small, the calculated difference in distensibility may be meaningless. In general, little or no measurable rise in pressure associated with a significant increase in volume indicates normal distensibility. A large pressure rise, on the other hand, suggests restricted distensibility (disproportionate elevation in the pressure), even when accompanied by an appreciable augmentation of volume.

Two of our three normal subjects were able to increase pulmonary blood flow without a significant change in the PBV or pressure. With more strenuous exercise, however, PBV increased appreciably with a slight rise in the P_d. The large coefficient of distensibility suggests that further augmentation of flow and volume would not have required much of a rise in pressure.

The distensibility characteristics of the pulmonary vascular bed in patients with predominant but compensated aortic regurgitation are similar to those in patients without cardiovascular abnormality, except, perhaps, for a slightly greater rise in the P_d with exercise. With left ventricular decompensation, however, as represented by patient T.M., the coefficient of distensibility was reduced. This patient had proven cystic medial necrosis of the aorta and his clinical condition deteriorated rapidly, a course which differed greatly from that of the other patients in the group.

In patients with predominant aortic stenosis, similar exercise resulted in a greater increase in the P_d with or without appreciable augmentation of the PBV. The calculated absolute volume distensibility and coefficient of distensibility were less than half the corresponding values in normal subjects. The P_d of most patients in this group was normal or only slightly elevated at rest, but the possibility of structural abnormality in the pulmonary vascular bed could not be ruled out. It is likely that chronic increase in resistance to filling of a concentrically hypertrophied, noncompliant left ventricle leads to structural changes in the pulmonary vascular bed similar to but less severe than those long recognized in association with mitral stenosis.[23] Supporting evidence for such a mechanism is provided by the left atrial hypertrophy

and the unusually large left atrial "a" wave frequently seen in these patients. In contrast, the relatively normal coefficient of distensibility in patients with compensated aortic regurgitation may be attributed to the compliant and dilated left ventricle, adapted to a volume load.

In patients with mitral valve disease the elevation in the LAm and PAm undoubtedly results from the physical consequence of altered blood flow through a deformed mitral valve orifice. The increased PBV, on the other hand, may be largely related to passive distention of the pulmonary

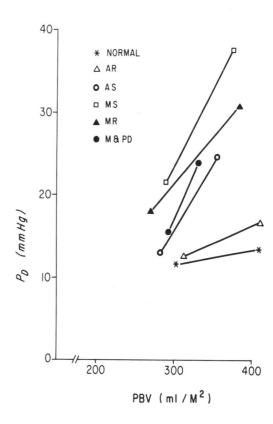

Figure 17-2. Segments of a family of pulmonary vascular pressure-volume curves observed at rest and during exercise in different groups of patients. See text discussion.

vascular bed by the elevated LAm and pulmonary venous pressure. The restricted pulmonary vascular system of these patients is probably primarily a manifestation of structural changes in the pulmonary vessels and in the pulmonary parenchyma, resulting from sustained pulmonary venous and arterial hypertension.[24-26]

In patients with primary myocardial or pericardial disease the work load during exercise was usually less than that performed by patients in other groups, as evidenced by the smaller oxygen uptake (Chapter 11). The coefficient of distensibility was much reduced, nevertheless, for reasons similar to those which explain the effect in patients with predominant aortic stenosis.

When the average pressure-volume change in the pulmonary vascular bed at rest and during exercise was plotted for the various groups of patients (Figure 17-2), the responses appeared to represent different segments of a family of pressure-volume curves analogous to the pattern of pulmonary relaxation pressure-volume curves in the normal dog as described by Sarnoff and Berglund.[6] The pressure-volume responses to exercise by normal subjects showed a significant increase in PBV with a minimal rise in P_d. The response in the group with predominant aortic regurgitation was similar to that observed in the normal subjects, although a slightly greater increase in P_d was associated with the same degree of augmented PBV. In patients with predominant aortic stenosis, in those with mitral valve disease and in those with primary myocardial or pericardial disease, the pressure-volume curves plotted progressively upward and to the left, indicating a disproportionate elevation of P_d associated with an equal or a smaller increase in PBV. The steep slope of the curve in these patients suggests overstretching of the pulmonary vessels and restricted pulmonary vascular distensibility.

REFERENCES

1. Burton, A.C.: Relation of structure to function of the tissues of the wall of blood vessels. Physiol. Rev., *34*, 617, 1954.

2. Roach, M.R., and Burton, A.C.: The reason for the shape of the distensibility curves of arteries. Canad. J. Biochem. & Physiol., *35*, 681, 1957.

3. Harris, P., and Heath, D.: *Human Pulmonary Circulation*, p. 28, Baltimore, Williams & Wilkins Company, 1962.

4. Burton, A.C.: *Physiology and Biophysics of the Circulation*, p. 72. Chicago, Year Book Medical Publishers, Inc., 1965.

5. Burton, A.C.: On the physical equilibrium of small vessels. Am. J. Physiol., *164*, 319, 1951.

6. Sarnoff, S.J., and Berglund, E.: Pressure volume characteristics and stress relaxation in the pulmonary vascular bed of the dog. Am. J. Physiol., *171*, 238, 1952.

7. Frasher, W.G., and Sobin, S.S.: Distensible behavior of pulmonary artery. Am. J. Physiol., *199*, 472, 1960.

8. Meyer, W.W., and Schollmeyer, P.: Die Volumendehnbarkeit und die Druck-Umfang-Beziehungen des Lungenschlagader-Windkessels in Abhangigkeit vom alter und pulmonalen Hochdruck. Klin. Wshr., *35*, 1070, 1957.

9. Deuchar, D.C., and Knebel, R.: The pulmonary and systemic circulations in congenital heart disease. Brit. Heart J., *14*, 225, 1952.

10. Patel, D.J., Schilder, D.P., and Mallos, A.J.: Mechanical properties and dimensions of the major pulmonary arteries. J. Appl. Physiol., *15*, 92, 1960.

11. Fleishner, F.G., Romano, F.J., and Luisada, A.A.: Studies of fluorocardiography in normal subjects. Proc. Soc. Exp. Biol. & Med., *67*, 535, 1948.

12. DuBois, A.B.: Instantaneous pulmonary capillary blood flow. *In* W.R. Adams and I. Veith (eds), *Pulmonary Circulation*, p. 36, New York, Grune & Stratton, 1959.

13. Lasser, R.P., and Amram, S.S.: Distensibility of pulmonary arterial tree in patients with mitral stenosis. Am. Heart J., *51*, 749, 1956.

14. Milnor, W.R., Jose, A.D., and McGaff, C.J.: Pulmonary vascular volume, resistance and compliance in man. Circulation, *22*, 130, 1960.

15. Freitas, F.M. de, Faraco, E.Z., Nedel, N., Azevedo, D.F. de, and Zaduchliver, J.: Determination of pulmonary blood volume by single intravenous injection of one indicator in patients with normal and high pulmonary vascular pressures. Circulation, *30*, 370, 1964.

16. Fishman, A.P.: Dynamics of the pulmonary circulation. *In* W.F. Hamilton and P. Dow (eds), *Handbook of Physiology*. Circulation, vol. 2, Chapter 48, p. 1667, Washington, D.C., American Physiological Society, 1964.

17. McCredie, M.: Measurement of pulmonary edema in valvular heart disease. Circulation, *36*, 381, 1967.

18. Yu, P.N., Murphy, G.W., Schreiner, B.F., and James, D.H.: Distensibility characteristics of the human pulmonary vascular bed. Study of pressure-volume response to exercise in patients with and without heart disease. Circulation, *35*, 710, 1967.

19. Burton, A.C.: *Physiology and Biophysics of the Circulation*, p. 153, Chicago, Year Book Medical Publishers, Inc., 1965.

20. Harris, P., and Heath, D.: *Human Pulmonary Circulation*, p. 337, Baltimore, Williams & Wilkins Company, 1962.

21. McIlroy, M.B., Marshall, R., and Christie, R.V.: The work of breathing in normal subjects. Clin. Sci., *13*, 127, 1954.

22. Marshall, R., McIlroy, M.B., and Christie, R.V.: The work of breathing in mitral stenosis. Clin. Sci., *13*, 137, 1954.

23. Smith, R.C., Burchell, H.B., and Edwards, J.E.: Pathology of the pulmonary vascular tree. IV. Structural changes in the pulmonary vessels in chronic left ventricular failure. Circulation, *10*, 801, 1954.

24. Parker, F., and Weiss, S.: The nature and significance of the structural changes in the lungs in mitral stenosis. Am. J. Pathol., *12*, 573, 1936.

25. Larrabee, W.F., Parker, R.L., and Edwards, J.E.: Pathology of intrapulmonary arteries and arterioles in mitral stenosis. Proc. Staff Meet. Mayo Clin., *24*, 316, 1949.

26. Heath, D., and Edwards, J.E.: Histological changes in the lung in diseases associated with pulmonary venous hypertension. Brit. J. Dis. Chest, *53*, 8, 1959.

Section V

CHAPTER 18

Summary and Comments

The first chapter of this monograph reviewed briefly the principles, history of the development, and clinical application of indicator-dilution techniques for the measurement of pulmonary blood volume (PBV). In the second chapter, the functional anatomy of the human pulmonary vascular bed was emphasized. The ensuing three chapters described (a) current techniques and methodology for the measurement of pulmonary blood flow, pulmonary vascular pressures, total blood volume and central blood volume; and (b) the importance and implications of pulmonary vascular pressure-flow-volume interrelationships.

The sixth chapter enumerated methods for estimating and partitioning the PBV in animals. The PBV is about 10% of the total blood volume. The distribution of blood in the three compartments of the pulmonary vascular bed (arteries, capillaries, and veins) is approximately 30, 20 and 50% respectively.

Various methods for measuring the PBV in man were reviewed in the seventh chapter. At present, almost all use either dye or a radioactive substance as an indicator. The former is usually measured in samples of blood withdrawn through a cuvette densitometer, whereas the latter indicator is suitable for the precordial counting technique. The merits, limitations, and potential errors of the various methods

were critically reviewed. In all the methods the estimated PBV is a virtual rather than an anatomic volume and includes an unknown amount of blood in one or more of the heart chambers. No presently available method is accurate enough to measure precisely the PBV in man.

The eighth chapter summarized data on PBV in man at rest obtained in our laboratory. The reproducibility of our method was demonstrated in a series of 57 patients in whom duplicate determinations of a number of parameters were made within periods of 10 to 15 minutes. The difference between the first and second determinations was always less than 45 ml/M² for PBV. Reproducibility of the method was further evident in the close agreement of the values of triplicate determinations of PBV in a series of 20 patients. Without exception, the PBV varied less than 50 ml/M² between any two of the three determinations.

In a group of 15 normal subjects the PBV varied from 204 to 314 ml/M² with a mean of 271 ml/M². In a group of 190 patients with mitral valve disease certain patterns of PBV changes were observed. The PBV was usually normal or slightly increased for class II patients, definitely increased for class III patients, and usually decreased for class IV patients. The increase in PBV in class II and III patients was most likely due to passive distention of pulmonary vessels as a result of elevated pulmonary venous and arterial pressures. In the advanced cases, the reduction of PBV was interpreted as a combination of several factors including structural thickening and reduced elasticity of the pulmonary vessels, functional vasoconstriction and thromboembolism.

In a group of 93 patients with aortic valve disease, the PBV was lower than in patients with mitral valve disease of corresponding functional classification. For example, the PBV was usually normal in class I and II patients, normal or slightly increased in class III patients, and definitely increased in a few class IV patients. One reason why the PBV was not reduced in class IV patients with aortic valve disease may be related to the relatively short period of pulmonary venous and arterial hypertension, and to the accordingly less severe structural changes and functional vasoconstriction in the pulmonary vessels.

In patients with idiopathic or thromboembolic pulmonary hypertension, the PBV was either normal or subnormal, a finding consistent with the invariable histologic demonstration of considerable obliteration of the pulmonary vessels, particularly the small arteries and arterioles.

With one exception the PBV was either normal or subnormal in a group of 24 patients with primary myocardial disease.

The ninth chapter described our studies of patients with congestive heart failure associated with either mitral stenosis or primary myocardial disease. The most surprising finding was the relatively normal PBV, most likely secondary to a restricted pulmonary vascular bed resulting from a variety of extra- and intra-luminal

pathophysiologic alterations. Notable examples include structural changes in the pulmonary arteries and veins, interstitial fibrosis and thromboembolism, and hypoxemic functional vasoconstriction. Pulmonary vascular pressure elevation rather than augmented PBV appeared to be the dominant hemodynamic feature of congestive heart failure. In other words, the pulmonary vascular pressure-volume characteristics in these patients were significantly displaced to the steep upper portion of the canine pulmonary vascular pressure-volume curve described by Sarnoff and Berglund. Thus, a large increase in pulmonary vascular pressure was associated with only a small increase in PBV. When pulmonary venous and capillary pressures exceed the colloid osmotic pressure, transudation of fluid into the alveoli and interstitial space would be expected. Therefore, the pulmonary "congestion" in congestive heart failure was considered to be more extravascular than intravascular.

In addition to alterations in the pulmonary vascular pressure-volume relationships, the importance of surfactant in controlling the elastic properties and compliance of the lungs in congestive heart failure was emphasized.

The relationship of the PBV to other variables in a large group of patients with heart disease was discussed in the tenth chapter. In general, no significant correlation was found between the PBV, cardiac output, stroke volume, pulmonary arterial pressure, left atrial pressure, pulmonary vascular resistance and left atrial volume. In certain classes of patients, the PBV correlated positively with total blood volume and pulmonary capillary blood volume. For most patients the PBV correlated positively with mean transit time through the pulmonary vascular bed, relative pulmonary vascular compliance, central blood volume and body surface area.

The eleventh chapter described changes in the PBV in man during physiologic, mechanical and chemical interventions. The evidence was convincing that inhalation of low oxygen caused pulmonary vasoconstriction. This was manifested by an increase in pulmonary arterial pressure associated with no change in pulmonary wedge or left atrial pressure and significantly decreased or unchanged PBV. The pressor effect probably occurred proximal to the pulmonary capillaries.

Recently, a rise in pulmonary arterial pressure has been reported during acute acidosis induced by intravenous infusion of lactic or hydrochloric acid, but no specific information was given concerning any changes in PBV. The available data suggest that the elevated pulmonary arterial pressure was due to pulmonary vasoconstriction.

Significant increase in pulmonary arterial pressure has been reported in many high altitude residents, but studies of the effects in PBV are scanty and inconclusive. Hypoxia was a likely major cause of the pulmonary hypertension, although other possible contributing factors such as increased total blood volume could not be ruled out.

Except for the active vasomotion observed during acute hypoxia or acute acidosis, the changes of PBV following most physiologic interventions were primarily passive in nature. In other words, a concordant change was usually observed in both pulmonary blood pressure and volume. PBV increased whenever pulmonary vascular or distending pressure rose (exercise, systemic vasoconstriction, impaired left ventricular function) or total blood volume was augmented (infusion of blood or fluid). PBV declined whenever pulmonary vascular or distending pressure fell (vasodepressor reactions, systemic vasodilatation or improved left ventricular function) or total blood volume was reduced (acute blood loss). Thus, the PBV changed passively in response to alterations in the distending or transmural pressures in the pulmonary vascular bed. Pressure changes in turn are governed partly by intrinsic pulmonary vasomotor activity and partly by such factors as the status of the systemic vessels and myocardium, the magnitude of pulmonary blood flow, the total blood volume, the perivascular air pressure, the alveolar surface tension, and the presence or absence of excessive interstitial fluid.

The effects or various pharmacologic agents on the PBV were summarized in the twelfth chapter. Three drugs, acetylcholine, isoproterenol and aminophylline, were found to produce active pulmonary vasodilation. Infusion of acetylcholine into the right heart or the main pulmonary artery usually caused a fall in pulmonary arterial pressure and an increase in PBV. The response was generally more pronounced in patients with moderate pulmonary hypertension than in normal subjects. Infusion of acetylcholine also counteracted the pulmonary hypertension induced by acute hypoxia. Which of the three compartments (arteries, capillaries or veins) actually participated in the vasodilation was uncertain, but the available data suggest that the pulmonary arteries were more actively involved than the pulmonary capillaries and veins. Intravenous infusion of isoproterenol or aminophylline also produced active dilatation of the pulmonary vascular bed, manifested by an increase in PBV and a decrease in pulmonary vascular pressure. Because the positive inotropic effects of these two drugs usually caused a decrease in PBV, however, the net effects of isoproterenol or aminophylline infusion were a decrease in pulmonary vascular pressure and a slight increase or no change in PBV.

Several pharmacologic agents induce pulmonary vasoconstriction. These include 5-hydroxytryptamine, histamine and possibly angiotensin and norepinephrine. Unfortunately, with the exception of angiotensin, little or no information concerning their effects on PBV is available.

Most of the other pharmacologic agents studied exerted their primary actions on structures other than the pulmonary vascular bed. For example, PBV and pulmonary vascular pressure decreased after the administration of digitalis glycosides which improved left ventricular function. Some adrenergic activators such as methoxamine and mephentermine produced systemic vasoconstriction resulting in an increase in both pulmonary vascular pressure and PBV. On the other hand, ganglionic blocking agents usually caused systemic vasodilatation, and both pulmonary vascular pressure and PBV declined. The changes in PBV under all these conditions were considered to be passive in nature, because the changes in both pressure and volume occurred together, and little or no pulmonary vasomotor activity was demonstrated.

The thirteenth chapter reviewed briefly the technique and methodology for estimating pulmonary diffusing capacity for carbon monoxide and pulmonary capillary blood volume (Vc). Two methods are frequently employed: (a) single breath and (b) steady state. The merits, limitations and potential errors of each method were discussed.

The Vc in normal subjects at rest and its changes in response to physiologic interventions and to pharmacologic agents were summarized in the fourteenth chapter. The mean Vc in a group of normal subjects was 50 ml/M². One of the most important factors affecting the Vc is the net pulmonary transmural pressure. Vc increased almost invariably when net pulmonary transmural pressure rose, as it did during head-down tilt, leg raising, inflation of pressure suit, immersion in water, negative pressure breathing, and exercise. On the other hand, Vc usually decreased in association with a decline in net pulmonary transmural pressure, such as occurred during head-up tilt, positive pressure breathing, forward acceleration, and forced expiration. Other factors which may be important in the regulation of Vc include total blood volume, left ventricular function, systemic vasomotor activity, lung volume, ventilation and alveolar pressure.

The responses of Vc to a few pharmacologic agents were included. Various mechanisms may be responsible, but the Vc was reported to decrease after the administration of 5-hydroxytryptamine, atropine and trimethaphan, and to increase after the infusion of acetylcholine, isoproterenol and norepinephrine.

The fifteenth chapter reported the Vc measured in patients with various types of cardiopulmonary disease. In patients with predominant mitral valve disease, Vc volume was usually normal or slightly increased in mild cases, moderately or markedly increased in more severely affected patients, and normal or decreased in those whose disease was most advanced. In patients with predominant aortic valve disease, Vc was usually normal or increased. Inasmuch as the structural abnormalities of the pulmonary vessels are usually less severe in patients with aortic disease than in those with mitral disease, less decrease in Vc would be expected.

Patients with congenital cardiovascular malformations, particularly in those with atrial septal defect, usually showed a significant increase in Vc.

Vc was usually subnormal in patients with chronic pulmonary disease and in those with thromboembolic or idiopathic pulmonary hypertension. No increase in Vc was found in patients with hyperthyroidism or in those with polycythemia vera.

Responses to inhalation of low oxygen and to acetylcholine infusion provided the basis of a detailed discussion of active pulmonary vasomotion in Chapter 16. Active vasoconstriction was observed during acute hypoxia and active vasodilatation occurred during acetylcholine infusion. At present, the changes in any specific compartment or segment of the pulmonary vascular bed cannot be differentiated. The evidence suggests, however, that the pulmonary arteries and arterioles are predominantly involved.

Pulmonary vascular pressure-volume responses during exercise led to a preliminary discussion of the distensibility characteristics of the human pulmonary vascular bed in the seventeenth chapter. In general, the coefficient of distensibility was large in normal subjects in whom an appreciable increase in PBV was accompanied by an insignificant change in the pulmonary vascular pressures. In patients with predominant aortic regurgitation and in the absence of cardiac failure, the response was similar to that observed in normal subjects. On the other hand, the coefficient of distensibility was significantly reduced in patients with predominant aortic stenosis, in those with mitral valve disease, and in those with primary myocardial or pericardial disease. In these three groups of patients a large rise in pulmonary vascular pressures was accompanied by an equal or smaller increase in PBV. The changes suggest overstretching of the pulmonary vessels resulting in restricted distensibility of the pulmonary vascular bed.

Despite increasing interest in the investigation of PBV in the past decade, many unresolved problems remain concerning the measurement, role and regulation of PBV in man. In a recent editorial, Fishman[1] listed four main lines of interest in the study of PBV at present: (a) the role of the lungs as a blood depot, (b) the blood reservoir in the lung as the site of stretch receptors, (c) the performance of the congested lungs, and (d) the partition of the PBV.

The volume of blood in the lungs at any moment depends upon the output of the right and left ventricles and on the distensibility characteristics of the pulmonary vascular bed. The PBV has been considered a depot for the blood supply to the left ventricle in the event of an acute reduction in the venous return and right ventricular output.[2] If total pulmonary inflow ceases for a few cardiac cycles, however, blood in the lungs will be insufficient to supply the left ventricle. Nevertheless, under certain conditions such as sudden postural changes, forced respiration, and exercise, a transient discrepancy between the left and right ventricular output may occur, and a portion of the PBV is probably available for maintenance or augmentation of the left ventricle output.

The neurohumoral control of the pulmonary circulation deserves emphasis. The vascular system containing the blood reservoir in the lungs has been suspected as the site of stretch receptors, stimulation of which may interact with neurohumoral effects related to the degree of atrial distention and vasomotor activity of the heart and systemic vessels.[3-5] Such relationships may be particularly pertinent when the lungs are acutely or chronically congested. Assessment of the precise functions and regulatory interactions of the stretch receptors will require precise study of the pressure-volume relationships in the total pulmonary vascular system as well as in its various segments under closely controlled conditions. Simpler and more reliable techniques are needed for the measurement of the total PBV and of the blood volume in each of the three vascular segments of the pulmonary vascular bed, again recalling that the PBV estimated by the currently available techniques invariably includes an unknown amount of blood in one or more of the cardiac chambers.

Simultaneous measurements of blood flow in a pulmonary artery and in a pulmonary vein by means of chronically implanted electromagnetic flow probes around the pulmonary vessels of dogs have been reported by several groups of investigators.[6-8] Recently, Brody and associates described a new and elegant method for the measurement of pressure and resistance to blood flow in pulmonary arteries, capillaries and veins in isolated lung lobes of dogs.[9,10] Such new approaches arouse hopes that more will be learned about instantaneous and longitudinal blood flow through the three pulmonary vascular segments in an individual lobe of the dog lung at rest, during physiological stress, and in response to pharmacologic agents. Whether similar techniques will be feasible and applicable to human subjects is uncertain.

We have emphasized that the PBV may not be increased in patients with chronic congestive heart failure and that so-called pulmonary congestion may be largely an effect of the accumulation of extravascular fluid in the lung. As recent studies of pulmonary extravascular fluid in patients with valvular heart disease are extended to those with congestive heart failure,[11-13] the relationships between the PBV and pulmonary extravascular fluid may be more precisely delineated.

REFERENCES

1. Fishman, A. P.: The volume of blood in the lungs. Circulation, *33*, 835, 1966.

2. Comroe, J.H.: Main functions of the pulmonary circulation. Circulation, *33*, 146, 1966.

3. Gauer, O.H., and Henry, J.P.: Circulatory basis of fluid control. Physiol. Rev., *43*, 423, 1963.

4. Ledmore, J.R., and Linden, R.J.: Reflex increase in heart rate from distension of the pulmonary vein-atrial function. J. Physiol., *170*, 456, 1964.

5. Shepherd, J.T.: Role of the veins in the circulation. Circulation, *33*, 484, 1966.

6. Morkin, E., Collins, J.A., Goldman, H.S., and Fishman, A.P.: Pattern of blood flow in the pulmonary veins of the dog. J. Appl. Physiol., *20*, 1118, 1965.

7. Morgan, B.C., Dillard, D.H., and Guntheroth, W.G.: Effect of cardiac and respiratory cycle on pulmonary vein flow, pressure and diameter. J. Appl. Physiol., *21*, 1276, 1966.

8. Kinnen, E., Stankus, A., and Yu, P.N.: Pulmonary venous blood flow characteristics. Proc. 20th Annual Conf. on Engr. in Med. & Biol., *9*: paper #16.7, 1967.

9. Brody, J.S., Stemmler, E.J., and DuBois, A.B.: Longitudinal distribution of vascular resistance in the pulmonary arteries, capillaries and veins. J. Clin. Invest., *47*, 783, 1968.

10. Brody, J.S., and Stemmler, E.J.: Differential reactivity in pulmonary circulation. J. Clin. Invest., *47*, 800, 1968.

11. Lilienfeld, L.S., Freis, E.D., Partenope, E.A., and Morowitz, H.J.: Transcapillary migration of heavy water and thiocyanate ion in the pulmonary circulation of normal subjects and patients with congestive heart failure. J. Clin. Invest., *34*, 1, 1955.

12. McCredie, M.: Measurement of pulmonary edema in valvular heart disease. Circulation, *36*, 381, 1967.

13. Korsgren, M., Luepker, R., Liander, B., and Varnauskas, E.: Pulmonary intra- and extra-vascular fluid changes with exercise. To be published.

AUTHOR INDEX

SUBJECT INDEX